# Health Care Management

# Health Care Management

Editor: Neil Perry

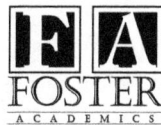

FA FOSTER
ACADEMICS

www.fosteracademics.com

www.fosteracademics.com

FA
FOSTER
ACADEMICS

**Cataloging-in-Publication Data**

Health care management / edited by Neil Perry.
    p. cm.
Includes bibliographical references and index.
ISBN 978-1-63242-669-7
1. Health services administration. 2. Public health administration. 3. Medical care.
4. Health planning. I. Perry, Neil.
RA971 .H43 2019
362.1068--dc23

Foster Academics,
118-35 Queens Blvd., Suite 400,
Forest Hills, NY 11375, USA

ISBN 978-1-63242-669-7 (Hardback)

# Contents

# Preface

This book has been an outcome of determined endeavour from a group of educationists in the field. The primary objective was to involve a broad spectrum of professionals from diverse cultural background involved in the field for developing new researches. The book not only targets students but also scholars pursuing higher research for further enhancement of the theoretical and practical applications of the subject.

The branch concerned with the general management, leadership and administration of hospitals, health care systems, hospital networks and public health systems is known as health care management. It is also called medical and health services management. It focuses on ensuring that all the required health outcomes are attained. Moreover, it ensures that the departments in a health institution are running smoothly and working towards the attainment of a common goal. Hospital administrators are the professionals dealing with the administration and management of hospitals and other health institutions. They are considered to be the central points of control within hospitals. This book includes some of the vital pieces of work being conducted across the world, on various topics related to healthcare management. Different approaches, evaluations, methodologies and advanced studies on healthcare management have been included in it. The extensive content of this book provides the readers with a thorough understanding of the subject.

It was an honour to edit such a profound book and also a challenging task to compile and examine all the relevant data for accuracy and originality. I wish to acknowledge the efforts of the contributors for submitting such brilliant and diverse chapters in the field and for endlessly working for the completion of the book. Last, but not the least; I thank my family for being a constant source of support in all my research endeavours.

**Editor**

# Digital Analysis of Sit-to-Stand in Masters Athletes, Healthy Old People, and Young Adults Using a Depth Sensor

Daniel Leightley [1],* [iD] and Moi Hoon Yap [2] [iD]

[1]   King's Centre for Military Health Research, Institute of Psychiatry, Psychology & Neuroscience, King's College London, London WC2R 2LS, UK

[2]   School of Computing, Mathematics and Digital Technology, Manchester Metropolitan University, Manchester M15 6BH, UK; m.yap@mmu.ac.uk

*   Correspondence: daniel.leightley@kcl.ac.uk

**Abstract:** The aim of this study was to compare the performance between young adults ($n = 15$), healthy old people ($n = 10$), and masters athletes ($n = 15$) using a depth sensor and automated digital assessment framework. Participants were asked to complete a clinically validated assessment of the sit-to-stand technique (five repetitions), which was recorded using a depth sensor. A feature encoding and evaluation framework to assess balance, core, and limb performance using time- and speed-related measurements was applied to markerless motion capture data. The associations between the measurements and participant groups were examined and used to evaluate the assessment framework suitability. The proposed framework could identify phases of sit-to-stand, stability, transition style, and performance between participant groups with a high degree of accuracy. In summary, we found that a depth sensor coupled with the proposed framework could identify performance subtleties between groups.

**Keywords:** kinect; depth sensor; motion capture; sit-to-stand; automated assessment; short physical performance battery

---

## 1. Introduction

There is a clear and advancing benefit to the development of digitised automated systems to evaluate human motion using depth sensor technology for use in the healthcare domain [1–3]. The general population is living longer; therefore, new and innovative means of quantifying and assessing a person's physical health are needed to better allocate resources and target interventions. While many in the ageing population will remain healthy, active, and engaged into later life, some studies have shown that a minority of older adults suffer from frailty and musculoskeletal disorders [4]. Focusing on frailty, it is not a single disease, but a combination of the natural ageing processes during which neuromuscular systems decline, and the accumulation of medical conditions leaves a person vulnerable to illness, trips, or falls [5]. Further, older adults have unstable balance and motion stability compared with the young, and the amount of body sway increases with more challenging motions [2,6].

Although in-person clinical assessment is vital, there is a need to develop more efficient clinical approaches that are suitable for the Internet-of-Things, assistive living [7], and Cloud Computing era [5,8,9]. There are many limitations in current assessment processes. First, clinician-led assessments are dependent on the skills, experiences, and judgement of the individual clinician, and therefore may not always be objective. Second, clinical assessments are open to subjective bias and contain inter-/intra-variance between assessments. Third, the entire process can be time-consuming considering the person's need to attend the appointment and undertake the assessment, and the need for clinics to arrange appointments and oversee the assessments. Fourth, people with physical mobility impairment increase their risk of further trauma by having to attend specialist clinics, so it would be preferable to undertake the assessment at home or a suitable location. Fifth, a person may exhibit different behavior because of the examination, which may alter the outcome and perceptions by the clinician.

Several studies have utilised depth sensor technology to analyse and quantify mobility to predict possible future declines in physical health [1,10,11]. Early identification could enable remedial clinician-led intervention to occur more quickly and thus improve patient outcomes [3,4,12]. Several attempts have been made to develop assessment systems to judge clinically relevant motions such as sit-to-stand, timed-up-and-go, and static balance [13–15]. While these systems have been shown to be useful in monitoring and quantifying balance, they fall short of assessing time- and speed-related measurements between distinct population groups which could be insightful to a clinician in the decision-making process.

There are several methods which seek to characterise sit-to-stand by decomposing the motion into phases to identify the start, middle, and end phase, and how the movement was performed [2,16,17]. Bennett et al. (2014) [16] used pressure sensors to gather movement data. The Centre of Mass was calculated and evaluated using a classifier to determine if different phases of motion could be identified. The authors could identify between slow, unstable sit-to-stand, and healthy transition phases. Ejupi et al. (2015) [13] used a depth sensor to examine the feasibility of detecting sit-to-stand motion between the elderly who may be prone to falling. By developing a system which uses time-and speed-related measurements, the authors could discriminate between those who were at high risk of falling and those who were not.

In this paper, we propose a non-invasive markerless digitalised and automated framework, using novel feature generation and motion decomposition, to analyse the performance of masters athletes, healthy old people, and young adults performing the sit-to-stand (five repetitions) motion, which is a functional test that is commonly used in a clinical setting to assess balance and stability [18]. The framework acquires motion capture (mocap) data from a single depth sensor, where the skeletal stream is de-noised using a heuristic algorithm, then decomposed into a set of novel time-and speed-related features. Analysis techniques are employed to identify the performance in execution, sitting, and stand-to-sitting, thus providing detailed insight into the stages of motion analysis for clinicians.

## 2. Materials and Methods

### 2.1. Data Collection

A comprehensive description of the data collection for the K3Da dataset has been previously reported in [19], but a summary is provided hereafter.

### 2.1.1. Participants

This study used the K3Da dataset [19], which consists of participants performing a range of clinically validated motions extracted from the Short Physical Performance Battery [18] under the supervision of a clinically trained individual and recorded using a markerless Microsoft Kinect One depth sensor (i.e., no devices are required to be affixed to the participant). Participants were recruited from staff at the Manchester Metropolitan University, a local athletics club, and elderly people from the general population. All reported that they had no history of neurological disorders or serious musculoskeletal injury, and each reported good upper and lower limb function.

The data collected was approved by the local ethics committee of the Manchester Metropolitan University (SE121308). Written informed consent was obtained for each participant.

### 2.1.2. Data Acquisition

Kinect data was captured using a custom application [20] which interfaced with a Microsoft Kinect One to record depth and mocap data at a 30 Hz sampling rate. The output, including depth and the skeleton model with 25 anatomical landmark locations, is shown in Figure 1. The sensor was placed on a tripod at a 70 cm height with a vertical angle of 0°. Room furniture was removed to enable maximum visibility and reduce occlusion, and lighting was standardised via lighting controls.

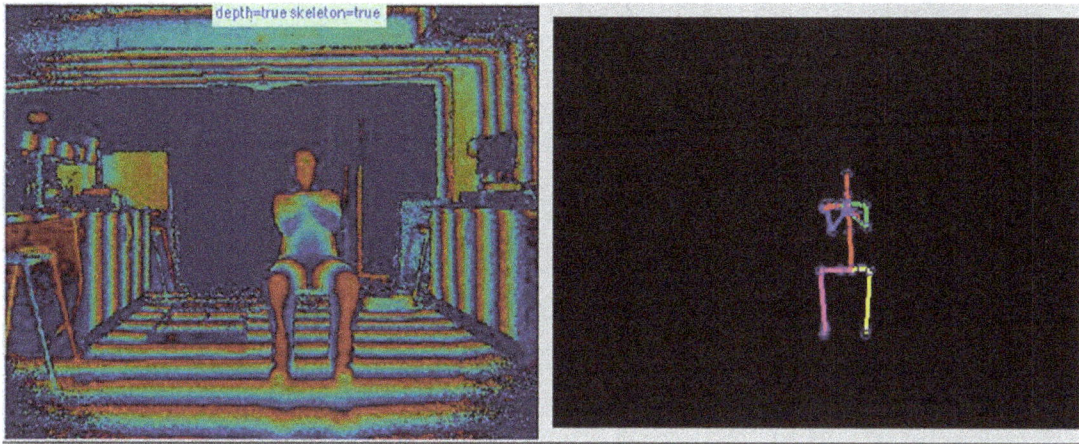

**Figure 1.** Example output of the Microsoft Kinect One depth sensor and skeleton model renders in MathWorks Matlab (2016B).

Each participant was asked to perform the sit-to-stand starting from a seated position. A chair with a seat height of 44 cm and secure back rest, without arm rests, was used (see Figure 2). When instructed, they had to stand up so that the legs were fully extended, and then sit down again. This was repeated five times with the aim to complete five complete stand/seat cycles within a 60 s period. The arms were held across the chest so that all the power needed to stand and sit was produced by the legs muscles. Each participant was provided with a maximum of three attempts to complete the motion within the time-limit.

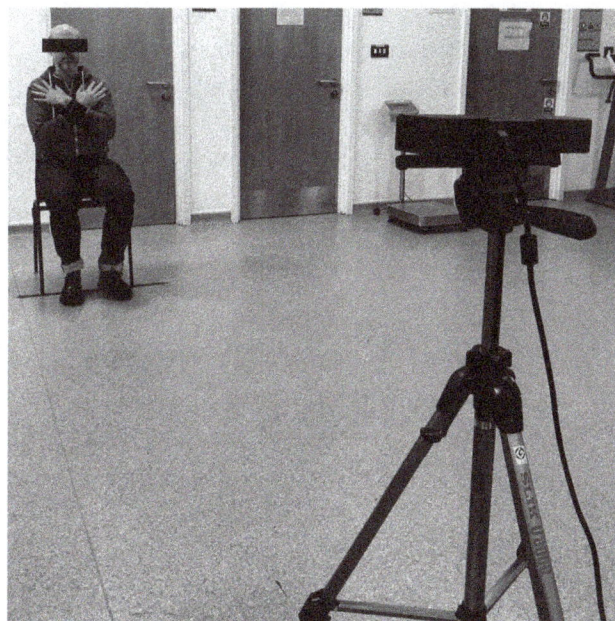

**Figure 2.** Example recording enviorment with the Microsoft Kinect One placed on a tripod at 70 cm.

### 2.1.3. Data Labelling

Two coders were recruited to annotate each motion sequence to identify specific points of interest using a video recording of the session. The following were coded:

1.  Peak of each sit-to-stand phase: The coder was asked to locate the minima and maxima of each peak of the standing and sitting repetition.
2.  Start and end of each sit-to-stand phase: The coder was asked to identify where they believe the start of the sit-to-stand and end (stand-to-sit) were located.
3.  Outlier frames: The K3Da dataset labelled each frame as a 'good' frame or 'outlier', which was reassessed by coders for agreement.

The locations were recorded for each motion and will be used as ground-truth when comparing the performance of the proposed framework. The inter-coder reliability ($\pm 10$ frames for each specific point of interest) was calculated at 0.84, and where differences occurred, the coders discussed their differences and came to an agreement (resulting in full agreement).

### 2.2. Assessment Framework

A single markerless depth sensor was used to record the sit-to-stand motion before the following phases were undertaken in an offline environment.

#### 2.2.1. Phase 1: Outlier Detection

Marker-less mocap systems can occasionally produce unreliable tracking of important anatomical locations (i.e., hand, arms, knees), for instance, an unorthodox body position (i.e., crouching down) or the occlusion of body parts (i.e., one leg hidden behind the other). These recording errors introduce noise in the mocap data, which can impact analysis of the sit-to-stand motion due to subtlety of motion differences [21]. To identify recording errors (outliers), we performed outlier detection based on the Euclidean distance and the principle that mutual Euclidean distances between any joint should not vary with time. A $k$-means clustering algorithm was used to detect outlier (noisy) frames, where mocap data of each frame are clustered into two groups; one which contains the good frames and the other containing the outlier, or poor quality frames.

A heuristic algorithm was employed to identify the centroid seed for both groups following the proposal of Arthur and Vassilvitskii (2017) [22]. After initialisation, $k$-means clustering is performed to identify and assign a group to the mocap frames. A goodness index is defined, Equation (1), based on the average $L2$ norm between the cluster centre (denoted as $c$) and a set of frames (denoted as $F$) assigned to the cluster, as proposed by [23,24]. The cluster which contains the highest $G_c$ value is selected as the *good* cluster, with the remaining cluster being identified as the outlier. This is given as:

$$G_c = \frac{\sum_{j=1}^{n} ||C_c - F_j||^2}{\max(n)}, \ 1 \leq c \leq 2. \tag{1}$$

where $n$ is the frame index and $j$ is the joint index. All frames which lie within the *good* cluster are used for all further analyses, and those labelled as *poor quality* frames are disregarded.

#### 2.2.2. Phase 2: Feature Generation

*Centre-of-Mass (CoM)*: The CoM [25,26] is encoded to describe the anterior-posterior (AP; i.e., forward and backward directional movement) and medio-lateral (ML; i.e., left and right directional movement) directional movement of the participant. Figure 3 demonstrates two-dimensional (2-D) examples of sit-to-stand motion sequences. Let *com* be the encoded CoM derived from three joints (*LeftHip, RightHip, SpineMid*) given as:

$$com = [\bar{x}, \bar{y}, \bar{z}]^n = \bar{x} = \frac{\sum_{j=1}^{3} F_{n,x}}{3}, \bar{y} = \frac{\sum_{j=1}^{3} F_{n,y}}{3}, \bar{z} = \frac{\sum_{j=1}^{3} F_{n,z}}{3}. \tag{2}$$

where $\bar{x}, \bar{y}, \bar{z}$ is the derived mean value, $n$ is a frame index, and *com* is a set of mean values.

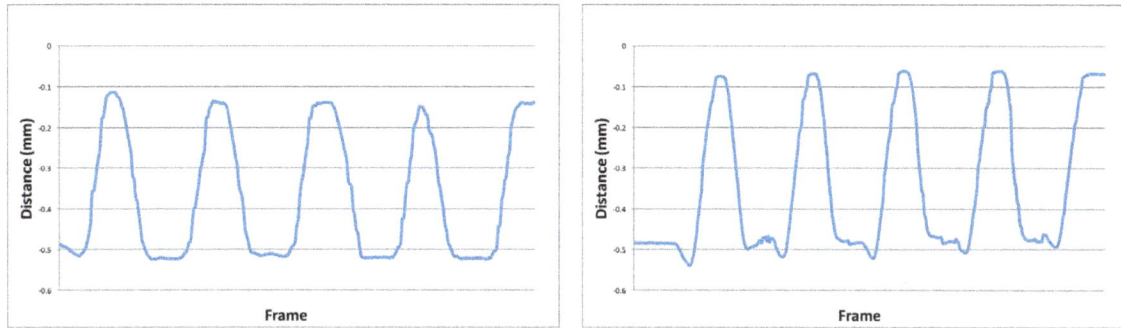

**Figure 3.** Visual 2-D (*y* axis) representation of the Centre-of-Mass feature encoded from two sequences of sit-to-stand. Left: motion performed by a healthy old participant. Right: motion performed by a young adults.

*Upper Body Flexion Angle (UBFA)*: Previous work has sought to represent the postural body *lean* by encoding the angle of the spine in relation to the floor plane [9,27]. However, implementing this type of computation for motions such as sit-to-stand will not suitably encode the upper body flexion of rising and sitting in a chair. In this work, we propose the Upper Body Flexion Angle (UBFA) to represent the *lean* of motions that require priority use of the upper torso. The UBFA is computed between the *SpineBase* and *Neck*, given as:

$$\theta = arc \cos \left( \frac{F_{SpineBase} \circ F_{Neck}}{||F_{SpineBase}||\ ||F_{Neck}||} \right)^n. \tag{3}$$

*Upper-frame Velocity (UfV)*: The Upper-frame Velocity (UfV) is encoded by computing the temporal difference of the motion in time sequential order between each frame ($n$–$n_{-1}$) of the CoM (*com*) feature defined earlier.

The CoM, UBFA, and UfV are concatenated into single matrices and used for analyses.

### 2.2.3. Phase 3: Transition Detection

The vertical displacement (*y-axis*) of the CoM (*com*) feature defined earlier was used to identify the transitions between sit-to-stand and stand-to-sit. Following a similar approach described by Ejupi et al. (2015) [13], an automatic identification technique was applied to identify the following phases: sitting, sit-to-peak-standing transition, and peak-standing-to-sitting transition. The automatic transition detection framework (Figure 4) is defined in the following three-step process:

1. Peak-standing and sitting: The *y-axis* of the CoM (*com*) feature was low-pass filtered using a Butterworth filter with a normalised cut-off frequency of six frames. Peak standing and sitting points were detected using the inverse maxima, to identify the local minima and maxima of the vector.

2. Start and end of each sit-to-stand phase: The start of the standing and sitting phase commenced when the following conditions were met; start of the sit-to-stand motion was defined as the first vertical increase above a threshold value, defined as the vertical mean (plus 15%), and the final stand-to-sit decreasing below the mean (minus 15%).

3.  Limitation: The maximum number of completed transitions was set at five, the required number for the sit-to-stand motion, meaning that if a participant performed more than five, they were not used in computation.

The motion was then divided into separate segments, sit-to-stand-to-sit, for analysis. The seated start and end of the sequence is removed and not factored into the analyses.

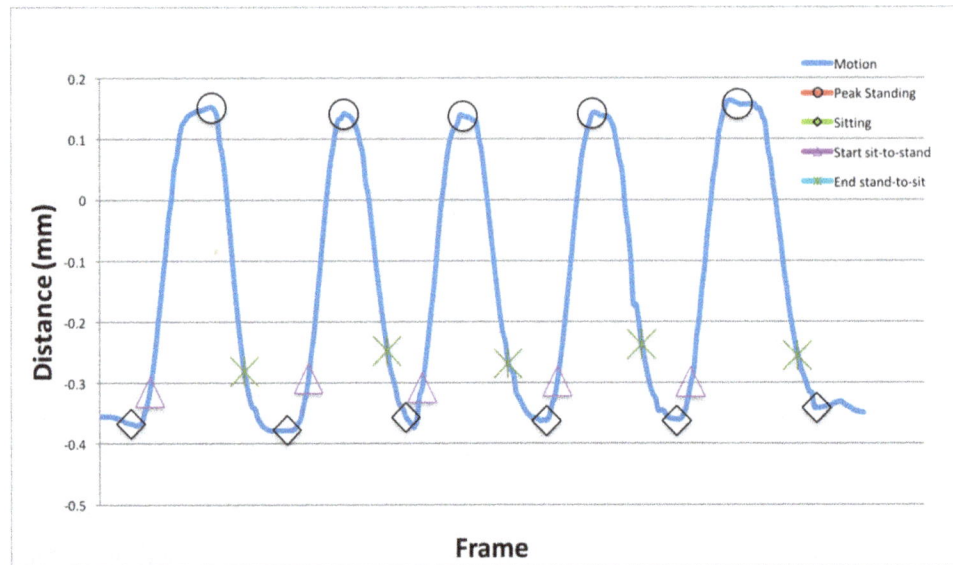

**Figure 4.** Example output of the proposed transition detection framework derived from the Centre-of-Mass feature vector.

### 2.3. Statistical Analyses

Analysis of Microsoft Kinect Data was performed using customised scripts in MathWorks Matlab (2016b) and statistical analyses were undertaken using the statistical software package STATA (version 14.0) with statistical significance defined as a $p$ value $< 0.05$. The AP, ML, UBFA, and UfV Sit/Stand values were presented as absolute values. Comparison between participant data was assed using Repeated Measures ANOVA to measure within-group differences. Where significant condition-by-group interaction was found, separate dependent sample $t$-tests were performed.

In addition, the following parameters are defined:

1.  Stand Time (s): The time taken between each peak-sitting to peak-standing.
2.  Sit Time (s): The time taken between each peak-standing to peak-sitting.
3.  CoM Stand ML (cm) and AP (cm): The directional movement observed during each peak-sitting to peak-standing.
4.  CoM Sit ML (cm) and AP (cm): The directional movement observed during each peak-standing to peak-sitting.
5.  Stand UfV (m/s): The velocity observed during each peak-sitting to peak-standing.
6.  Sit UfV (m/s): The velocity observed during each peak-standing to peak-sitting.
7.  Stand UBFA (deg): The angle of the torso observed during each peak-sitting to peak-standing.
8.  Sit UBFA (deg): The angle of the torso observed during each peak-standing to peak-sitting.
9.  Total Time (s): The total time is computed from the first peak-sitting to the last peak-sitting (5 repetitions).

## 3. Results

The participants ($n = 40$) are divided into three groups based on their age and self-reported physical performance ability; young adult ($n = 15$), healthy old person ($n = 10$), and masters athletes ($n = 15$). There was a statistical difference between age, height, and body mass index between groups (see Table 1). Each participant typically took no longer than 15 s (450 frames, 30 Hz recording rate) to complete the movement, and no participant required and/or requested a second attempt.

**Table 1.** Characteristics of participants divided by group.

| Parameter (SD) | Young Adult | Healthy Old | Masters Athletes | $p$-Value |
|---|---|---|---|---|
| Age, years | 26.40 ($\pm$3.16) | 74.90 ($\pm$4.11) | 66.93 ($\pm$5.03) [a,b] | 0.00 |
| Height, cm | 176.47 ($\pm$8.59) | 170.30 ($\pm$5.97) [c] | 166.01 ($\pm$10.07) | 0.04 |
| Weight, kg | 77.93 ($\pm$18.11) | 80.25 ($\pm$15.32) | 61.90 ($\pm$9.39) | 0.594 |
| Body mass index | 23.01 ($\pm$5.70) [b,c] | 22.65 ($\pm$5.38) | 19.14 ($\pm$2.11) | 0.04 |

The $p$-value represents the main effect obtained from the ANOVA. Results from dependent comparisons are included as [a] significantly different from Young; [b] significantly different from healthy old; [c] significantly different from masters athletes.

### 3.1. Outlier Detection

The proposed outlier detection method performed strongly when assessed on the ability to detect individual outlier frames when compared to manual annotation (as annotated in [19]). Overall detection accuracy was 93.87% ($\pm$8.84), and each participant group obtained the following results; young adult obtained 96.47% ($\pm$2.96), healthy old obtained 87.16 ($\pm$12.40), and masters athletes obtained 95.77% ($\pm$7.52). The reasons behind misclassification were explored further, and it was found that this was due to occlusion of the body, noisy outer limbs due to inaccurate tracking, and loose clothing causing tracking inaccuracies.

### 3.2. Transition Detection

Detection of the peak standing point, sitting, start of sit-to-stand, and end of stand-to-sit was compared to manual annotation to compute the accuracy and reliability of detection. Points of interest were determined as correct if they lay within $\pm$10 frames of the manual annotation. The rates for points of interest are presented in Table 2 alongside the accuracy results in Figure 5. Detection rates across the transition phases was high, and the framework can identify the sitting phase; however, there was misclassification between sitting and end of stand-to-sit due to similarities between both phases.

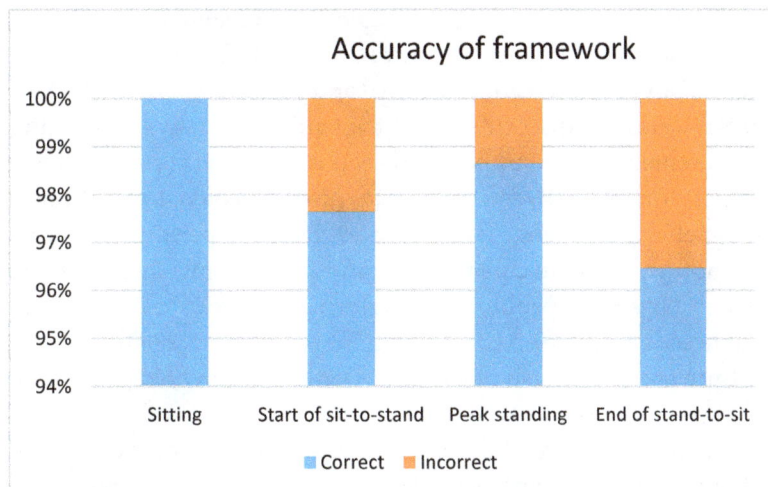

**Figure 5.** Classification results for each phase. Correct classifications versus incorrect classifications.

**Table 2.** Transition detection rates for each point of interest.

| Parameter | Average Detection Rate (SD) |
|---|---|
| Sitting | 6 ($\pm$0) |
| Start of sit-to-stand | 4.76 ($\pm$0.48) |
| Peak standing | 4.93 ($\pm$0.35) |
| End of stand-to-sit | 4.34 ($\pm$0.63) |

### 3.3. Identifying Subtle Differences

The framework was able to detect subtle differences between participant groups based on an automated detection of the points of interest (see Table 3); the results are in-line with the literature and indicate the potential use in a healthcare setting [2]. Young adults could complete the sit-to-stand (five repetitions) in less than 8 s compared with healthy old people, who took an average of 12 s. It was observed that for Stand time, Sit UBFA, and UfV, there were significant differences between the young adults and masters athletes.

**Table 3.** Computed results for the sit-to-stand motion for each participant group.

| Parameter | Young Adults | Healthy Old | Masters Athletes | $p$-Value |
|---|---|---|---|---|
| Stand Time (s) | 1.02 ($\pm$0.18) | 2.02 ($\pm$0.21) | 1.51 ($\pm$0.19) [a] | 0.02 |
| CoM Stand ML (cm) | 0.24 (0.05) | 0.03 (0.26) | 0.17 (0.06) | 0.56 |
| CoM Stand AP (cm) | 0.21 ($\pm$0.01) [b] | 0.01 ($\pm$0.19) | 0.04 ($\pm$0.14) | 0.04 |
| Stand UBFA (deg) | 12 ($\pm$2.86) | 18 ($\pm$4.09) | 14 ($\pm$3.58) | 0.62 |
| Stand UfV (m/s) | 0.82 ($\pm$0.19) | 0.71 ($\pm$0.38) | 0.73 ($\pm$0.19) | 0.16 |
| Sit Time (s) | 0.92 ($\pm$0.23) | 1.47 ($\pm$0.73) | 0.98 ($\pm$0.35) | 0.23 |
| CoM Sit ML (cm) | 0.22 (0.06) | 0.04 (0.28) [a,c] | 0.22 (0.09) | 0.00 |
| CoM Sit AP (cm) | 0.22 ($\pm$0.03) | 0.03 ($\pm$0.17) | 0.05 ($\pm$0.16) | 0.53 |
| Sit UBFA (deg) | 17 ($\pm$3.19) | 16 ($\pm$3.71) [a] | 10 ($\pm$2.38) [a] | 0.05 |
| Sit UfV (m/s) | 0.98 ($\pm$0.19) | 0.78 ($\pm$0.58) | 0.83 ($\pm$0.21) [a] | 0.04 |
| Total time (s) | 7.98 ($\pm$2.09) | 12.18 ($\pm$3.76) | 9.28 ($\pm$0.94) | 0.24 |

The $p$-value represents the main effect obtained from the ANOVA. Results from dependent comparisons are included as a significantly different from Young; b significantly different from healthy old; c significantly different from masters athletes.

## 4. Discussion and Conclusions

In this work, we utilise a depth sensor and automated framework to identify a range of clinically relevant outcome features that may be useful to a clinician in providing greater insight into the performance capability of a participant. Unique insights were obtained for each group. Young adults could execute the sit-to-stand, but presented large AP and ML. The healthy old group were able to execute the sit-to-stand, but presented a reduced AP and ML sway and an increase in time taken to stand and sit. Masters athletes could execute the sit-to-stand with relative ease, with little impediment to their motion, but presented reduced upper body lean when standing and sitting.

Comparing the performance between participant groups demonstrates the ability of the system to distinguish between effects of ageing. The young adults could perform the sit-to-stand with little impediment to their motion and were able to maintain control. While there is no doubt that masters athletes maintain a high physical capability [28], performance nevertheless declines with advancing age alongside loss of muscle power and cardiopulmonary function [29–31], so it is possible that the balance and performance of movements such as sit-to-stand in healthy old people and masters athletes decline with increasing age and loss of muscular control.

This work exclusively focused on the use of depth sensor technology due to its ability to track human motion without any physical anatomical landmarks, sensors, or devices being placed on the participant's body. There are several studies that have utilised wearable technology (i.e., mobile devices, accelerometer, and gravity sensors) to track balance and sit-to-stand motions successfully;

however, they are only capable of providing outcomes in relation to where the device/marker has been located, which means that the body itself is not being assessed, and they are expensive to implement widely [32–34]. However, future work should explore uniting both modalities to provide a holistic overview of the execution of balance and sit-to-stand motions.

There are several limitations in this study, most of which relate to the use of technology in making a clinical judgement. First, the Kinect is sensitive to light, occlusion, and placement, which could impact the tracking of the skeletal joints and the outcomes from the framework. Future studies are needed to improve tracking in different environments. Second, this study relied on labelling annotated by human coders, and there is a potential that bias may impact coding. Future studies are needed to explore the relationship between human coding and computerised coding comparisons. Third, the detection of outlier frames may have impacted the detection of phases. Future work should seek to explore the use and reliability of interpolation methods, such as [35], to replace outlier frames with an estimation of the correct frame. Finally, this study presented multiple analyses; however, we should consider how a clinician would interpret these results. Future work should seek to explore how we should present data in a clinical context.

We have proposed a framework which unites depth sensor technology and feature extraction to assess the sit-to-stand motion sequence. The framework has been shown to be reliable and accurate in evaluating the transition phases and providing clinical outcome measures. Future work will focus on future clinical validation, increase the number of participants, improve reliability, and extend the framework to analyse a wide range of motions.

**Author Contributions:** D.L. designed the study, undertook data preparation and data analysis, and wrote all drafts of the manuscript. M.H.Y. contributed to the study design and data analysis, and assisted in writing all drafts of the manuscript. All authors have read and approved the final manuscript.

## References

1. Leightley, D.; McPhee, J.S.; Yap, M.H. Automated Analysis and Quantification of Human Mobility Using a Depth Sensor. *IEEE J. Biomed. Health Inform.* **2017**, *21*, 939–948. [CrossRef] [PubMed]

2. Leightley, D.; Yap, M.H.; Coulson, J.; Piasecki, M.; Cameron, J.; Barnouin, Y.; Tobias, J.; McPhee, J.S. Postural Stability during Standing Balance and Sit-to-Stand in Master Athlete Runners Compared with Nonathletic Old and Young Adults. *J. Aging Phys. Act.* **2017**, *25*, 345–350. [CrossRef] [PubMed]

3. Clark, R.; Pua, Y.-H.; Fortin, K.; Ritchie, C.; Webster, K.; Denehy, L.; Bryant, A. Validity of the Microsoft Kinect for assessment of postural control. *Gait Posture* **2012**, *36*, 372–377. [CrossRef] [PubMed]

4. Collard, R.M.; Boter, H.; Schoevers, R.A.; Oude Voshaar, R.C. Prevalence of frailty in community-dwelling older persons: A systematic review. *J. Am. Geriatr. Soc.* **2012**, *60*, 1487–1492. [CrossRef] [PubMed]

5. Practitoners, G. *Fit for Frailty: Consensus Best Practice Guidance for the Care of Older People Living with Frailty in Community and Outpatient Settings*; British Geriatrics Society Tech Report; British Geriatrics Society: London, UK, 2014.

6. Gill, J.; Allum, J.H.J.; Carpenter, M.G.; Held-Ziolkowska, M.; Adkin, A.L.; Honegger, F.; Pierchala, K. Trunk Sway Measures of Postural Stability during Clinical Balance Tests: Effects of Age. *J. Gerontol. A Biol. Sci. Med. Sci.* **2001**, *56*, M438–M447. [CrossRef] [PubMed]

7. Fortino, G.; Gravina, R.; Guerrieri, A.; di Fatta, G. Engineering Large-Scale Body Area Networks Applications. In Proceedings of the 8th International Conference on Body Area Networks, Boston, MA, USA, 30 September–2 October 2013.

8. Gregory, P.; Alexander, J.; Satinksky, J. Clinical Telerehabilitation: Applications for Physiatrists. *Am. Acad. Phys. Med. Rehabil.* **2011**, *3*, 647–656. [CrossRef] [PubMed]

9. Leightley, D.; Yap, M.H.; Hewitt, B.M.; McPhee, J.S. Sensing Behaviour using the Kinect: Identifying Characteristic Features of Instability and Poor Performance during Challenging Balancing Tasks. In Proceedings of the Measuring Behavior 2016, Dublin, Ireland, 25–27 May 2016.

10.  Dehbandi, B.; Barachant, A.; Smeragliuolo, A.H.; Long, J.D.; Bumanlag, S.J.; He, V.; Lampe, A.; Putrino, D. Using data from the Microsoft Kinect 2 to determine postural stability in healthy subjects: A feasibility trial. *PLoS ONE* **2017**, *12*, e0170890. [CrossRef] [PubMed]

11.  Guenterberg, E.; Ostadabbas, S.; Ghasemzadeh, H.; Jafari, R. An Automatic Segmentation Technique in Body Sensor Networks based on Signal Energy. In Proceedings of the 4th International ICST Conference on Body Area Networks, Los Angeles, CA, USA, 1–3 April 2009.

12.  Mentiplay, B.F.; Perraton, L.G.; Bower, K.J.; Pua, Y.H.; McGaw, R.; Heywood, S.; Clark, R.A. Gait assessment using the Microsoft Xbox One Kinect: Concurrent validity and inter-day reliability of spatiotemporal and kinematic variables. *J. Biomech.* **2015**, *48*, 2166–2170. [CrossRef] [PubMed]

13.  Ejupi, A.; Brodie, M.; Gschwind, Y.J.; Lord, S.R.; Zagler, W.L.; Delbaere, K. Kinect-Based Five-Times-Sit-to-Stand Test for Clinical and In-Home Assessment of Fall Risk in Older People. *Gerontology* **2015**, *62*, 118–124. [CrossRef] [PubMed]

14.  Vernon, S.; Paterson, K.; Bower, K.; McGinley, J.; Miller, K.; Pua, Y.-H.; Clark, R.A. Quantifying Individual Components of the Timed up and Go Using the Kinect in People Living with Stroke. *Neurorehabil. Neural Repair* **2015**, *29*, 48–53. [CrossRef] [PubMed]

15.  Agethen, P.; Otto, M.; Mengel, S.; Rukzio, E. Using Marker-less Motion Capture Systems for Walk Path Analysis in Paced Assembly Flow Lines. *Procedia CIRP* **2016**, *54*, 152–157. [CrossRef]

16.  Bennett, S.L.; Goubran, R.; Rockwood, K.; Knoefel, F. Distinguishing between stable and unstable sit-to-stand transfers using pressure sensors. In Proceedings of the 2014 IEEE International Symposium on Medical Measurements and Applications (MeMeA), Lisbon, Portugal, 11–12 June 2014; pp. 1–4.

17.  Acorn, E.; Dipsis, N.; Pincus, T.; Stathis, K. Sit-to-Stand Movement Recognition Using Kinect. *Stat. Learn. Data Sci.* **2015**, *9047*, 179–192.

18.  Guralnik, J.; Simonsick, E.; Ferrucci, L.; Glynn, R.; Berkman, L.; Blazer, D.; Scherr, P.; Wallace, R. A Short Physical Performance Battery Assessing Lower Extremity Function: Association with Self-Reported Disability and Prediction of Mortality and Nursing Home Admission. *J. Gerontol.* **1994**, *49*, 85–93. [CrossRef]

19.  Leightley, D.; Yap, M.H.; Coulson, Y.B.J.; Mcphee, J.S. Benchmarking Human Motion Analysis Using Kinect One: An open source dataset. In Proceedings of the IEEE Conference of Asia-Pacific Signal and Information Processing Association, Chicago, IL, USA, 16–19 December 2015.

20.  Leightley, D. Recording Kinect One Stream Using C#. 2016. Available online: https://leightley.com/recording-kinect-one-streams-using-c/ (accessed on 11 July 2017).

21.  Blumrosen, G.; Miron, Y.; Intrator, N.; Plotnik, M. A Real-Time Kinect Signature-Based Patient Home Monitoring System. *Sensors* **2016**, *16*, 1965. [CrossRef] [PubMed]

22.  Arthur, D.; Vassilvitskii, S. K-means++: The Advantages of Careful Seeding. In Proceedings of the Eighteenth Annual ACM-SIAM Symposium on Discrete Algorithms, New Orleans, LA, USA, 7–9 January 2007; pp. 1027–1035.

23.  Sinha, A.; Chakravarty, K. Pose Based Person Identification Using Kinect. In Proceedings of the International Conference on Systems, Man and Cybernetics, Manchester, UK, 13–16 October 2013; pp. 497–503.

24.  Leightley, D.; Li, B.; McPhee, J.S.; Yap, M.H.; Darby, J. Exemplar-based Human Action Recognition with Template Matching from a Stream of Motion Capture. *Image Anal. Recognit.* **2014**, *8815*, 12–20.

25.  Gonzalez, A.; Fraisse, P.; Hayashibe, M. A personalized balance measurement for home-based rehabilitation. In Proceedings of the IEEE Conference on Neural Engineering, Paris, France, 22–24 April 2015; pp. 711–714.

26.  Gonzalez, A.; Hayashibe, M.; Fraisse, P. Estimation of the center of mass with Kinect and Wii balance board. In Proceedings of the International Conference on Intelligent Robots and Systems, Vilamoura-Algarve, Portugal, 7–12 October 2012; pp. 1023–1028.

27.  Bó, A.P.L.; Hayashibe, M.; Poignet, P. Joint angle estimation in rehabilitation with inertial sensors and its integration with Kinect. In Proceedings of the 2011 Annual International Conference of the IEEE Engineering in Medicine and Biology Society, Boston, MA, USA, 30 August–3 September 2011; pp. 3479–3483.

28.  Rittweger, J.; di Prampero, P.E.; Maffulli, N.; Narici, M.V. Sprint and endurance power and ageing: An analysis of master athletic world records. *Proc. R. Soc. Lond. B Biol. Sci.* **2009**, *276*, 683–689. [CrossRef] [PubMed]

29.  Degens, H.; Maden-Wilkinson, T.M.; Ireland, A.; Korhonen, M.T.; Suominen; Heinonen, A.; Radak, Z.; McPhee, J.S.; Rittweger, J. Relationship between ventilatory function and age in master athletes and a sedentary reference population. *J. Age* **2013**, *35*, 1007–1015. [CrossRef] [PubMed]

30. Michaelis, I.; Kwiet, A.; Gast, U.; Boshof, A.; Antvorskov, T.; Jung, T.; Rittweger, J.; Felsenberg, D. Decline of specific peak jumping power with age in master runners. *J. Musculoskelet. Neuronal Interact.* **2008**, *8*, 64–70. [PubMed]

31. Runge, M.; Rittweger, J.; Russo, C.R.; Schiessl, H.; Felsenberg, D. Is muscle power output a key factor in the age-related decline in physical performance? A comparison of muscle cross section, chair-rising test and jumping power. *Clin. Physiol. Funct. Imaging* **2004**, *24*, 335–340. [CrossRef] [PubMed]

32. Adusumilli, G.; Joseph, S.E.; Samaan, M.A.; Schultz, B.; Popovic, T.; Souza, R.B.; Majumdar, S. iPhone Sensors in Tracking Outcome Variables of the 30-Second Chair Stand Test and Stair Climb Test to Evaluate Disability: Cross-Sectional Pilot Study. *JMIR Mhealth Uhealth* **2017**, *5*, e166. [CrossRef] [PubMed]

33. Bonato, P. Advances in wearable technology and its medical applications. In Proceedings of the 2010 Annual International Conference of the IEEE Engineering in Medicine and Biology Society (EMBC), Buenos Aires, Argentina, 31 August–4 September 2010; pp. 2021–2024.

34. Papi, E.; Koh, W.S.; McGregor, A.H. Wearable technology for spine movement assessment: A systematic review. *J. Biomech.* **2017**, *64*, 186–197. [CrossRef] [PubMed]

35. Milani, S.; Calvagno, G. Joint denoising and interpolation of depth maps for MS Kinect sensors. In Proceedings of the 2012 IEEE International Conference on Acoustics, Speech and Signal Processing (ICASSP), Kyoto, Japan, 25–30 March 2012; pp. 797–800.

# Laying Anchor: Inserting Precision Health into a Public Health Genetics Policy Course

Stephen M. Modell [1,*], Toby Citrin [1] and Sharon L. R. Kardia [2]

[1] Department of Health Management and Policy, University of Michigan School of Public Health, 1415 Washington Heights, Ann Arbor, MI 48109-2029, USA; tcitrin@umich.edu

[2] Department of Epidemiology, University of Michigan School of Public Health, M5174, SPH II, 1415 Washington Heights, Ann Arbor, MI 48109-2029, USA; skardia@umich.edu

* Correspondence: mod@umich.edu

**Abstract:** The United States Precision Medicine Initiative (PMI) was announced by then President Barack Obama in January 2015. It is a national effort designed to take into account genetic, environmental, and lifestyle differences in the development of individually tailored forms of treatment and prevention. This goal was implemented in March 2015 with the formation of an advisory committee working group to provide a framework for the proposed national research cohort of one million or more participants. The working group further held a public workshop on participant engagement and health equity, focusing on the design of an inclusive cohort, building public trust, and identifying active participant engagement features for the national cohort. Precision techniques offer medical and public health practitioners the opportunity to personally tailor preventive and therapeutic regimens based on informatics applied to large volume genotypic and phenotypic data. The PMI's (*All of Us* Research Program's) medical and public health promise, its balanced attention to technical and ethical issues, and its nuanced advisory structure made it a natural choice for inclusion in the University of Michigan course "Issues in Public Health Genetics" (HMP 517), offered each fall by the University's School of Public Health. In 2015, the instructors included the PMI as the recurrent case study introduced at the beginning and referred to throughout the course, and as a class exercise allowing students to translate issues into policy. In 2016, an entire class session was devoted to precision medicine and precision public health. In this article, we examine the dialogues that transpired in these three course components, evaluate session impact on student ability to formulate PMI policy, and share our vision for next-generation courses dealing with precision health. *Methodology*: Class materials (class notes, oral exercise transcripts, class exercise written hand-ins) from the three course components were inspected and analyzed for issues and policy content. The purpose of the analysis was to assess the extent to which course components have enabled our students to formulate policy in the precision public health area. Analysis of student comments responding to questions posed during the initial case study comprised the initial or "pre-" categories. Analysis of student responses to the class exercise assignment, which included the same set of questions, formed the "post-" categories. Categories were validated by cross-comparison among the three authors, and inspected for frequency with which they appeared in student responses. Frequencies steered the selection of illustrative quotations, revealing the extent to which students were able to convert issue areas into actual policies. Lecture content and student comments in the precision health didactic session were inspected for degree to which they reinforced and extended the derived categories. *Results*: The case study inspection yielded four overarching categories: (1) assurance (access, equity, disparities); (2) participation (involvement, representativeness); (3) ethics (consent, privacy, benefit sharing); and (4) treatment of people (stigmatization, discrimination). Class exercise inspection and analysis yielded three additional categories: (5) financial; (6) educational; and (7) trust-building. The first three categories exceeded the others in terms of number of student mentions (8–14 vs. 4–6 mentions). Three other categories were considered and excluded because of infrequent mention. Students suggested several means of trust-building, including PMI personnel working with community leaders, stakeholder consultation, networking, and use of social media. Student representatives prioritized participant and research institution access to PMI information over commercial access. Multiple schemes were proposed for participant consent and return of results. Both pricing policy and Medicaid coverage were touched on. During the didactic session, students commented on the importance of provider training in precision health. Course evaluation highlighted the need for clarity on the organizations involved in the PMI, and leaving time for student-student interaction. *Conclusions*: While some student responses during the exercise were terse, an evolution was detectable over the three course components in student ability to suggest tangible policies and steps for implementation. Students also gained surety in presenting policy positions to a peer audience. Students came up with some very creative suggestions, such as use of an electronic platform to assure participant involvement in the disposition of their biological sample and personal health information, and alternate examples of ways to manage large volumes of data. An examination of socio-ethical issues and policies can strengthen student understanding of the directions the Precision Medicine Initiative is taking, and aid in training for the application of more varied precision medicine and public health techniques, such as tier 1 genetic testing and whole genome and exome sequencing. Future course development may reflect additional features of the ongoing *All of Us* Research Program, and further articulate precision public health approaches applying to populations as opposed to single individuals.

**Keywords:** precision medicine; precision public health; education; genetics; cancer; cardiovascular disease; population health; race; health disparities; health policy

---

## 1. Introduction: The Precision Medicine Initiative—Its Expansion and Course Insertion

### 1.1. Course Structure and Prior Precision Health Components

The Precision Medicine Initiative (PMI) was created as a collaboration between the U.S. National Institutes of Health, health-related institutions and organizations, and the American public to research and develop individually tailored forms of therapy and prevention based on the amassing of genetic, environmental, and lifestyle data. The PMI has made news headlines and is now a solid part of the health-related literature, but its breadth and implications need translation to the professional educational level. In the pages to follow, we describe an innovative effort to include the PMI and precision health in a public health genetics policy course. "Issues in Public Health Genetics" (HMP 517) has now been taught at the University of Michigan School of Public Health for more than fifteen years. The instructors' backgrounds are in law (Toby Citrin, J.D., chief instructor) and medicine and public health (Stephen M. Modell, M.D., M.S., co-instructor). The course is designed to acquaint students, typically of public health and genetic counseling, with the array of technical, ethical, and social issues facing professionals in the area of public health genetics, and with methods to convert issues into health policy [1]. We define policy as decisions made by public, private, professional, and community groups and organizations to affect behavior and direct resources. The policies focused on in the course range from the implementation of genetic screening programs to changes needing to take place at the state and federal levels to allow implementation and regulation of new genetic technologies to occur.

The "Issues in Public Health Genetics" semester consists of twenty-five one and a half hour long classroom sessions. The course as a whole is divided into four segments: A. "Policy Development" (nine sessions covering alternative methods of policymaking and their socio-ethical bases, from the fundamentals of the policymaking process to genetics law and legislation); B. "Individual, Community, and Professional Issues" (frameworks different professionals use in the design of genetic testing and screening programs, including consideration of race-ethnicity and health disparities—seven sessions);

C. "Health Industry Issues" (issue areas and policy tools relating to genetics and the health industry, such as marketing issues, technology transfer, and consumer perspectives—five sessions); and D. "Looking Back and Looking Forward" (historical and cutting edge developments from eugenics to gene therapy—five sessions).

The sessions follow a seminar format, allowing considerable give-and-take and mutual discovery between its two instructors and students, as well as between the students themselves. Before class begins, the professors post on Canvas, the electronic curricular system, an average of three pertinent assigned readings, a number of supplementary readings, and a sheet with two to three questions to be discussed in class for the particular session. Typical questions ask how students would launch a program or policy, and how they would implement it. By the second session, a two- to three-page case study is circulated to the students (past examples: epigenetic research, biobanks, direct-to-consumer genetic testing). The case study for the semester presents the students with a larger number of socio-ethical and policy questions than a typical session, generally in the neighborhood of ten, which are discussed by session 3 in combination with an instructor presentation on policy frameworks. The case study is referred to recurrently throughout the course, and thus binds the course together thematically for the semester.

The one and a half hour sessions generally start out with 10 to 15 slides presented by the two instructors. Examples provided are brief, in comparison to the larger recurrent case study. Throughout, the intention is to move the students beyond just the scientific techniques being employed and the ethical issues they generate, to consider professional, institutional, and governmental policies and how they could be implemented. The goal of the course is to enable to students to formulate policy in the genetics area. To promote this goal, the instructors stop at various points in their presentation and ask for general thoughts, issues the students might see as important, and how an issue raised by students could be translated into policy. This formal presentation period, however, lasts no more than half the class period. The rest of the period is devoted to class discussion of the questions placed on Canvas for the session. This portion of every class allows a flow of questions, suggestions, and comments between students and instructors, with occasional probing questions offered by the instructors. Class composition, consisting of 10 to 20 students per year, remains constant throughout the semester. The students become familiar with each other and the course protocol fairly quickly. The first several class sessions are whole group, later evolving into alternating use of whole group and break-out group discussion, depending on the particular session. The break-outs are achieved either by dividing the classroom longitudinally, or allowing the students to self-assign themselves to one of three to four possible groups. Fifteen percent of a student's grade is based on class participation and their follow-up postings in Canvas discussions. Thirty percent of the grade is based on two class exercises, one of which follows the theme of the recurrent case study. One of the class exercises involves individual student presentations; the other group presentations. Students self-assign themselves to roles for both varieties of class exercise format. The exercises are mostly occupied by the students presenting in response to a two to three-page class exercise sheet provided to them well in advance. The instructors also briefly introduce the exercise at the beginning, and conclude each individual or group presentation with a spontaneous question or two.

In terms of course content, the "Genetic Tools for Public Health Practice" session within segment B looks at various examples of genetic screening (prenatal, newborn, and adult, including use of family health history) and the ethical issues involved. The U.S. Centers for Disease Control and Prevention Office of Public Health Genomics (CDC-OPHG) has developed a framework of genetic conditions based on a three-tiered structure. Tier 1 conditions have techniques of genetic risk assessment that have been systematically validated [2]. We describe how screening newly diagnosed cases of colorectal cancer for Lynch syndrome, the most common heritable form of colorectal and endometrial cancer, can identify both index cases and their relatives requiring further attention. Low-density lipoprotein receptor (LDLR) mutation testing, and in some cases, APOB and PCSK9 testing, is called for in adults whose cholesterol measures have passed a critical threshold, and in children where family testing for familial hypercholesterolemia has identified a mutation. Genetic testing in these instances is criterion-based and aimed at the individual, bypassing testing of a wider clinical or general subpopulation (conventional testing for cholesterol lipoproteins has been advocated by some professional organizations for all children 21 years of age or younger). Tier 1 genetic testing for rare, high penetrance conditions, where either use of family history or genetic testing has been fully validated, is an important constituent of precision public health [3]. These forms of testing are not without controversy, such as whether testing should be "universal" among those at risk, availability of coverage, and privacy issues connected with contact of other family members. We bring these areas to the attention of our students so they can become acquainted with the considerations going into genetic testing implementation.

Each year, the syllabus is revised to reflect the latest genetic developments. In 2013, the American College of Medical Genetics and Genomics came out with policy recommendations on the reporting of incidental (secondary) findings in whole exome (WES) and whole genome (WGS) sequencing [4]. These forms of next-generation sequencing are especially valuable for the study of rare Mendelian conditions, and for identifying the genetic variants in all of a person's genes (genome) and genetic coding regions (exome). Next generation sequencing has allowed clinicians to identify rare, private mutations, undetectable by standard genetic testing, in adult cancer and cardiovascular cases [5,6], and previously insoluble childhood cases involving conditions that would otherwise be fatal [7]. Serious mutations of mutual interest to the medical and public health communities that were detectable by sequencing include hereditary breast and ovarian cancer, Lynch syndrome (hereditary nonpolyposis colorectal cancer), hypertrophic cardiomyopathy, and long QT syndrome, a potentially fatal heart arrhythmia characterized by Q-T interval elongation on the electrocardiogram. In the clinical domain, whole genome and exome sequencing represent significant techniques in the burgeoning field of precision medicine, as the genes detected have allowed administration of life-saving personalized regimens. Use in the public health domain for newborn screening remains a contentious possibility, which is not yet realized [8,9]. Ethical issues involving right not-to-know, age of testing and reporting in pediatric cases, and "Who should decide?" arise [10,11]. In 2014, Wendy Uhlmann, a clinical associate professor and genetic counselor in internal medicine and human genetics at the University of Michigan, introduced the topic of disclosure of incidental findings in WGS into segment B of the course.

## 1.2. Advent of the U.S. Precision Medicine Initiative

In January 2015, then President Barack Obama announced the "Precision Medicine Initiative", which was touted as "a bold new research effort to revolutionize how we improve health and treat disease" [12]. Efforts were underway to bring about new opportunities for individualized interventions through sponsored PMI research at major academic institutions and the establishment of a million person cohort for conducting this research. The seedbed for the initiative lay in the fruits of prior personalized medicine efforts, which had yielded now heavily used pharmacogenomic regimens such as Gleevec for chronic myelogenous leukemia and other tyrosine kinase inhibitors such as gefitinib for non-small-cell lung cancer [13]. The ongoing creation of new biobanks and genome-wide study consortia internationally, both public and private, were forerunners. Indeed, eight years prior the U.S. Health and Human Services Secretary's Advisory Committee on Genetics, Health, and Society had issued a report on the feasibility of a large U.S. population cohort study of genes, environment, and disease [14]. The unique opportunity now taking place was that large amounts of genotypic information on rare and more common (single nucleotide polymorphism—SNP) variants could be collected. New targeted therapies could be developed based on the resources of an immense pooled repository of genetic and other health information, in the hopes that the outgoing discoveries could be applied in a highly personalized way in real time.

The President's announcement inaugurated a string of events that proceeded at a fast clip as we were planning our course syllabus for fall 2015 and again for 2016. In March 2015, the U.S. National Institutes of Health (NIH) announced the formation of the Precision Medicine Initiative Working

Group of the Advisory Committee to the (U.S. National Institutes of Health; NIH) Director [15]. In July, the working group held a public workshop on participant engagement and health equity as they related to the proposed national research cohort [16]. On 17 September (nine days after our course start-up for 2015), the PMI Working Group delivered to the Advisory Committee a report providing the framework for building a national research cohort of one million or more Americans [17].

The public health community was attuned to the start-up of the Precision Medicine Initiative. Muin Khoury of the U.S. Centers for Disease Control and Prevention Office of Public Health Genomics (CDC-OPHG) and colleagues published nine articles in the span of 2015–2016 touching on the relationship of precision medicine to public health and cancer screening [18–21]. In addition, in 2015, the *American Journal of Public Health* (AJPH) carried a major editorial on precision medicine and health disparities [22]. The equity concern has been an integral part of our course, as the public health code of ethics is deeply concerned with the health and empowerment of disenfranchised community members [23].

The leadership of the PMI has shown a great willingness to enroll as broad a swath of 1 million plus participants as possible, with inclusion of participants from varied racial-ethnic and socio-economic backgrounds. Its recently stated goal is to enroll 70 to 75% of the participants from individuals traditionally underrepresented in biomedical research [24]. The NYC Consortium, a PMI research center sub-awardee consisting of Columbia, Weill Cornell, New York–Presbyterian, and NYC Health + Hospitals/Harlem, for example, has a goal of "deliver[ing] equitable and culturally responsive care to the city's most vulnerable populations" [25]. Its precision medicine program is applying an individualized approach to treating cancers; genetic diseases; and a broad range of other illnesses across an ethnically, culturally, and socioeconomically diverse population. In 2017, the PMI expanded its national network of provider organizations from the deep South to Wisconsin in the North, and from regional medical centers to local community health centers. Blue Cross Blue Shield and Walgreens are two of the organizations helping to enroll participants.

In segment A of the class, we have a "public deliberation" session that acquaints students with examples from a variety of settings of rational democratic deliberation—reasoned discussion on key values taking place in an atmosphere of mutual respect [26]. One such instance was the Oregon Health Experiment, "Oregon Health Priorities for the 1990s", aimed at determining the health services citizens considered most important and, therefore, of highest priority for government funding [27]. A laudable number of local citizen forums, that is, nineteen, were held throughout the state, with 560 people completing the priorities survey, the results of which went to the Oregon legislature. A gender balance of 196 male and 358 female individuals participated. However, 56% of the participants worked in healthcare, and it has been observed that the preponderance of participants were white and well-educated. The PMI seems to have overcome this demographic limitation through vigorous efforts at expanding its enrollee provider network.

We felt it essential to integrate the Precision Medicine Initiative into the course, in a way that fulfills the public health concern with the health of the community and the rights and welfare of its members. Initially, we included the PMI in the course as a case study and class exercise (fall 2015), then integrated it as a full didactic session in fall 2016. This article reviews the three PMI educational components, with special attention paid to student involvement and the issues that were discussed and deliberated over. In the center is a brief qualitative analysis of student responses in one of those components—a class exercise. Our piece ends with a glimpse of future possibilities for inclusion of precision medicine and precision public health in the curricula experienced by budding health professionals.

## 2. Methods

Our analysis of the three Precision Medicine and Public Health course components resembles a "nested case-control design", which situates a case-control study in the context of a cohort study [28]. Here, we nest a brief qualitative study of the student responses in the Precision Medicine and Public

Health case study and class exercise between the above narrative description of previous course elements touching on precision health, and an examination of the precision medicine and public health topics covered and student comments rendered in the Precision Medicine Initiative didactic session. The two aims of this analysis are the following: (1) show how precision health, the PMI in particular, can be incorporated into a public health genetics policy course; and (2) assess the extent to which this inclusion has allowed our students to formulate policy in the precision public health area.

Knowing that precision public health was a new area with lasting implications, the course instructors took extensive notes on student–instructor and student–student dialogue during the three course components. Verbatim records of student presentations are kept during class exercises to enable accurated grading. The instructors have inspected and analyzed for issues and policy content relevant data for the three Precision Medicine Initiative-related sessions: (1) class notes containing what each participant said—for all three sessions; (2) student hand-ins for the class exercise; and (3) the topical areas covered in the class materials of the didactic session. The didactic session topical areas were inspected, following analysis of the case study and class exercise, for content that reinforces and extends the themes elicited by the case study and class exercise, and illustrative student comments.

In the analysis, student responses for the case study and class exercise, both oral and written, were categorized into thematic areas. The pre-categories were formed by assorting themes in the ten shared case study/class exercise questions (page 3 of the case study and class exercise hand-outs) into issue and policy areas. The post-categories were formed by manually labeling sentences in the case study and class exercise student responses for major themes. Categories were cross-checked by the three authors. The authors recorded frequency of mentions in the pre-and post-categories for the following: (1) case study student responses; (2) in-class exercise student responses; and (3) class exercise hand-ins, which were used to select exemplary quotations within the major categories. In keeping with the course policy orientation, we have analyzed student responses to determine our students' ability to formulate issue areas into policy, that is, to satisfy aim 2, rather than to systematically explore the various categories of responses. We also include student comments on the Precision Medicine and Public Health class exercise, collected as part of the overall end-of-semester course evaluation, to show whether students felt the class exercise was useful and what changes could be made in the future. The evaluation did not include questions on the case study and didactic session.

In writing this piece, the authors have inspected the precision medicine and precision public health technical, program-related, and socio-ethical literature we collected at the time of the 2015/2016 classes, and supplemented this inspection with additional current PubMed and NIH website searches. The PMI has evolved into the NIH *All of Us* Research Program, which began beta testing in June 2017 and had a full national roll-out of the cohort-based program and extensive provider network in Spring 2018. This article is written from the standpoint of what has taken place in the national program as of June 2018.

## 3. Results

### 3.1. Course Moorings: Findings from the Precision Medicine and Public Health Case Study

"Issues in Public Health Genetics" uses the case study approach in session 3 to ground students in principles of policymaking, and the different bodies and phases involved [29]. For the fall 2015 Case Study in Precision Medicine and Public Health, students were provided in advance with a two-page description of the PMI, 10 ethical-legal-social implications (ELSI)/policy-related questions, a policy types sheet, two assigned and two supplementary readings on precision medicine and public health and the PMI, and a number of general and genomics-specific policy readings. The case study begins with former U.S. President Barack Obama's announcement of the Precision Medicine Initiative. The Initiative announcement envisioned a new era of medicine wedding together novel research, technology, and policies aimed at the development of innovative treatments [12]. The instructor-provided description distinguishes PMI near-term and long-term goals. In the near-term, the PMI was directed at supporting clinical trials in partnership with pharmaceutical companies to test combinations of targeted therapies. The therapies being tested together with enabling diagnostic tests have focused especially on cancer and tumor molecular signatures [30]. The PMI's longer term goal, now proceeding at a brisk pace, is the creation of a national cohort study of one million or more Americans. Students read the ambitious description of the million person enterprise as it originally appeared on the National Institutes of Health website:

"Each voluntary participant will share their genomic information and biological specimens. This information, along with important clinical data from electronic health records, such as laboratory test results and magnetic resonance imaging (MRI) scans, and lifestyle data, such as calorie consumption and environmental exposures tracked through mobile health devices, will help researchers understand how genomic variations and other health factors affect the development of disease. Through the consent process, participants will control how the information is used in research and shared. As active participants, they also will have access to their own health data, as well as research using their data, to help inform their own health decisions" [31].

One can see that the PMI's goals are laden with both immense potential and equally large design challenges. We capitalize on the challenges to allow our students to analytically move through the ELSI and policy considerations necessary for accomplishing the PMI's stated goals. We ask our students to consider the 10 questions posted on the course Canvas website before class and to be prepared to discuss in class relate to the following: (1) assurance of services (access to data and results, maintaining equity, minimizing health disparities); (2) participation in the PMI (involvement, representativeness); (3) ethical issues (consent, privacy, and benefit sharing); and (4) treatment of people (stigmatization, discrimination). These four overarching "pre-" categories follow from a direct inspection of the questions in Table 1, as performed by the three authors.

**Table 1.** Questions posed to students for the precision medicine and public health class exercise.

---

- How can we assure that the large longitudinal cohort study will enlist volunteers representative of the demographic groups most relevant to addressing our major health problems?
- What kind of consent should be obtained for those participating in the cohort?
- How can we assure that the Initiative reduces and does not widen health disparities?
- How can we assure access to the drugs and therapies resulting from the Initiative by those for whom they will provide most benefit?
- How can we prevent the development and marketing of drugs targeting specific racial or ethnic groups from stigmatizing these groups?
- What privacy safeguards need to be built into the large cohort study?
- How might we achieve adequate involvement in the development and implementation of the Initiative by appropriate stakeholder groups?
- Who should have access to the database created by the large cohort study, and for what purposes?
- Should those receiving financial benefits from utilizing the database have an obligation to share the benefits for public health purposes?
- How can we prevent the increase in individualized health information from being used to discriminate in employment or insurance?

---

Following instructor presentation of policymaking frameworks, the case study discussion began with give-and-take between instructors and students to lay-out the process of realizing the PMI's goals. The class envisioned the process as containing four steps: (1) announcement of the PMI's near-term and longer-term goals (which students had read about); (2) incorporation of these plans into the Congressional budget; (3) NIH director to map-out the division of money for the PMI and its various needs; and (4) formation of an advisory group, with subgroups as needed and a stakeholder group (suggested by the chief instructor, who was privy to their activities in the months before class began). The instructors noticed that the students were not accustomed to connecting policymaking steps in this manner, but expected them to gain familiarity with this mode of thinking as the semester proceeded.

The students were then asked for those issues they found most pressing. Student responses to the case study fell into two of the four preliminary categories above—participation (2 responses) and ethics (privacy—3 responses; consent—2 responses). One student felt consent was a priority, given that it would be needed for use of the samples. The student mentioned that consent was a part of the U.S. Office for Human Research Protections (OHRP) regulations. She was asked for examples, and offered the ongoing debates about dried blood spots being stored by states as instances where government programs were likely to benefit from more structured consent policy. In the case of the PMI, an advisory commission could start with recommendations, and then government agencies (Secretary of Health and Human Services, NIH, or state health departments, she suggested) could firm up the consent policies. The student proposed researchers and public groups working together early on to fashion policy.

A second student felt that the need for privacy safeguards was paramount. He remarked, "These have changed the last ten years with the Internet. Does the federal government have the capacity to handle million person data?" This class member took a practical approach to the problem—"Hire the right people; pull lessons from the U.S. census". On being asked whether a federal agency could be granted authority over the privacy of samples and personal health information, he suggested that responsible private vendors could be used. Students and instructors then explored whether and how the data could be de-identified.

Towards the end of the discussion, the instructors asked the class how diversity of the national cohort could be assured. The conversation over this topic needed more instructor prompting than previously, suggesting that the students, either at the undergraduate or graduate level, had received more exposure to ethical than social dilemma problem-solving. Representativeness of the cohort would not only make it more technically useful, but also improve trust among groups that had been either ignored or mistreated by past biomedical research. Students were further asked to consider, "Who gets the benefits?" Would private sector biotech be the primary beneficiary? Should consumers' interests not be considered foremost? The class was reminded that public health was not well represented in the advisory groups convened by NIH, and that the public health community was a stakeholder as well.

All of these lines of inquiry elicited fairly detailed and pragmatic student responses, more so than the instructors had expected. However, it was clear, as demonstrated in the questioning about participant representativeness questioning, that the discussion could be taken further after additional student exploration. The student responses had also been somewhat scattershot in terms of the steps in policymaking that would be needed. The case presentation, therefore, provided a scaffolding for a more incisive precision medicine and public health exercise that would appear further down the road in the course. The questions students grappled with would be revisited. Introduction of the case study at this early point in the course also allowed periodic reference to precision medicine and public health considerations throughout the course.

### 3.2. *Setting Sail: Findings from the Precision Medicine and Public Health Class Exercise*

The questions posed to our students in the session 3 case study on precision medicine and public health provided an initial exposure to the relevant issues and the chance for students to loosely consider positions on the issues leading to policies. The session 16 precision medicine and public health class exercise took place slightly after the course midpoint. Students would now have the opportunity to offer individual recommendations and to defend them. At this stage in the course, students had been exposed to sessions on the policymaking process, genetics legislation, public deliberation, ethical perspectives, issues of race and ethnicity, and tools for public health practice. Although not always the case in the years we have taught the course, we designed the narrative to be usable in both the case study and exercise sessions in order to maintain student familiarity with it. Other than the specific assignment, the descriptive narrative and 10 questions were identical in both the case study and class exercise hand-outs, the latter being distributed several weeks in advance. In addition, by the time of the class exercise, mention of the Precision Medicine Initiative (PMI) had been made recurrently throughout the prior sessions.

The individual class exercise added a context to the questions posed in the case study. In the class exercise scenario contained in the advance hand-out, students learned that the NIH had established a working group on precision medicine as a component of the NIH advisory committee to the Director. The actual PMI working group had delivered its culminating report on a framework for a one million plus research cohort to the advisory committee to the NIH Director four weeks before the class exercise. The student involvement in decision-making thus paralleled what was taking place in the real world. In the hand-out, the working group on precision medicine was to convene a meeting to hear testimony from invited stakeholders recommending policies to address ELSI aspects of the Precision Medicine Initiative. Students were asked to choose in advance from a list of 19 possible professional, industry-based, and civic organizations. One student reminded us in the end-of-course evaluation that "an overview of what the organizations are beforehand would save time for additional research on the actual policy issues". This suggestion could be honored by supplying a one to two sentence description plus a web site for each organization. The supplementary readings we place on Canvas are broken down by organization category, thus reflect different stances that might be taken.

Before the class session, student stakeholders were required to submit a one to two-page memorandum describing their organization's recommendations (the written exercise) online. During the in-class portion, each stakeholder was allotted 10 min to present their positions on relevant issues, and respond to one to two professor (advisory committee "chair" and "co-chair") questions (the in-class exercise). Students self-assigned themselves to represent the following organizations: CDC's Office of Public Health Genomics, American Society of Human Genetics (ASHG), National Society of Genetic Counselors (NSGC), Pharmaceutical Research and Manufacturers of America (PhRMA), Genetic Alliance, Council for Responsible Genetics, and the National Urban League. One student commented in the end-of-semester course evaluation, "I think it would be good for a student to perhaps be expected to take on both a governing/regulatory body and an advising group in order to see both roles". While time constraints do not permit a student's adopting two roles, we have added more time for open discussion, sometimes up to 15 min, in past class exercises. Dawning multiple perspectives for purposes of open discussion is a valuable suggestion, and might grant students a chance to voice positions that most represent how they personally feel. This conclusion is backed up by a second student's evaluation comment: "I think maybe a shorter presentation (5 min) and more in character discussion would have been interesting".

Assurance (14 oral responses; 13 written responses), participation (13 oral; 6 written), and ethics (26 oral—11 consent, 6 privacy, 9 benefit sharing; 19 written—8 consent, 6 privacy, 5 benefit sharing) were the three most frequent categories of student responses in both the oral and written exercise. New "post-" categories of responses also appeared, which we added to the four "pre-" categories from the case study: financial considerations, education, and trust-building. Treatment of people (stigmatization, discrimination), an earlier category, fell midway among these new categories in terms of frequency of mention; financial and educational considerations only received four to six responses, respectively. Low number of mentions in student responses prompted eventual exclusion of three contemplated categories: ethics-ownership, regulation, and translation.

In attending to the student responses, the chair and co-chair were checking to make sure that students had an appreciation of the advancements and challenges posed by the PMI, and that their proposals would positively and not negatively impact the participants according to the role they adopted. A 2018 report by Data & Society, *Fairness in Precision Medicine*, notes that large-scale precision medicine research studies, such as the *All of Us* Research Program, Project Baseline, and New York University's Human Project, have made strides in prioritizing a diverse enrollment, a major step towards ensuring that benefits could be equitably distributed [32]. Data & Society conducted interviews with 21 individuals. The resultant report "stressed that varying sources of data would need to be used, but that harnessing these different sources would require tackling similar [historical and analytical] concerns regarding the potential for bias" (p. 24). The potential for sampling bias, due to the history of biomedical research studies focusing on volunteers of European descent, was voiced by our National Urban League student representative. The Genetic Alliance representative in our class exercise proposed: "We must connect and engage with community and advocacy groups, and then reach out to the public with the help of those groups and their web sites and means of communication". These comments confirmed to us that our students had an appropriate level of attention for group hopes and concerns, which goes beyond simply being focused on the program or intervention itself. The students suggested the use of social media, such as Facebook and Twitter, as ways to create diverse involvement (Table 2). A means of avoiding recruitment bias is to allow the participants themselves to tap into the study description and self-enroll, rather than being enrolled according to fixed quotas that the study professionals have arranged.

**Table 2.** Student responses in key precision medicine and public health class exercise areas.

---

Trust-Building

- Shareholder consultation before the implementation of a new treatment into clinical settings. (U.S. Centers for Disease Control and Prevention (CDC) Office of Public Health Genomics student representative);
- Researchers and participants being equally involved would establish trust. (National Society of Genetic Counselors student representative);
- A large number of people surveyed indicated they would be more likely to participate knowing their health information would be returned (National Society of Genetic Counselors student representative);
- The key to enrolling a diverse population is to work transparently with and gain the trust of communities and groups to utilize pre-existing networks. We must connect and engage with community and advocacy groups and then reach out to the public with the help of those groups and their websites and means of communication. We are also supportive of using social media such as Facebook and Twitter to increase diverse involvement (Genetic Alliance student representative);
- To build trust in the community, the PMI will need to work with community leaders, develop adequate privacy and data use agreements, and host focus groups to ensure vulnerable populations' voices are heard in the development of recruitment and consent materials (National Urban League student representative).

---

Assuring access and equity

- Emphasis should be put into reaching out to members of disadvantaged communities who would not otherwise become informed about participating in the Precision Medicine Initiative (CDC Office of Public Health Genomics student representative);
- Both the design of new drug trials, and the 1M+ cohort must include individuals from underserved groups. . . . Expanding payment policies to cover new therapies that serve the underserved (Pharmaceutical Research and Manufacturers of America (PhRMA) student representative);
- New technologies must meet social needs. Problems rooted in poverty, racism, and other forms of inequality cannot be remedied by technology alone (Council for Responsible Genetics student representative);
- The development of new pharmacogenomics drugs and tests must not widen health disparities or support differential access to care. Current trends can be exacerbated by the pricing out of individuals from receiving appropriate health care needs (National Urban League student representative).

---

**Table 2.** *Cont.*

Ethics—Benefit sharing

- We believe that the data, particularly the genetic data from the one million person cohort, should be freely available to the public through online databases (American Society of Human Genetics student representative);
- There is an overwhelming need for resources to be made available to help individuals understand the meaning of genetic results to prevent harm (National Society of Genetic Counselors student representative);
- The dataset should be available for research purposes only, but available for all qualified academic, industry, and government workers (Pharmaceutical Research and Manufacturers of America (PhRMA) student representative);
- We strongly support open access and believe that all researchers should have access to this data. Furthermore, the public should have open access to published articles using this data (Genetic Alliance student representative);
- Determine how the genome interacts with exposures. The findings should focus on the individual and not on industry—the goal is what benefits people (Council for Responsible Genetics student representative);
- By reporting information on genetics in a manner in which the average person can understand, the project runners will not only be fulfilling a duty to the American people, but also facilitating the continuation of their research (Council for Responsible Genetics student representative).

Ethics—Consent and privacy

- What kind of consent should be obtained for those participating in the cohort? We should seek the broadest possible consent. Such a dataset does not fit the model of "here is exactly what I plan to do with the data", but must be mined for insight. Consent should be established by a central IRB (institutional review board) committee composed of members representing all stakeholders (Pharmaceutical Research and Manufacturers of America (PhRMA) student representative);
- Anonymized data can be made available online to the public through VCF (variant call formatted) files like the 1000 Genomes Project with single nucleotide polymorphism (SNP) frequencies, genotypes and haplotypes. Non-genetic information—lifestyles and phenotypic data—can be made available by consent through appropriate controlled channels. NIH (the U.S. National Institutes of Health agency) has policy outlines for data sharing in genome-wide association studies. These need to be revamped and updated (American Society of Human Genetics student representative);
- They [participants] should also know who will have access to their data and whether it may be sold or transferred to outside groups, a concern which has become particularly important given the recent efforts to network biobanks and the sale by 23 and Me of genetic information to corporations. In addition, participants should be informed about whether their data will be "anonymized" (no identifying information available) or "de-identified" (no identifying information directly attached, but still accessible), and made aware that . . . it may still be possible to determine with some degree of certainty one's identity from their genome. (Council for Responsible Genetics student representative).

The U.S. Precision Medicine Initiative initiated by former President Obama in 2015 has hoped to avoid the fate of the National Children's Study (NCS), which planned to track 100,000 children from birth to adulthood [33]. This effort entailed a longitudinal study examining the influences of a range of factors, from chemical to psychosocial, on child development and health. Among the reasons for the study's termination were a cumbersome recruitment plan, based on enrolling pregnant women by knocking on doors in a random sample of about 100 counties [34]. With a surge in costs, NIH dropped the 40 NCS sites at academic institutions, and transferred management of enrollees to several large contractors. More socially-based means can be used to propel recruitment, along the lines of the plans proposed by our students and through the type of network expansion being undertaken by the *All of Us* Research Program.

Success in enrollment and in the conduct of a research study is dependent on the trust of the participants. The Genetic Alliance student representative felt that operating through pre-established channels within community organizations, which requires a period of familiarization between public constituents and the research team, is a valuable way of engaging in trust building. In his oral presentation, the Pharmaceutical Research and Manufacturers of America (PhRMA) student representative suggested a "trust of stakeholders—public, provider, and industry". The trust concept, consisting of an umbrella organization charged with fiduciary responsibility for seeing to the best interests of the participants, was first proposed by Howard University in 2003 for a biobank to investigate diseases that predominantly affect African Americans. Samples housed in the Genomic Research in African Diaspora (GRAD) biobank were to be managed by a private company with a fiduciary duty to the enrollees, the First Genetic Trust in Chicago [35]. The Michigan BioTrust for Health was created to enable research on the four million dried blood spots stored from newborn screening by the state of Michigan before 2010 [36]. A combination of retroactive opt-out and proactive informed consent policies have enabled the biobank to go forward with investigations as far ranging as epigenetic exposure and childhood brain tumor risk, to lab-on-a-chip for newborn metabolic disorders [37]. The Michigan BioTrust is overseen by both a scientific advisory board, and a community values advisory board. The latter provides advice on what types of research are ethically acceptable, and methods for engaging and informing the public. Similarly, the *All of Us* Research Program's advisory panel and its working group of the advisory committee to the NIH Director formed to provide external oversight and expert advice on the program's goals and operations. The July 2015 open workshop allowed outside public representation on the design of an inclusive cohort, building and sustaining public trust, and active and effective participant engagement [6]. Our National Society of Genetic Counselors (NSGC) student representative stated that, "Researchers and participants being equally involved would establish trust". The ideal, as expressed by our students, would be an ongoing collaboration between experts and lay people. The 2015 open workshop and the continued presence of advocacy leaders on the program advisory committees are partial reflections of this shared student suggestion.

We were surprised that the number of ethics-related comments during the oral presentations exceeded the number of stigmatization/discrimination comments by a ratio of 5:1. This imbalance could be due to student's previous exposure to bioethics, because as undergraduates, they were eying health fields, but it also serves as a wake-up call to medical and public health educators charged with communicating the implications of precision tools. The NSGC student representative cited the need to ensure ethical directions for the research so as to avoid discrimination. The student acknowledged the existence of the Genetic Information Nondiscrimination Act (GINA), at the same time recognizing its being limited to health insurance and not covering life or disability insurance. Considering the case of BiDil, which its manufacturer NitroMed, after a retrospective revisiting of the data, decided to market exclusively for heart failure in African Americans, forgoing other groups in its prescribing [38], the concern over discrimination is justified. Many authorities view BiDil as a forerunner to race-based pharmacogenomics. In an effort to give people control over the uses to which donated biological samples and personal health information were being put, two of our groups recommended utilization of the "platform for engaging everyone responsibly" (PEER) system. PEER is the product of a collaboration between Genetic Alliance and Private Access [39]. The system allows the health consumer to decide which types of research and research organizations will have access to their biological samples and personal information. Instructions can be changed at any time, making PEER's operation dynamic through time. The PEER system is quite reasonable for applying to a moderate size biobank, such as the Genetic Alliance's registry and biobank devoted to research on Pseudoxanthoma Elasticum, but can it serve a one million plus cohort? Because the *All of Us* Research Program cohort and provider networks are so immense, application of PEER might be too unwieldy. It should be noted, however, that *All of Us* Research Program research center sub-awardees have as their goal the examination of samples and health data on a much more limited scale. The Illinois Precision Medicine Consortium has launched a longitudinal research cohort of 125,000 participants, and the University of Michigan's "Michigan Genome Initiative" has accumulated genomic and electronic health record data on 35,000 plus non-emergency surgical patients (The University of Michigan supplies tools and methodology to the *All of Us* Research Program's Data and Research Support Center; its overall precision health activities are part of an institutional initiative). It would be feasible to either employ PEER at the sub-awardee level, or have participant input in an advisory sense help in establishing community trust concerning the directions the research is taking.

The ethics behind the million person cohort are based on maximization of benefit and avoiding maleficence-untoward, detrimental consequences. Our students portrayed benefit to research cohort participants as falling under two headings: (1) information to be received back by participants; and (2) treatments that might ultimately benefit participants or participant groups. Several student representatives mentioned the importance of new pharmacogenomics regimens being available to individuals of diverse socio-economic backgrounds. One representative stated in response to instructor questioning that the government should be responsible for payment of drugs, a suggestion that was simply too terse. We agree with a course evaluation comment asking us to "Encourage students to take concrete positions on issues". Part of this role is fulfilled by asking the student to clarify their response during the question and answer session. Other students suggested institutional policies that would avoid excluding individuals because of prohibitory prices, and more specific governmental policies, such as continued expansion of Medicaid, to support cost-effective implementation of precision medicine. The National Urban League student representative suggested local groups, networks, and Genetic Alliance associated advocacy organizations could monitor and investigate potential health disparities. We look for student awareness of the need to include communities and community-based organizations in the research process, and commended this idea.

Comments regarding access to information from the PMI addressed both consumer and non-consumer needs. The PhRMA student representative felt that PMI information should be available only for research purposes, to qualified individuals from academia, government, and industry. Lifestyle information was viewed as more sensitive, with one group suggesting it should be released judiciously through "controlled channels". While this point was well taken, we felt the distinction between sharing of genotypic and lifestyle plus phenotypic data, and their means of release by NIH, could have been further articulated. Our advocacy group student representatives endorsed open access, which would also allow participants to gain access to PMI information. A distinction needs to be made between accessing general information from the PMI, and one's own information. In her oral presentation, the NSGC student representative cited a concern with non-return of results, and indicated that "98% of participants want their information back". A large number of people surveyed by the Foundation for the National Institutes of Health indicated they would be more likely to participate knowing their health information would be returned [17]. The Center for Responsible Genetics (CRG) student representative discussed a "reverse identification" scheme for linking participant scientific and medical historical data back together to enable such personalized disclosure. The National Society of Genetic Counselors made a very insightful connection with results returned to individuals by direct-to-consumer genetic testing companies; adequate counseling resources would need to be in place.

The ability to report back to the patient, particularly after his or her biospecimen has been analyzed and compared with other comparables within a precision medicine database, is a real-time goal of precision medicine. Leaders such as Francis Collins of NIH and Muin Khoury of CDC have discussed such an ambition for diabetes treatment and smoking cessation [21,30]. In dialogues on the fruits of the Human Genome Project with the African American and Latino participants in our *Communities of Color and Genetics Policy* Project, we found that participants were interested in both maintaining privacy of results, and receiving their own genetic testing results back, even if it meant not anonymizing their sample [40]. In part, the reason against disclosure of individual results is ethical—results at the research stage are uncertain. This leaning differs from medical practice once a given diagnostic test has entered the medical mainstream after due validation. In addition, the re-linking of human subjects' data, which no longer involves preliminary data but now research results, would be administratively impractical on a widespread scale. The CDC-OPHG does describe a process of aggregate result bidirectional reporting between state disease registries, for example, in the cancer field, and those institutions that contributed data to the registry [41]. Such information could be highly useful to providers and their patients for those groups being seen at a particular healthcare site. Accordingly, the Genetic Alliance student representative advocated public open access for articles published using million person cohort data.

Among our groups, PhRMA was the most optimistic in terms of the pay-off of the Precision Medicine Initiative. In addition to its student representative's suggestion that the PMI's goals could be maximized by allowing data to be shared with a variety of research stakeholders, he felt the "broadest possible consent" (blanket consent) should be obtained from participants. This viewpoint was counterbalanced by the perspective of the American Society of Human Genetics (ASHG) student representative, who wrote that any benefits of the publicly available data should be used "to benefit the overall health of the public", a view that deemphasized institutional benefits. The Council for Responsible Genetics student representative was concerned about biobanks sharing information with corporations and the sale of personalized information by 23 and Me, implying that potential benefit and risk must both be considered when lifting confidentiality. The PhRMA and professional/advocacy viewpoints both had the health consumer in mind, but the circle of benefit was prioritized differently. The exercise was intended to draw out a spectrum or polarity of responses to the ethical, legal, and social issues inherent in precision medicine and public health. It appeared this interchange accomplished our purpose. We received a student course evaluation comment that "I know time is a constraint, but I was ready to have a discussion, in the role I was in, with the other stakeholders, and to try to hash out a policy. I wished there had been time for that". Occasionally we have asked students or groups with likely contrasting positions to present sequentially, and incorporated a point raised by one group into a question aimed at the other group. Another technique is to allow a student to ask the second or third question during an individual's or group's question and answer session. Often, the question is based on a differing position. The time after presentations generally allows for student give-and take, but not for more thoroughgoing consensus building. Afterwards, class conversion via the electronic Canvas Discussion helps to fill this need.

### 3.3. Charting a Course: Findings from the Precision Medicine and Public Health Class Didactic Session

Upon inspecting the student responses within the 2015 case study and class exercise, we felt that our attendees should be provided with a more distinct definition of precision public health, as the PMI tends to focus on amelioration of the later stages of disease. In fact, the distinction between prevention-oriented and treatment-oriented precision techniques was a question we had asked our students, with one replying that where a condition lies along a "range of risk" could help to differentiate the model to adopt. In addition, several of our students in the exercise issued comments on the need to guarantee equity in the fruits of precision medicine, which strengthened our belief that a didactic class session emphasizing this topic should added. Session 12 in the fall 2016 curriculum occupied this intellectual space.

A Precision Public Health Summit was held on the 6–7 June 2016 at the University of California San Francisco. The Summit's aim identified two major aspects of precision public health: "to look at ways that vast amounts of data can be used to benefit the health and well-being of larger populations, as well as to decrease health disparities" [42]. In the class, we present four characteristics molding precision health into the public health context: by utilizing (1) an ecological model of health; (2) principles of population screening; (3) evidence-based decision-making; and (4) public health policy and practice [21]. The U.S. National Academy of Medicine's 2003 report *The Future of the Public's Health in the 21st Century* defines an ecological model as one based "on understanding the ecology of health and the interconnectedness of the biological, behavioral, physical, and socio-environmental domains" [43,44]. The last domain introduces consideration of equity and class in connection with health.

The National Urban League student representative during the 2015 class exercise stated her support of the social determinants of health model, which emulates a public health ecological framework, and felt it should be a part of professional education. These models provide a rationale, when translated into effectiveness research, for targeting disparities in marginalized populations. She stated, "We have reservations about the huge costs of the Precision Medicine Initiative taking away resources and public interest from other policies that would be more impactful on these [urban] populations". The student cited the *National Healthcare Quality and Disparities Report* indicating that across a range of measures of healthcare access, Latinos received equivalent care to whites in only 17% of healthcare measures [45]. African Americans and Latinos received poorer quality care than whites on 73% and 77%, respectively, of those measures. As we tell our students, improvements in health often demand more than medical attention. Ronald Bayer and Sandro Galea, whose writings on precision medicine and social justice we include in the course, cite the findings of the British Civil Service's Whitehall Study. This investigation found that even when healthcare services were provided as a matter of right and the cost of care was no longer a barrier to treatment, a marked social gradient persisted [46]. A substantial proportion of the population fared poorly on health indicators. Bayer and Galea view targeting of public health efforts as optimal when they are broad-based and cross-sectoral. These considerations do not mitigate the value of the PMI, but they do indicate that for full effect, targeting will need to go beyond the individual level and take into account social determinants.

We asked the students in our class session, "Will precision medicine increase or decrease health disparities?" Part of the answer to minimizing disparities was addressed during the exercise by one student's suggestion to make sure an adequate number of racial-ethnic minorities are recruited into studies and study centers being awarded by the NIH, especially when conditions disproportionately suffered by minorities, such as prostate cancer and asthma, are being investigated. Other healthcare reform era solutions, such as expanded coverage under the Affordable Care Act, are important. The outcomes of the *All of Us* Research Program will not always exist at the research stage. Targeted interventions will need to be paid for. To be avoided is "a high-tech personalized approach that [is] only available to those with means or platinum/Cadillac insurance plans" [42]. Our students brought up the wise point that in the case of regimens going beyond simply taking a pill at home, assurance of basic transportation to the health center through whatever arrangements can be made is fundamentally important.

Built into the original description of the PMI are means of engaging potentially marginalized populations: "The Obama Administration will forge strong partnerships with existing research cohorts, patient groups, and the private sector to develop the infrastructure that will be needed" [31]. Of course, it is to be hoped that the White House and the President's Secretary of Health and Human Services will continue to support the PMI, regardless of which administration is in office. We cite the value of incentives, such as giving participants wearable health monitoring technology, and providing an interactive web site for people [47]. Like many biobanks, the Norwegian Nord-Trondelag Health (HUNT) Study biobank makes commercial use of its human biological samples, but an upfront public contribution fee from each project and financial return to the research and health communities are also fixtures in its sample management strategy [48]. Involving representatives of the research participants in governance is an important ingredient in furthering buy-in, and has taken place to some extent within the PMI working group and advisory structure. These representatives may hail from an advocacy group, or be members of a board, or even individuals from industry or academe, so long as they can serve as and are viewed as trusted representatives.

The last big issue that we entertain with our students, a logistical one, is the vast amount of information that will pour out of the PMI. Recall that the plan is to recruit more than one million Americans, and to capture genotypic, phenotypic, lifestyle, and environmental information on each. Whole-genome sequencing alone produces an immense amount of information. The question we naturally pose to our students is, "How can we deal adequately with the flood of information given the lack of time or expertise to interpret and apply the knowledge?" One instructor suggestion was to be sure the information trickling down from the Initiative is valid and not subject to misinterpretation. An astute pupil brought to the class's attention the point that The Cancer Genome Atlas (TCGA), a collaboration between the National Cancer Institute and the National Human Genome Research Institute, could serve as an example. TCGA has a biospecimen core resource (BCR) that serves as the interface between the TCGA program and the various tissue source sites collecting tumor samples [49]. The BCR also ensures that human subjects protections and guidelines are adhered to at each of the collection sites. However, it is also the case that the TCGA program office does not provide to investigators help with bioinformatics or guidance on research projects using the data. We noted a student comment that the best way to ensure that precision medicine and public health do not widen health disparities would be to enable adequate provider training of and education of the involved public. Suitable expertise must exist at the clinician level, which will likely be the state of affairs for information flowing out of the PMI, too. The didactic session provided a useful capstone to the previous year's precision public health activities, translating the major issues in consolidated form for our students.

*3.4. Final Arrival: Summary of Findings for the Three Course Components*

For the most part, we would give our students a positive rating in terms of their responses to instructor questions and thoughtfulness during class discussion. It was gratifying to hear their policy suggestions both for the process of policymaking (e.g., work with community leaders, conduct stakeholder consultations, engage IRBs to establish consent policy) and its substance (dynamic consent, data de-identification and anonymization, expanded payment policies). In so doing, the students came up with some very creative suggestions, such as use of the PEER electronic platform to assure participant involvement in the disposition of their biological sample and personal health information. We also heard a lot of timely responses involving research program-participant collaboration, and a suggestion for using social media to disseminate awareness of the program, which made us wish our students could have been there at the NIH public workshop. Students quite appropriately articulated the need for attention to consent and privacy policies. We did detect at the beginning of the course more student competence in solving ethical dilemmas than reasoning-out steps for implementing policies and narrowing social gaps in proposed programs, such as assuring representativeness. While some students gave overly concise replies to "chair" and "co-chair" queries during the exercise, for the most part, responses were practically grounded and reflected useful policy measures. Student weaknesses, including not knowing how to concisely articulate points to an audience under a fixed time limit, seemed diminished by the end of the exercise session. In terms of evaluation of the Precision Medicine and Public Health exercise by students who returned our internal questionnaire, five students rated it as very valuable (compared to four for the second, CRISPR class exercise); one rated it as somewhat valuable; and one circled "N/A". The students in our class, largely health science-oriented, often broach in our final class debriefing that they do not feel completely at home in public health policymaking, but admit they have gained useful familiarity with the process, and that the class exercises have helped. The precision medicine and public health exercise furthered the course's policymaking goal and motivated the students to want to collaborate with each other in designing policy. A limitation of the analysis we have performed is that because of its retrospective nature, we lack the capacity to evaluate student perceptions of the case study and didactic session.

## 4. Conclusions: A Look to the Horizon of Precision Public Health Education

In the didactic session, we have one slide with the straightforward title "Training Necessary". Certainly, one solution for dealing with the plethora of information stemming from the Precision Medicine Initiative is to train the clinicians and young public health investigators who will feed the results back into their own research, and the medical and public health practitioners who will be using the information for their patients and community members. Mirnezami and colleagues foresaw the need for new training paradigms for doctors, "who will benefit from a deeper, more holistic view of illness integrating traditional pathophysiology-based models with emerging molecular mechanisms" [50]. This training requirement is engendered both by the new gene-disease associations that will be detected, and the volume of information the national cohort will generate. Though the educational level at which the training must take place may be uncertain, its necessity becomes manifest well before the time the provider is ready to apply a precision medicine intervention to his or her patient.

Much of the medical view of the PMI is pharmacogenomic, albeit with greatly enhanced informational and real-time capabilities. In May 2018, the *All of Us* Research Program announced funds to attain whole-genome sequencing of 200,000 people per year [24]. Whole-genome and exome sequencing can be of great utility in identifying new pharmacogenomic targets and solutions for medically refractory cases, particularly when big data aids the search [51,52]. These techniques are beginning to make their way into medical, other graduate level, and genetic counseling education [53]. A postgraduate program in clinical pharmacology and pharmacogenomics at the University of Chicago offers training in personalized therapeutics, and includes the ethics and economics of pharmacogenomics, as well as limited service aboard an IRB [54]. Web resources also exist to support practitioner utilization of pharmacogenomic information to guide drug therapy [55]. Genetic epidemiology courses in schools of public health include WGS and WES as research techniques. Public health practitioners are currently most likely to encounter WGS and WES in the epidemiologic tracking of virulent pathogens, which requires professional training [3]. Use in newborn screening remains under investigation. Our study suggests that training in these techniques can also benefit from an awareness of costs and accessibility by different consumer groups.

As our course lays out, public health practitioners are especially concerned with the health of the family, community, and population. Muin Khoury and Sandro Galea write that to-date, "substantial evidence indicates that a genetically targeted approach to health has demonstrated a population [not just an individual] health benefit" [18]. The example they supply is evidence-based tier 1 (tests fully validated) genomic interventions, which includes both index case and family cascade testing. Tier 1 genetic testing is already a solid topic in public health genetics courses like ours. The CDC has made available tool kits containing informational and technical resources for the implementation of tier 1 genetic testing [41].

A second precision approach medicine and public health are likely to adopt as the PMI proceeds is the use of polygenic risk scores, which incorporate genetic variants of both small and large effect size. Researchers at the University of Michigan School of Public Health and the Fred Hutchinson Cancer Research Center in Seattle, WA have combined risk information from 19 lifestyle and environmental factors and 63 genetic variants ("E-scores" and "G-scores") with family history to yield an overall risk score for colorectal cancer [56]. Medical investigators in the United States and Canada have employed polygenic risk scores in the identification of individuals with a high burden of subclinical coronary atherosclerosis, and for genotypic analysis of individuals with extreme levels of high-density lipoprotein cholesterol [57,58]. Development of such scoring systems is likely to accelerate as further genotype-phenotype associations emerge from the *All of Us* Research Program and investigators connected with it. Training in genome-wide association studies is a major part of public health epidemiology coursework here at University of Michigan; the topic of "phenome-wide association studies" will follow as these studies increase in number [59]. Both techniques are used in the formation of risk scores. The American Public Health Association policy statement on genetic and genomic literacy indicates that provider training needs to include familiarity with risk stratification and its proper interpretation, and an awareness of circumstances for resorting to lifestyle modification versus pharmacologic measures [60].

The two approaches—(1) tier 1 genetic testing, and use of WGS and WES; and (2) use of polygenic risk scores—are basically the major genetic mutation and SNP versions of targeted interventions for at-risk populations. The use of such interventions requires education, ideally starting at the graduate level and extending to workforce training [60]. More will be asked of the patient or health consumer than in prior forms of testing. Education for future practitioners should contain elements of consent, confidentiality and data sharing, group sensitivity to informatics-based testing, costs, and coverage. As our students demonstrated, absorbing material related to these topics requires time and multiple didactic experiences.

A final distinction to be made is between precision public health applied to individuals and groups, such as families, and precision public health applied to populations. Professionals employ cascade screening to hunt down further family members who are at risk for infectious or genetic disease. Although, socially-minded authorities have also viewed it important to target geographic areas or populations based on basic healthcare needs, such as the need for nutritional supplementation, HIV therapy, or to address the problems of racial residential segregation [46,61]. Indeed, county of residence, with data obtained from the National Center for Health Statistics and population counts from the Census Bureau, may be the most telling indicator of mortality risk [62]. The collective approach to targeted health is only lightly if at all touched on by the PMI, but is critical to a complete precision public health approach to disease risk.

The *All of Us* Research Program stands at an equilibrium point between two wave fronts—precision medicine and precision public health. Its products will be used to develop new targeted therapies, and new predictive measures such as risk scores. It is an energetic lead for both, with more developments yet to come. Inclusion of the Precision Medicine Initiative in a public health course like HMP 517 lays the anchor on what needs to be taught and discussed. We are very pleased to have been able to incorporate this unique point in time capturing the start of a national precision medicine project into the course. The techniques that comprise precision medicine and precision public health stand to be strengthened by the PMI in the same way that the arsenal of useful genetic tests was boosted by the Human Genome Project. A broader vision for curriculum development includes early-stage disease pharmacogenomics [63], cascade screening [64], and targeted social interventions in the same vessel. Once the full chest of precision health tools is packed, it's "anchors away!" for the next-generation of teaching precision public health.

**Author Contributions:** S.M.M. is the paper's principal author. T.C. and S.L.R.K. participated in identifying qualitative categories, provided major guidance on paper themes, helped with draft editing, and suggested references.

## References

1. Modell, S.M.; Citrin, T. Ethics instruction in an issues-oriented course on public health genetics. *Health Educ. Behav.* **2002**, *29*, 43–60. [CrossRef] [PubMed]
2. Centers for Disease Control and Prevention, Office of Public Health Genomics. Public Health Genomics Knowledge Base (v4.0): Tier Table Database. Available online: https://phgkb.cdc.gov/PHGKB/topicStartPage.action (accessed on 22 July 2018).
3. Khoury, M.J.; Bowen, M.S.; Clyne, M.; Dotson, W.D.; Gwinn, M.L.; Green, R.F.; Kolor, K.; Rodriguez, J.L.; Wulf, A.; Yu, W. From public health genomics to precision public health: A 20-year journey. *Genet. Med.* **2018**, *20*, 574–582. [CrossRef] [PubMed]
4. Green, R.C.; Berg, J.S.; Grody, W.W.; Kalia, S.S.; Korf, B.R.; Martin, C.L.; McGuire, A.L.; Nussbaum, R.L.; O'Daniel, J.M.; Ormond, K.E.; et al. ACMG recommendations for reporting of incidental findings in clinical exome and genome sequencing. *Genet. Med.* **2013**, *15*, 565–574. [CrossRef] [PubMed]
5. Biswas, A.; Das, S.; Kapoor, M.; Shamsudheen, K.V.; Jayarajan, R.; Verma, A.; Seth, S.; Bhargava, B.; Scaria, V.; Sivasubbu, S.; et al. Familial hypertrophic cardiomyopathy—Identification of cause and risk stratification through exome sequencing. *Gene* **2018**, *660*, 151–156. [CrossRef] [PubMed]
6. Purshouse, K.; Schuh, A.; Fairfax, B.P.; Knight, S.; Antoniou, P.; Dreau, H.; Popitsch, N.; Gatter, K.; Roberts, I.; Browning, L.; et al. Whole-genome sequencing identifies homozygous *BRCA2* deletion guiding treatment in dedifferentiated prostate cancer. *Cold Spring Harb. Mol. Case Stud.* **2017**, *3*, a001362. [CrossRef] [PubMed]

7.    Sawyer, S.L.; Hartley, T.; Dyment, D.A.; Beaulieu, C.L.; Schwartzentruber, J.; Smith, A.; Bedford, H.M.;
      Bernard, G.; Bernier, F.P.; Brais, B.; et al. Utility of whole-exome sequencing for those near the end of the
      diagnostic odyssey: Time to address gaps in care. *Clin. Genet.* **2016**, *89*, 275–284. [CrossRef] [PubMed]

8.    Knoppers, B.M.; Senecal, K.; Borry, P.; Avard, D. Whole-genome sequencing in newborn screening programs.
      *Sci. Transl. Med.* **2014**, *6*, 229cm2. [CrossRef] [PubMed]

9.    Fleischer, J.A.; Lockwood, C.M. Newborn screening by whole-genome sequencing: Ready for prime time?
      *Clin. Chem.* **2014**, *60*, 1243–1244. [CrossRef] [PubMed]

10.   ACMG Board of Directors. Points to consider for informed consent for genome/exome sequencing.
      *Genet. Med.* **2013**, *15*, 748–749. [CrossRef] [PubMed]

11.   American College of Medical Genetics and Genomics. Incidental findings in clinical genomics: A clarification.
      *Genet. Med.* **2013**, *15*, 664–666. [CrossRef] [PubMed]

12.   Whitehouse. The Precision Medicine Initiative. Available online: https://obamawhitehouse.archives.gov/
      precision-medicine (accessed on 29 May 2018).

13.   Modell, S.M.; Kardia, S.L.R.; Citrin, T. The precision medicine and precision public health approaches to
      cancer treatment and prevention: A cross-comparison. *Adv. Genet. Res. (Nova Biomed.)* **2017**, *17*, 107–138.

14.   Secretary's Advisory Committee on Genetics, Health, and Society. Policy Issues Associated with Undertaking
      a New Large U.S. Population Cohort Study of Genes, Environment, and Disease. Available online: https:
      //osp.od.nih.gov/wp-content/uploads/2013/11/SACGHS_LPS_report.pdf (accessed on 30 May 2018).

15.   National Institutes of Health. *All of Us* Research Program. PMI Working Group of the Advisory Committee to
      the Director. Available online: https://allofus.nih.gov/about/who-we-are/pmi-working-group-advisory-
      committee-director (accessed on 25 May 2018).

16.   National Institutes of Health. *All of Us* Research Program. ACD Precision Medicine Initiative Working Group
      Public Workshop: Participant Engagement and Health Equity Workshop. Available online: www.nih.gov/
      allofus-research-program/participant-engagement-health-equity-workshop (accessed on 25 May 2018).

17.   National Institutes of Health. *All of Us* Research Program. The Precision Medicine Initiative Cohort
      Program—Building a Research Foundation for 21st Century Medicine: Precision Medicine Initiative
      (PMI) Working Group Report to the Advisory Committee to the Director, NIH. 17 September 2015.
      Available online: www.nih.gov/sites/default/files/research-training/initiatives/pmi/pmi-working-group-
      report-20150917-2.pdf (accessed on 29 May 2018).

18.   Khoury, M.J.; Galea, S. Will precision medicine improve population health? *JAMA* **2016**, *316*, 1357–1358.
      [CrossRef] [PubMed]

19.   Marcus, P.M.; Pashayan, N.; Church, T.R.; Doria-Rose, V.P.; Gould, M.K.; Hubbard, R.A.; Marrone, M.;
      Miglioretti, D.L.; Pharoah, P.D.; Pinsky, P.F.; et al. Population-based precision cancer screening: A symposium
      on evidence, epidemiology, and next steps. *Cancer Epidemiol. Biomark. Prev.* **2016**, *25*, 1449–1455. [CrossRef]
      [PubMed]

20.   Green, R.F.; Dotson, W.D.; Bowen, S.; Kolor, K.; Khoury, M.J. Genomics in public health: Perspective from
      the Office of Public Health Genomics at the Centers for Disease Control and Prevention (CDC). *Healthcare*
      **2015**, *3*, 830–837. [CrossRef] [PubMed]

21.   Khoury, M.J.; Evans, J.P. A public health perspective on a national precision medicine cohort: Balancing
      long-term knowledge generation with early health benefit. *JAMA* **2015**, *313*, 2117–2118. [CrossRef] [PubMed]

22.   Dankwa-Mullan, I.; Bull, J.; Sy, F. Precision medicine and health disparities: Advancing the science of
      individualizing patient care. *Am. J. Public Health* **2015**, *105* (Suppl. 3), S368. [CrossRef]

23.   Thomas, J.C.; Irwin, D.E.; Zuiker, E.S.; Millikan, R.C. Genomics and the public health code of ethics. *Am. J.
      Public Health* **2005**, *95*, 2139–2143. [CrossRef] [PubMed]

24.   National Institutes of Health. *All of Us* Research Program. Genome Centers Funding Announcement
      (FA) Webinar Questions & Answers (Q&A). Available online: https://allofus.nih.gov/sites/default/files/
      genome_webinar_qa.pdf (accessed on 19 July 2018).

25.   Eskenazi, K. Four NYC Medical Centers Receive New NIH Precision Medicine Grant. Available online:
      http://newsroom.cumc.columbia.edu/blog/2016/07/08/four-nyc-medical-centers-receive-new-nih-
      precision-medicine-grant (accessed on 16 March 2018).

26.   Gutmann, A.; Thompson, D. Deliberating about bioethics. *Hastings Cent. Rep.* **1997**, *27*, 38–41. [CrossRef]
      [PubMed]

27. Crawshaw, R.; Garland, M.; Hines, B.; Anderson, B. Developing principles for prudent health care allocation—The continuing Oregon experiment. *West. J. Med.* **1990**, *152*, 441–446. [PubMed]

28. Hennekins, C.H.; Buring, J.E. *Epidemiology in Medicine*; Mayrent, S.L., Ed.; Little, Brown and Company: Boston, MA, USA, 1987; pp. 153–177.

29. Erskine, J.A.; Leenders, M.R.; Mauffette-Leenders, L.A. *Teaching with Cases*, 3rd ed.; Ivey Publishing: London, ON, Canada, 2003.

30. Collins, F.S.; Varmus, H. A new initiative on precision medicine. *N. Engl. J. Med.* **2015**, *372*, 793–795. [CrossRef] [PubMed]

31. White House, Office of the Press Secretary. FACT SHEET: President Obama's Precision Medicine Initiative. Available online: https://obamawhitehouse.archives.gov/the-press-office/2015/01/30/fact-sheet-president-obama-s-precision-medicine-initiative (accessed on 29 May 2018).

32. Ferryman, K.; Pitcan, M. Data & Society. Fairness in Precision Medicine. Available online: https://datasociety.net/wp-content/uploads/2018/02/Data.Society.Fairness.In_.Precision.Medicine.Feb2018.FINAL-2.26.18.pdf (accessed on 16 March 2018).

33. Reardon, S. US tailored-medicine project aims for ethnic balance. *Nature* **2015**, *523*, 391–392. [CrossRef] [PubMed]

34. Kaiser, J. NIH Cancels Massive U.S. Children's Study. Available online: www.sciencemag.org/news/2014/12/nih-cancels-massive-us-children-s-study (accessed on 25 May 2018).

35. Dalke, K. African-American Biobank: Who Will Be in It? Available online: www.genomenewsnetwork.org/articles/05_03/biobank.shtml (accessed on 26 May 2018).

36. Modell, S.M.; Citrin, T.; Platt, J.E.; Kardia, S.L.R. Distinctive Features of Public Health Ethics in the Domain of Expanded Genetic Screening and Population Biobanking. In *Patient Rights: Ethical Perspectives, Emerging Developments and Global Challenges*; Pope, J., Ed.; Nova Science Publishers: Hauppauge, NY, USA, 2015; pp. 1–27.

37. Michigan Department of Health and Human Services, Michigan BioTrust for Health. Research Use of Michigan's Residual Blood Spots. Available online: www.michigan.gov/documents/mdch/Dried_Blood_Spot_Research_Table_Public_Report_347898_7.pdf (accessed on 30 May 2018).

38. Brody, H.; Hunt, L.M. BiDil: Assessing a race-based pharmaceutical. *Ann. Fam. Med.* **2006**, *4*, 556–560. [CrossRef] [PubMed]

39. Genetic Alliance. Platform for Engaging Everyone Responsibly (PEER). Available online: www.geneticalliance.org/programs/biotrust/peer (accessed on 30 May 2018).

40. Bonham, V.L.; Citrin, T.; Modell, S.M.; Franklin, T.H.; Bleicher, E.W.B.; Fleck, L.M. Community-based dialogue: Engaging communities of color in the United States' genetics policy conversation. *J. Health Politics Policy Law* **2009**, *34*, 325–359. [CrossRef] [PubMed]

41. Office of Public Health Genomics, Centers for Disease Control and Prevention. Lynch Syndrome Phase 1. Available online: www.cdc.gov/genomics/implementation/toolkit/lynch_2.htm (accessed on 30 May 2018).

42. San Francisco Medical Center, University of California. About the Precision Health Summit. Available online: https://precisionmedicine.ucsf.edu/programs/precision-population-health/summit (accessed on 29 May 2018).

43. Institute of Medicine, Committee on Assuring the Health of the Public in the 21st Century. *The Future of the Public's Health in the 21st Century*; National Academies Press: Washington, DC, USA, 2013.

44. Payne, P.W., Jr.; Royal, C.; Kardia, S.L. Genetic and social environment interactions and their impact on health policy. *J. Am. Acad. Orthop. Surg.* **2007**, *15* (Suppl. 1), S95–S98. [CrossRef] [PubMed]

45. U.S. Department of Health and Human Services, Agency for Healthcare Research and Quality (AHRQ). 2016 National Healthcare Quality and Disparities Report. Available online: www.ahrq.gov/research/findings/nhqrdr/nhqdr16/index.html (accessed on 30 May 2018).

46. Bayer, R.; Galea, S. Public health in the precision-medicine era. *N. Engl. J. Med.* **2015**, *373*, 499–501. [CrossRef] [PubMed]

47. Jaffe, S. Planning for US Precision Medicine Initiative underway. *Lancet* **2015**, *385*, 2448–2449. [CrossRef]

48. Steinsbekk, K.S.; Ursin, L.O.; Skolbekken, J.-A.; Solberg, B. We're not in it for the money—Lay people's moral intuitions on commercial use of 'their' biobank. *Med. Health Care Philos.* **2013**, *16*, 151–162. [CrossRef] [PubMed]

49. National Institutes of Health. The Cancer Genome Atlas. Biospecimen Core Resource. Available online: https://cancergenome.nih.gov/abouttcga/overview/howitworks/bcr (accessed on 29 May 2018).

50. Mirnezami, R.; Nicholson, J.; Darzi, A. Preparing for precision medicine. *N. Engl. J. Med.* **2012**, *366*, 489–491. [CrossRef] [PubMed]

51. Hemingway, H.; Asselbergs, F.W.; Danesh, J.; Dobson, R.; Maniadakis, N.; Maggioni, A.; van Thiel, G.J.M.; Cronin, M.; Brobert, G.; Vardas, P.; et al. Big data from electronic health records for early and late translational cardiovascular research: Challenges and potential. *Eur. Heart J.* **2018**, *39*, 1481–1495. [CrossRef] [PubMed]

52. Katsila, T.; Patrinos, G.P. Whole genome sequencing in pharmacogenomics. *Front. Pharmacol.* **2015**, *6*, 61. [CrossRef] [PubMed]

53. Linderman, M.D.; Sanderson, S.C.; Bashir, A.; Diaz, G.A.; Kasarskis, A.; Zinberg, R.; Mahajan, M.; Suckiel, S.A.; Zweig, M.; Schadt, E.E. Impacts of incorporating personal genome sequencing into graduate genomics education: A longitudinal study over three course years. *BMC Med. Genom.* **2018**, *11*, 5. [CrossRef] [PubMed]

54. Dolan, M.E.; Maitland, M.L.; O'Donnell, P.H.; Nakamura, Y.; Cox, N.J.; Ratain, M.J. University of Chicago Center for Personalized Therapeutics: Research, education and implementation science. *Pharmacogenomics* **2013**, *14*, 1383–1387. [CrossRef] [PubMed]

55. Chang, K.-L.; Weitzel, K.; Schmidt, S. Pharmacogenetics: Using genetic information to guide drug therapy. *Am. Fam. Physican* **2015**, *92*, 588–594.

56. Thomas, L. Colorectal Cancer: Screening Should Include Environment, Genetic Factors. Available online: https://news.umich.edu/colorectal-cancer-screening-should-include-environment-genetic-factors (accessed on 16 March 2018).

57. Natarajan, P.; Young, R.; Stitziel, N.O.; Padmanabhan, S.; Baber, U.; Mehran, R.; Sartori, S.; Fuster, V.; Reilly, D.F.; Butterworth, A.; et al. Polygenic risk score identifies subgroup with higher burden of atherosclerosis and greater relative benefit from statin therapy in the primary prevention setting. *Circulation* **2017**, *135*, 2091–2101. [CrossRef] [PubMed]

58. Dron, J.S.; Wang, J.; Low-Kam, C.; Khetarpal, S.A.; Robinson, J.F.; McIntyre, A.D.; Ban, M.R.; Cao, H.; Rhainds, D.; Dube, M.P.; et al. Polygenic determinants in extremes of high-density lipoprotein cholesterol. *J. Lipid Res.* **2017**, *58*, 2162–2170. [CrossRef] [PubMed]

59. Denny, J.C.; Bastarache, L.; Roden, D.M. Phenome-wide association studies as a tool to advance precisions medicine. *Annu. Rev. Genom. Hum. Genet.* **2016**, *17*, 353–373. [CrossRef] [PubMed]

60. American Public Health Association. Strengthening Genetic and Genomic Literacy. (APHA Policy # 201012). Available online: https://apha.org/policies-and-advocacy/public-health-policy-statements/policy-database/2014/07/30/16/37/strengthening-genetic-and-genomic-literacy (accessed on 30 May 2018).

61. Desmond-Hellmann, S. Progress lies in precision. *Science* **2016**, *353*, 731. [CrossRef] [PubMed]

62. Mokdad, A.H.; Dwyer-Lindgren, L.; Fitzmaurice, C.; Stubbs, R.W.; Bertozzi-Villa, A.; Morozoff, C.; Charara, R.; Allen, C.; Naghavi, M.; Murray, C.J.L. Trends and patterns of disparities in cancer mortality among US counties, 1980–2104. *JAMA* **2017**, *317*, 388–406. [CrossRef] [PubMed]

63. Ritchie, M.D. The success of pharmacogenomics in moving genetic association studies from bench to bedside: Study design and implementation of precision medicine in the post-GWAS era. *Hum. Genet.* **2012**, *131*, 1615–1626. [CrossRef] [PubMed]

64. Roberts, M.C.; Dotson, W.D.; DeVore, C.S.; Bednar, E.M.; Bowen, D.J.; Ganiats, T.G.; Green, R.F.; Hurst, G.M.; Philp, A.R.; Ricker, C.N.; et al. Delivery of cascade screening for hereditary conditions: A scoping review of the literature. *Health Aff.* **2018**, *37*, 801–808. [CrossRef] [PubMed]

# 3

# From Inpatient to Ambulatory Care: The Introduction of a Rapid Access Transient Ischaemic Attack Service

**Mohana Maddula \*, Laura Adams and Jonathan Donnelly**

Tauranga Hospital, Bay of Plenty District Health Board, Tauranga 3112, New Zealand;
laura.adams@bopdhb.govt.nz (L.A.); jonathan.donnelly@bopdhb.govt.nz (J.D.)
\* Correspondence: mohana.maddula1981@gmail.com

**Abstract:** *Background*: Transient Ischaemic Attacks (TIA) should be treated as a medical emergency. While high-risk TIAs have higher stroke risks than low-risk patients, there is an inherent limitation to this risk stratification, as some low-risk patients may have undiagnosed high-risk conditions. Inequity of care for TIA patients was observed, such that high-risk patients received urgent assessment through acute admission, while low-risk patients faced long waits for clinical consultation. A redesign of the TIA service was planned to offer timely assessment for all patients and avoid acute admission for high-risk patients. *Methods*: Service reconfiguration was undertaken to set up a daily weekday rapid access TIA clinic where patients would be assessed, investigated, and treated. *Results*: A re-audit of clinic performance showed a significant increase in the number of patients seen in the ages of 18 to 52. The median time from referral to clinical consultation improved from 10 days to 1. There were similar significant improvements seen in median time to brain imaging (from 10.5 days to 1), and carotid ultrasound (from 10 days to all scans being performed on the same day). *Conclusions*: The redesigned service achieved the objective of offering urgent assessment and investigations for all TIA patients, including low-risk patients, while avoiding the acute admission for high-risk patients. We share our experience of establishing a successful rapid access ambulatory service without any additional resources.

**Keywords:** transient ischaemic attack; TIA; stroke

## 1. Introduction

Strokes are an important cause of death and long-term adult disability, and many strokes can be prevented with appropriate medical intervention. A Transient Ischaemic Attack (TIA) is defined as an abrupt onset of a focal neurological deficit as a result of focal ischaemia lasting less than 24 h and without radiological evidence of acute ischaemia. TIAs herald high risks of stroke over the next few hours and days, and should therefore be treated as a medical emergency. Urgent clinical assessment, investigation, and initiation of secondary preventive measures have been shown to significantly reduce the risk of stroke [1,2].

A previous New-Zealand-wide audit in 2013 showed evidence of significant improvements in the provision of care for patients with suspected TIA, with a shift to assessment in an ambulatory care setting, rather than acute admission. There was however much variation in practice and service set-up [3]. Management in specialized rapid access TIA clinics results in reduced stroke risk [4]. Moreover, a non-admission-based approach with outpatient clinic follow-up has been shown to be better at stroke prevention and cost-effectiveness, compared with admission-based care [5].

The Tauranga hospital serves a population of about 46,000 in the western Bay of Plenty region of New Zealand. At the time of review, the TIA clinic ran concurrently with the general Stroke & TIA outpatient service, encompassing follow-ups from the inpatient wards and new patient referrals from primary care. 'High-risk' TIA patients (those with ABCD2 score > 3, atrial fibrillation or carotid stenosis, crescendo TIAs, and those on anticoagulation) were admitted for urgent investigation and treatment, while 'low-risk' TIAs (ABCD2 score < 4) would be mostly managed by GPs, with a follow-up in the hospital TIA clinic.

An audit over two months in 2016 showed unacceptably long delays for review of patients in the TIA clinic and subsequent investigations. There was a concern of underutilization of the service, with the observation that many 'low-risk' TIA patients were completely managed by General Practitioners (GPs), contrary to current recommendations. There was also an overreliance on the ABCD2 score, with referring clinicians often incorrectly applying this risk-stratification tool to make a TIA diagnosis. The ABCD2 score has low sensitivity and specificity when used by non-specialists in the community or emergency department [6,7]. One in five patients with an ABCD2 score < 4 have symptomatic carotid stenosis of >50% or atrial fibrillation [8]. Over the last few years, there has been a shift away from solely using the ABCD2 score to reliably discriminate between high- and low-risk TIAs. The 2017 Australian & NZ stroke guidelines make a weak recommendation that the ABCD2 score should not be used in isolation when determining the urgency of an assessment, as this may delay the recognition of atrial fibrillation and carotid stenosis [9]. The UK stroke guidelines take one step further and completely abandon use of the ABCD2 score [10].

With this in mind, the TIA service at Tauranga Hospital was redesigned to provide a timely assessment and equity of care for all suspected TIAs, including 'low-risk' patients who may have undiagnosed high-risk factors (such as carotid stenosis). Another objective of the new service was to provide rapid ambulatory assessment for 'high-risk' patients in place of acute admission.

## 2. Methods

Service reconfiguration was undertaken to set up a daily weekday one-stop rapid access TIA clinic, where patients would be assessed, investigated (on the same day where necessary), and treated. A daily weekday clinic was felt to be needed in order to meet fluctuations in the numbers of referrals. Although desirable to provide a seven days service, this did not prove feasible, as the service was run by only one stroke physician and registrar. Only suspected high-risk TIAs would be admitted during the weekends.

All service improvement projects can face challenges; Table 1 illustrates some of these and how solutions were found. General Practitioner and in-hospital referral pathways were modified, such that high-risk TIA patients would be offered TIA clinic consult within 24–48 h of referral, and low-risk patients within seven days.

**Table 1.** Challenges faced by the service improvement project and how solutions were found.

| Challenges/Barriers to Change | Solutions |
|---|---|
| In-hospital processing of referrals was taking a few days as this was reliant on several administrative steps. | The referral process was streamlined; the stroke physician was accessible by phone during working hours and received email alerts of inpatient referrals and electronic General Practitioner referrals, enabling prompt triaging of referrals and early allocation of clinic slots. |
| Limited outpatient clinic space to see patients at short notice and review after same day investigations. | A single room on the stroke ward was converted into a consultation room. This enabled an easy oversight of clinic patients and a review after investigations. |
| Limited clinician time. No additional staff were provided. | The Stroke Physician and Registrar dropped one weekly outpatient clinic each and was this time redistributed to provide daily weekday TIA (Transient Ishcaemic Attack) clinics. |

**Table 1.** *Cont.*

| Challenges/Barriers to Change | Solutions |
|---|---|
| Limited Radiology resources. No additional funding to increase carotid or brain imaging appointments. | Referral pathway for carotid imaging was modified, such that only the stroke team could request carotid ultrasound in order to filter out inappropriate investigations (e.g., where imaging was unlikely to change overall management). This allowed for the allocation of two fixed carotid ultrasound appointments per day for TIA clinic patients. Same-day brain imaging was also available. |
| Need for urgent cardiac monitoring to identify patients with paroxysmal atrial fibrillation/flutter in place of inpatient telemetry. | The Stroke service purchased Holter monitor units to be used for the sole purpose of TIA clinic patients. Patients would have them fitted the same day and wear them for at least 48 h. These would get analysed urgently, and results were forwarded to Stroke physician. |

## 3. Results

The redesigned TIA service came into effect on 1 May 2017. Referrals were triaged the same way, although the emphasis was put on prompt review of the electronic referral and administrative processes, such as allocation of clinic appointment (Table 1). During the triage, two referrals (both from GPs) were declined following a review of the clinical information, as the likelihood of a neurovascular event or any other serious pathology was felt to be extremely unlikely. In both cases, the referrers were sent prompt written correspondence with advice and signposting of other hospital services if the GP still wanted to a second opinion. Table 2 shows audit results of equivalent time periods before and following the implementation of changes. There was a significant increase in the number of patients seen in the new TIA clinic. Most referrals were from GPs ($n$ = 24), followed by ED (Emergency Department) ($n$ = 15), other inpatient teams ($n$ = 12), and Ophthalmology ($n$ = 1). Twenty-four patients and 12 patients were diagnosed with TIA and stroke, respectively; the rest were TIA 'mimics', such as syncope, migraine and postural hypotension. Carotid ultrasound imaging was indicated in 25 patients, and in all cases this was performed on the same day. Where indicated, brain imaging was performed on 35 patients: 26 patients had CT (Computed Tomography) scans, and nine had MRIs (Magnetic Resonance Imaging), with a median time of one day. One patient waited 39 days for brain imaging; this was felt to be a non-urgent scan for the evaluation of suspected mild dementia.

**Table 2.** Audit cycle results before and after implementation of the redesigned service.

| | Before 1st Audit Cycle Oct.–Nov. 2016 | After 2nd Audit Cycle May–June 2017 |
|---|---|---|
| Number of patients seen in TIA clinic | 18 | 52 |
| Median time (days) from referral to clinic consult—All referrals | 10 (range 0 *–40) | 1 (range 0 *–4) |
| Median time (days) to brain imaging where indicated | 10.5 (range 2–64) | 1 (range 0 *–39) |
| Median time (days) to carotid US imaging where indicated | 10 (range 1–143) | 0 * (all patients imaged on same day) |

\* same day.

There were 21 patients included in the audit classified as high-risk according to the aforementioned criteria, and 31 low-risk patients. For both high- and low-risk patients, the median time to review was one day. No patients were admitted to the hospital with a stroke or TIA within 90 days of their review. Feedback from patients was excellent (Figure 1), despite concern that some may be displeased about having to wait around in the clinic for same-day investigations.

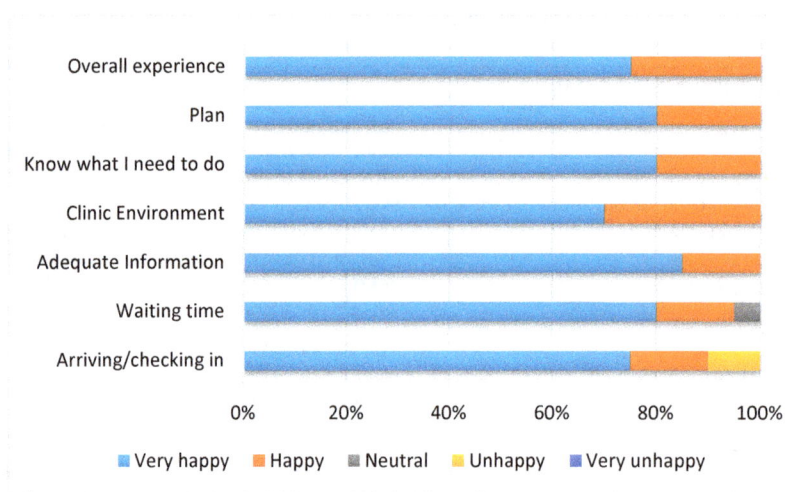

**Figure 1.** Patient feedback.

## 4. Discussion

The establishment of rapid access TIA clinic centres across in North America the UK, and Australia has shifted the focus of TIA care from inpatient to outpatient management. In our new rapid access service, all suspected TIA patients were provided with an early consult and underwent timely investigations where needed. We achieved the objective of improving access to specialist assessment for all TIAs, even those deemed to be low-risk, some of which may have yet unknown high-risk conditions. This was achieved while providing timely assessment for high-risk patients without acute admission.

The data shows that there is a substantial reduction in time until specialist consult, time for imaging where required (both brain and carotid), and hospital admissions for high-risk TIAs. Utilisation of the service increased due to an organisation-wide awareness and a shift from community management to rapid specialist referral. A total of 69% of patients seen had a confirmed diagnosis of TIA or stroke, which is in line with similar data obtained from other TIA clinic studies [11]. This would suggest that appropriate patients were being referred to the service, that the triage process worked well to allow prompt clinic review and avoid inappropriate use of the service (two referrals were declined as stated above), and that clinical reasoning and diagnostic accuracy was consistent with standard practice at other centres. One area of concern is the number of patients diagnosed with stroke (12; 23%). While it may be reasonable to provide an outpatient clinic review to those patients who have had a minor stroke, there is a possibility that some patients with acute stroke may not receive the benefit of multidisciplinary team input in a stroke unit if there were seen in clinic. Feedback was provided to GPs and Emergency Department doctors about the importance of referring patients with persisting neurological symptoms for admission, rather than referral to the TIA clinic.

We achieved this service improvement in the provision of timely specialist care for patients with suspected TIA without any additional resources. This was achieved through the redesign of the service, which included the use of electronic systems (such as emails for receipt of referrals instead of hard copy referrals), reducing the inappropriate use of investigations (such as filtering out unnecessary carotid doppler ultrasound requests), and redistribution of existing resource (dropping existing outpatient clinics and using this clinician time to provide the daily TIA service). Although we have not performed a cost-benefit analysis as part of the service redesign, we expect to find cost-saving through the management of suspected high-risk TIA patients through this ambulatory setting instead of hospital admission.

With the ever-increasing burden of healthcare expenditure and demand for hospital beds around the world, healthcare systems are increasingly looking at ambulatory models for the management of various health conditions as an alternative to hospital admission. In the development of our Rapid

Access TIA service, we have shared our experience of developing this service together with the challenges we faced and how solutions were found.

## 5. Conclusions

We were able to successfully introduce a rapid access ambulatory clinic for assessment and management of patients with suspected TIA through service redesign. During this process we encountered some challenges, however we were able to find successful solutions without the need for any additional resource.

**Author Contributions:** The conceptualization, writing, review, and editing were done by M.M., formal analysis was done by L.A., and the original draft preparation was done by both L.A. and J.D.

**Funding:** This research received no external funding.

**Acknowledgments:** Suzanne Board (Quality Improvement, Bay of Plenty District Health Board), Trish Blattmann (Clinical Nurse Specialist, Bay of Plenty District Health Board).

## References

1. Lavallee, P.C.; Meseguer, E.; Abboud, H.; Cabrejo, L.; Olivot, J.M.; Simon, O.; Mazighi, M.; Nifle, C.; Niclot, P.; Lapergue, B.; et al. A transient ischaemic attack clinic with round-the-clock access (SOS-TIA): Feasibility and effects. *Lancet Neurol.* **2007**, *6*, 953–960. [CrossRef]

2. Rothwell, P.M.; Giles, M.F.; Chandratheva, A.; Marquardt, L.; Geraghty, O.; Redgrave, J.N.; Lovelock, C.E.; Binney, L.E.; Bull, L.M.; Cuthbertson, F.C.; et al. Effect of urgent treatment of transient ischaemic attack and minor stroke on early recurrent stroke (EXPRESS study): A prospective population-based sequential compression. *Lancet* **2007**, *370*, 1432–1442. [CrossRef]

3. Brownlee, W.; Ranta, A.; Dale-Gandar, J.; Bennett, P.; Gommans, J.; Fink, J.; Barber, P.A. Changes in the provision of transient ischaemic attack services in New Zealand 2008 to 2013. *N. Z. Med. J.* **2014**, *127*, 23–29. [PubMed]

4. Sehatzadeh, S. Is transient ischemic attack a medical emergency? An evidenced-based analysis. *Ont. Health Technol. Assess. Ser.* **2015**, *15*, 1–45. [PubMed]

5. Sanders, L.M.; Cadilhac, D.A.; Srikanth, V.K.; Chong, C.P.; Phan, T.G. Is nonadmission-based care for TIA patients cost-effective? *Neurol. Clin. Pract.* **2015**, *5*, 58–66. [CrossRef] [PubMed]

6. Bradley, D.; Cronin, S.; Kinsella, J.A.; Tobin, W.O.; Mahon, C.; O'Brien, M.; Lonergan, R.; Cooney, M.T.; Kennelly, S.; Collins, D.R.; et al. Frequent inaccuracies in ABCD2 scoring in non-stroke specialists' referrals to a daily rapid access stroke prevention service. *J. Neurol. Sci.* **2013**, *332*, 30–34. [CrossRef] [PubMed]

7. Ghia, D.; Thomas, P.; Cordato, D.; Epstein, D.; Beran, R.G.; Cappelen-Smith, C.; Griffith, N.; Hanna, I.; McDougall, A.; Hodgkinson, S.J.; et al. Low positive predictive value of the ABCD2 score in emergency department transient ischaemic attack diagnoses: The south western Sydney transient ischaemic attack study. *Intern. Med. J.* **2012**, *42*, 913–918. [CrossRef] [PubMed]

8. Wardlow, J.A.; Brazzelli, M.; Chappell, F.M.; Miranda, H.; Shuler, K.; Sandercock, P.A.; Dennis, M.S. ABCD2 score and secondary stroke prevention. *Neurology* **2015**, *85*, 373–380. [CrossRef] [PubMed]

9. Stroke Foundation. *Clinical Guidelines for Stroke Management 2017*; Stroke Foundation: Melbourne, Australia, 2017.

10. Royal College of Physicians. *National Clinical Guideline for Stroke 2016*, 5th ed.; Royal College of Physicians: London, UK, 2016.

11. Martin, P.J.; Young, G.; Enevoldson, T.P.; Humphrey, P.R. Overdiagnosis of TIA and minor stroke: Experience at a regional neurovascular clinic. *QJM* **1997**, *90*, 759–763. [CrossRef] [PubMed]

# 4

# Functionality in Middle-Aged and Older Overweight and Obese Individuals with Knee Osteoarthritis

Neda S. Akhavan [1,2], Lauren Ormsbee [1,2], Sarah A. Johnson [3], Kelli S. George [1,2], Elizabeth M. Foley [1,2], Marcus L. Elam [4], Zahra Ezzat-Zadeh [1], Lynn B. Panton [1,2] and Bahram H. Arjmandi [1,2,*] (iD)

[1] Department of Nutrition, Food and Exercise Sciences, Florida State University, Tallahassee, FL 32306-4310, USA; nsa08@my.fsu.edu (N.S.A.); lormsbee@fsu.edu (L.O.); ksg15c@my.fsu.edu (K.S.G.); ef15c@my.fsu.edu (E.M.F.); ze09@fsu.edu (Z.E.-Z.); lpanton@admin.fsu.edu (L.B.P.)

[2] Center for Advancing Exercise and Nutrition Research on Aging (CAENRA), College of Human Sciences, Florida State University, Tallahassee, FL 32306-4310, USA

[3] Department of Food Science and Human Nutrition, Colorado State University, Fort Collins, CO 80523-1571, USA; Sarah.Johnson@colostate.edu

[4] Department of Human Nutrition and Food Science, California State Polytechnic University, Pomona, CA 91768-2557, USA; mlelam@cpp.edu

* Correspondence: barjmandi@fsu.edu

**Abstract:** Patients with knee osteoarthritis (OA) suffer from immobility and pain. The objective of this cross-sectional study was to investigate the relationship between pain and functionality in middle-aged and older overweight and obese individuals with mild-to-moderate knee OA. Overall pattern, physical activity, and total energy expenditure (TEE) were assessed in 83 participants. The Western Ontario McMaster Universities Arthritis Index (WOMAC) was used to assess lower extremity pain and function. The six-minute walk test (6-MWT) and range of motion (ROM) were also assessed. Results indicated that age was inversely associated with body mass index (BMI) ($r = 0.349$) and total WOMAC scores ($r = 0.247$). BMI was positively associated with TEE ($r = 0.430$) and WOMAC scores ($r = 0.268$), while ROM was positively associated with the 6-MWT ($r = 0.561$) and negatively associated with WOMAC ($r = 0.338$) and pain scores ($r = 0.222$). Furthermore, women had significantly greater WOMAC scores ($p = 0.046$) than men. Older participants ($\geq 65$ years old) had significantly lower BMI ($p = 0.002$), and distance traveled during the 6-MWT ($p = 0.013$). Our findings indicate that older individuals in this population with knee OA had lower BMI, greater ROM, and less pain and stiffness and walked slower than middle-aged individuals. Women reported greater pain, stiffness, and reduced functionality, indicating that the manifestation of OA may vary due to gender.

**Keywords:** pain; joint; body mass index (BMI); men; women; Western Ontario McMaster Universities Arthritis Index (WOMAC); exercise

---

## 1. Introduction

Osteoarthritis (OA) is the most common joint disorder in the world and one of the leading causes of disability worldwide [1]. According to reports by the United Nations, 15% of the world's population over the age of 60 years will have symptomatic OA by the year 2050 [2]. This is also true of developed countries, including the United States of America (US). It is estimated that 72 million Americans are at or approaching retirement age. As the US population increases in age, the prevalence of musculoskeletal conditions associated with functional disability and pain is increasing [3]. Over 20 million Americans have knee OA, a progressive degenerative disease, and suffer from complications including immobility and joint pain [4]. The prevalence is expected to parallel increases in the aging population. OA is characterized by the breakdown of articular cartilage in a synovial joint coupled with the thickening and remodeling of adjacent bone, as well as the growth of osteophytes and bone spurs [5]. OA can also be characterized as a chronic inflammatory disease which affects the whole joint, damaging cartilage and remodeling the subchondral bone structure [6]. Although the symptomatic results of OA are relatively known, the causes of OA are not well established. Quality of life is a major concern for individuals with OA as 80% of individuals with OA have some degree of restriction to their daily activities and 25% suffer from major immobility [7]. The annual costs of care for individuals with OA in the US is estimated to be anywhere between $15 and $26 billion per year, and therefore represents a large economic burden. There is no cure for OA; rather, treatment focuses on delaying the progression of the disease and symptom management [8].

A major modifiable risk factor for the development of OA is excess body weight [9–12]. Overweight and obese individuals have a greater prevalence of knee OA in comparison with normal weight individuals due, in part, to cartilage degeneration caused by excess body weight [9]. In fact, individuals with a body mass index (BMI) greater than $30.0 \, kg/m^2$ are 6.8 times more likely to develop knee OA compared to men and women of normal weight BMI between 18.5 and $24.9 \, kg/m^2$ [9]. Overweight and obese individuals with OA suffer from structural damage of the joints due to increased mechanical load, decreased muscle strength, as well as metabolic changes and inflammation [10]. Body composition is of particular importance in overweight and obese individuals with OA where a 1 kg increase in fat mass (androidal, trunk, or total body) is associated with an increase in tibiofemoral cartilage degeneration [11]. Adipose tissue is a metabolic endocrine organ which can secrete adipokines that can promote inflammation and are detrimental in individuals with OA [12]. Thus, a state of increased inflammation and increased mechanical loading due to obesity may exacerbate pain and stiffness in individuals with knee OA.

The risk for development of OA increases with age; older individuals are at a greater risk for progression of OA due to musculoskeletal changes commonly observed in this population contributing to alterations outside and within the joints [13]. OA typically becomes symptomatic in many individuals after the age of 50 years, possibly due to increases in age-related changes such as increased systemic inflammation, sarcopenia, reduced physical activity, and increased joint stiffness [14]. Particularly in individuals over the age of 65 years, quality of life can be compromised in individuals with OA, and postmenopausal women may manifest, present, and develop the disease differently than men due to anatomic, genetic, and hormonal differences, due to the loss of estrogen [15]. In a meta-analysis by Srikanth et al. [16], women over the age of 55 years tended to have more severe OA particularly in the knee as opposed to other sites in comparison to men, in addition to greater prevalence and incidence of OA.

In addition to pain and inflammation, functionality is a serious problem in individuals with OA and assessment of joint functionality is critical to management and treatment of patients with OA. Reduced range of motion (ROM) and impaired joint mobility are major indicators of disability in individuals with knee or hip OA [17]. The Western Ontario McMaster Universities Arthritis Index (WOMAC) is a widely used clinical questionnaire for assessing the state of individuals with OA, which includes subsections examining pain, stiffness, and physical functioning of the joints [18]. Due to either over- or under-estimation of self-reported functional capacity, objective measures of functionality such as the six-minute walk test (6-MWT) are used to evaluate exercise capacity as well as morbidity and mortality in obese and diseased populations [19]. Establishing the association between knee functionality and disability in this population can provide insight for the assessment as well as the management of symptoms associated with OA.

The exact etiology of OA is unknown and there is a paucity of research examining functionality in overweight and obese individuals who have mild-to-moderate knee OA. Investigating the relationship between pain and functionality in middle-aged and older, overweight and obese men and women with mild-to-moderate knee OA provides insight into potential interventions for reducing the progression and symptoms of OA within this population. Thus, the hypothesis of this cross-sectional study was that BMI would be positively associated with WOMAC, total energy expenditure (TEE), 6-MWT, and pain scores, and negatively associated with ROM and overall functionality measured from the WOMAC in overweight and obese individuals with mild-to-moderate knee OA. We also hypothesized that women and older individuals in the study would have greater WOMAC and pain scores, while having reduced ROM and distance traveled from the 6-MWT.

## 2. Materials and Methods

### 2.1. Participants

Overweight or obese (BMI $\geq$ 25.0 kg/m$^2$), otherwise healthy men and women between the ages of 40 and 90 years with clinically diagnosed mild-to-moderate bilateral or unilateral OA of the knee were recruited for screening from the greater Tallahassee, Florida, and surrounding areas using flyers, radio, and online listings. A Kellgren–Lawrence radiological score of 1–3 was used for diagnosis of knee OA from previous medical records. Participants were excluded if they had a history of severe liver and/or kidney disease or any other chronic or acute diseases that may affect OA, knee surgery (including arthroscopy) or significant injury of the target knee joint within 6 months prior to the start of the study, and any hyaluronan or cortisone injections within 2 months prior to study enrollment. This study was approved by the Florida State University Institutional Review Board. After initial pre-screening over the telephone, eligible participants were asked to come to the Human Performance Laboratory in the Department of Nutrition, Food and Exercise Sciences at Florida State University for an onsite screening and to provide written informed consent. Included participants were able to walk unassisted and had experienced knee pain for at least six months.

### 2.2. Study Overview

After the screening visit and enrollment, participants came for a subsequent visit to the Human Performance Laboratory in the morning seven days later. Basic anthropometric assessments were performed including measurement of height and weight to calculate BMI. Physical activity recalls [20] were performed to assess participants' physical activity patterns and TEE. ROM, WOMAC, pain assessments, and 6-MWT were used to measure function and levels of pain.

### 2.3. Assessment of Physical Activity

TEE and overall trend of physical activity of participants from the past seven days (with weekdays separately calculated from weekend days) were assessed using Five-City Project Physical Activity Recall [20]. The level of physical activity was based on either moderate (3–5 metabolic equivalents [METs], e.g., mopping and brisk walking), hard (5.1–6.9 METs, e.g., scrubbing floors and jogging), or very hard activities ($\geq$7.0 METs, e.g., cross-country skiing and high-impact aerobics). METs were calculated as follows: 24 h $-$ (time spent sleeping + time doing moderate intensity activity + time doing hard intensity activity + time in very hard intensity activity). The weighted METs/h average was taken and converted to kcal/d.

### 2.4. Assessment of Range of Motion, Functionality, and Lower Extremity Pain

Knee ROM ($^\circ$) was assessed using a computerized isokinetic dynamometer (Biodex, Shirley, NY, USA). The leg that was most affected by OA was used for ROM testing. Participants were seated in an upright position with the test leg secured at 90$^\circ$, and the dynamometer arm rotor aligned to the lateral side of the knee joint. Each participant was instructed to raise the leg as high as he/she could for a period of approximately 2 s, long enough for a steady ROM value to be reached. Three repetitions were performed, and an average ROM was recorded. The WOMAC assessment form was presented to each participant for measuring lower extremity pain and function [21]. Participants reported subscale scores from 0 (no pain, stiffness, or difficulty) and 1 (mild) to 4 (extreme) for pain, stiffness, and difficulty in performing basic physical tasks during the previous 48 h. A total score (0–100) was then derived from the tallying of subscale scores. Each participant completed a 6-MWT based on a standardized protocol [22]. The participants were instructed to walk as quickly as possible without causing pain or discomfort to their knees for six minutes on a flat surface while wearing comfortable shoes. During testing, research personnel refrained from walking alongside or in front of the participants to avoid influencing their pace. The total distance covered (meters) was measured using a trundle wheel.

### 2.5. Statistical Analysis

Data were analyzed using Pearson-product moment correlations, where degree of relationships between anthropometric assessments, physical activity, TEE, ROM, WOMAC, and the 6-MWT were determined. The Pearson correlation coefficient r was used to examine the relationship between variables. The magnitudes of correlation coefficients were considered as very small to none ($r < 0.1$), small ($0.1 \leq r < 0.3$), moderate ($0.3 \leq r < 0.5$), large ($0.5 \leq r < 0.7$), very large ($0.7 \leq r < 0.9$), nearly perfect ($0.9 \leq r < 1.0$), and perfect ($r = 1.0$) [23]. Independent-sample t-tests were performed to determine if there were differences within this population in BMI, WOMAC, pain scores, ROM, and 6-MWT between males and females as well as older ($\geq 65$ years of age) and middle-aged individuals. Statistical analyses were performed with the IBM (International Business Machines) SPSS (Statistical Package for the Social Sciences) computer program (version 22). All data are presented using means $\pm$ standard deviation. All significance was accepted at $p \leq 0.05$.

### 3. Results

A total of 137 participants were determined to be eligible for an in-person screening (Figure 1) through an initial telephone screening of 252 participants. From the 252 participants who were telephone screened, 100 participants did not meet the inclusion criteria and 15 did not return calls. From the 137 participants who were screened on-site, there were 83 participants, 66 females and 17 males who met the age inclusion criteria, that were diagnosed with mild-to-moderate bilateral or unilateral OA of the knee and a Kellgren–Lawrence radiological score of 1–3 who met the inclusion criteria and were enrolled in this cross-sectional study. Common causes for participant exclusion were non-physician approval of mild-to-moderate knee OA, not meeting the BMI criteria (BMI $\leq 24.9$ kg/m$^2$), traveling, and not being interested in participating in the study.

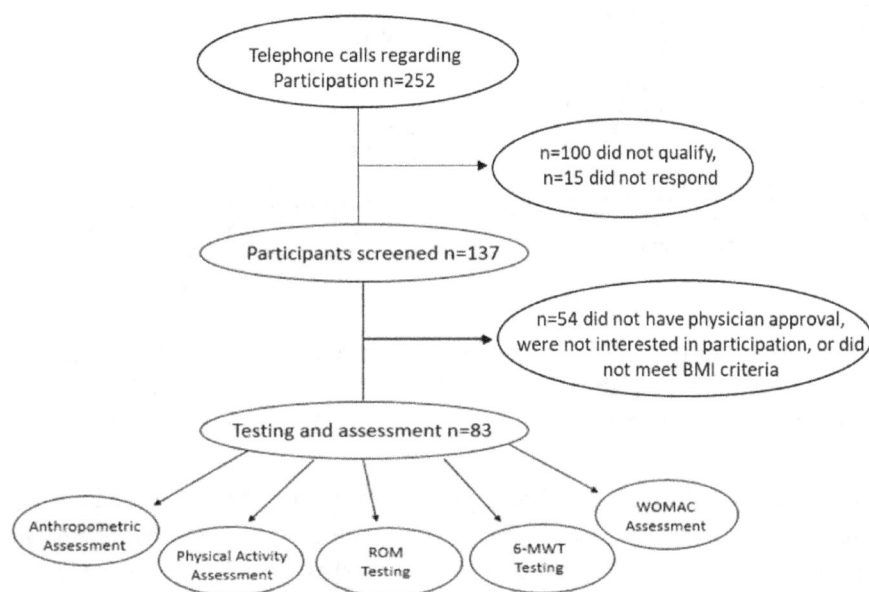

**Figure 1.** Study flowchart.

## 3.1. Baseline Characteristics

The mean age of participants was $62.0 \pm 9.2$ years old with an average height of $167.0 \pm 8.4$ cm, weight of $90.0 \pm 19.5$ kg, and BMI of $32.5 \pm 6.2$ kg/m$^2$ (Table 1). The mean for ROM, 6-MWT, and WOMAC scores were $68.2 \pm 13.4°$, $407.6 \pm 88.1$ m, and $53.4 \pm 15.4$, respectively (Table 1). The mean number of hours per day for moderate, hard, and very hard activity was $2.78 \pm 2.74$, $1.07 \pm 0.52$, and $0.13 \pm 0.04$ h/day, respectively, with a mean TEE of $3809 \pm 1120$ kcals/day (Table 1).

**Table 1.** Participant characteristics ($n = 83$).

|                     | All ($n = 83$) | Female ($n = 66$) | Male ($n = 17$) | Range        |
|---------------------|---------------|-------------------|-----------------|--------------|
| **Age (years)**     | 62.0 (9.0)    | 61.2 (8.6)        | 64.8 (8.8)      | 52.8–71.2    |
| **Weight (kg)**     | 90.0 (19.5)   | 88.6 (20.0)       | 99.4 (15.7)     | 70.5–109.5   |
| **Height (cm)**     | 167.0 (8.4)   | 164.6 (7.1)       | 176.5 (6.5)     | 158.6–175.4  |
| **BMI (kg/m$^2$)**  | 32. (6.2)     | 32.6 (6.6)        | 31.9 (4.9)      | 26.3–38.7    |
| **ROM (°)**         | 68.2 (13.4)   | 64.1 (13.9)       | 68.4 (11.7)     | 54.8–81.6    |
| **6-MWT (meters)**  | 407.6 (88.1)  | 404.1 (87.6)      | 421.3 (91.3)    | 319.5–495.7  |
| **WOMAC**           | 53.4 (15.4)   | 60.1 (14.9)       | 51.8 (15.7)     | 38.0–68.7    |
| **Moderate (hours)**| 2.8 (2.8)     | 2.7 (2.7)         | 2.8 (3.0)       | 0.0–5.6      |
| **Hard (hours)**    | 0.5 (1.0)     | 0.5 (1.1)         | 0.7 (0.8)       | 0.0–1.5      |
| **Very Hard (hours)**| 0.04 (0.14)  | 0.05 (0.15)       | 0.02 (0.06)     | 0.0–0.18     |
| **TEE (kcals)**     | 3809 (1120)   | 3707 (1105)       | 4201 (1120)     | 2688–4929    |

Values are shown as means and standard deviations (SD). Range of motion (ROM); six-minute walk test (6-MWT); Western Ontario McMaster Universities Arthritis Index (WOMAC); moderate, hard, and very hard physical activity (PA); total energy expenditure (TEE).

## 3.2. Age

Significant negative correlations were found between age and weight ($r = -0.299$, $p = 0.006$), BMI ($r = -0.349$, $p = 0.001$), and total WOMAC scores ($r = -0.247$, $p = 0.025$) (Figure 2). These results indicate that as age increases, body weight decreases and knee functionality increases.

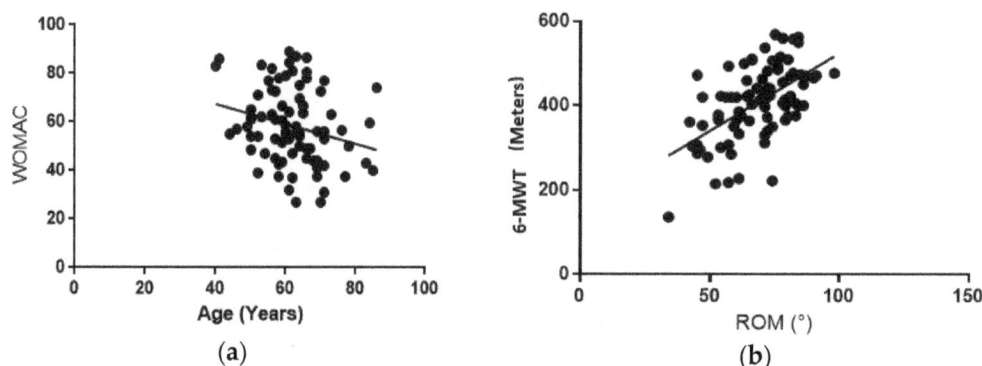

(a)                                            (b)

**Figure 2.** Right panel (**a**): WOMAC score vs. age. As participants aged, WOMAC scores decreased, ($r = -0.247$, $p = 0.025$). Left panel (**b**): 6-MWT vs. ROM. Regardless of age or gender, those who were able to walk further during the 6-MWT had a greater knee ROM ($r = 0.561$, $p < 0.001$).

Older participants ($\geq 65$ years old) had significantly lower BMI ($p = 0.002$), and less distance traveled during the 6-MWT ($p = 0.013$) in comparison to middle-aged participants ($<65$ years old) who had no significant differences in ROM ($p = 0.118$) and WOMAC scores ($p = 0.091$) (Table 2).

**Table 2.** Body mass index (BMI) and physical functionality outcomes ($n = 83$).

| | Female ($n = 66$) | Male ($n = 17$) | $p$-Value | <65 years ($n = 55$) | ≥65 years ($n = 28$) | $p$-Value |
|---|---|---|---|---|---|---|
| **BMI (kg/m$^2$)** | 32.9 (6.7) | 31.2 (4.8) | $p > 0.05$ | 43.0 (6.7) | 29.6 (4.0) [t] | $p = 0.002$ |
| **ROM (°)** | 64.8 (12.8) | 78.1 (9.8) | $p > 0.05$ | 69.8 (12.6) | 65.0 (14.6) | $p > 0.05$ |
| **WOMAC** | 60.1 (14.9) * | 51.8 (15.7) | $p = 0.046$ * | 54.4 (15.8) | 60.4 (14.9) [t] | $p > 0.05$ |
| **6-MWT** | 388.0 (85.8) | 465.4 (65.3) | $p > 0.05$ | 424. 5 (84.2) | 374.0 (87.6) [t] | $p = 0.013$ [t] |

Values are shown as means and standard deviations (SD). Total WOMAC scores for females were significantly greater than male values. Additionally, BMI, distance traveled for the 6-MWT were significantly lower in older (≥65 years) individuals when compared to those of middle age, regardless of gender. (*) Indicates significant differences between females and males; ([t]) indicates significant differences between individuals <65 years and ≥65 years.

### 3.3. Body Mass Index (BMI)

BMI was positively correlated with TEE ($r = 0.430$, $p < 0.001$ and WOMAC scores ($r = 0.268$, $p = 0.014$). This indicates that higher BMI's are associated with increased energy expenditure and decreased functionality.

### 3.4. Range of Motion (ROM)

ROM was positively associated with the 6-MWT ($r = 0.561$, $p < 0.001$ (Figure 3) and negatively associated with WOMAC ($r = -0.338$, and $p = 0.002$) and pain scores ($r = -0.222$, $p = 0.002$) (Figure 4).

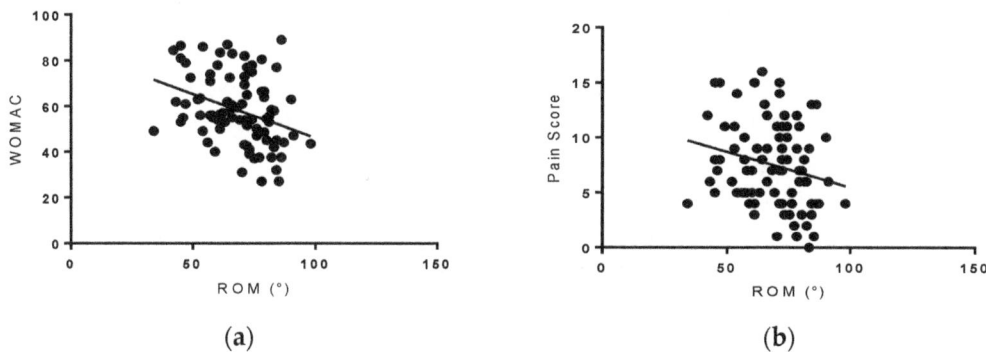

(a)    (b)

**Figure 3.** Right panel (**a**): WOMAC score vs. ROM. Individuals with a lower WOMAC score had greater knee ROM ($r = -0.338$, $p = 0.002$). Left panel (**b**): pain score vs. ROM. Individuals with a lower pain score had a greater knee ROM ($r = -0.222$, $p = 0.002$).

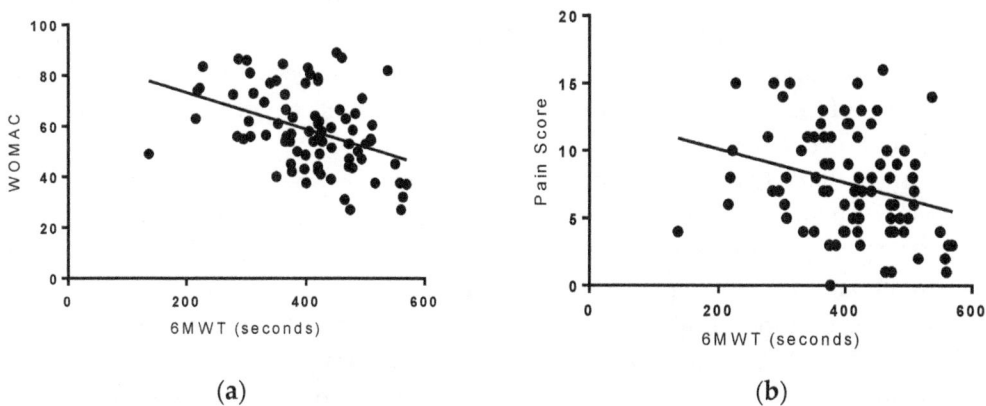

(a)    (b)

**Figure 4.** Right panel (**a**): WOMAC score vs. 6-MWT. While WOMAC scores decreased, distance walked during the 6-MWT increased ($r = -0.413$, $p < 0.001$). Left panel (**b**): pain score vs. 6-MWT. As pain scores decreased, distance walked during the 6-MWT increased ($r = -0.222$, $p = 0.010$).

### 3.5. Six-Minute Walk Test (6-MWT)

The 6-MWT negatively correlated with WOMAC scores ($r = -0.413$, $p < 0.001$ and pain scores ($r = -0.222$, $p = 0.010$) (Figure 4), while positively correlating with very hard activity ($r = 0.238$, $p = 0.030$). These results indicate that participants who were able to go a longer distance with the 6-MWT, tended to have lower pain and higher functionality scores.

### 3.6. Total Energy Expenditure (TEE)

TEE was positively associated with weight ($r = 0.476$, $p < 0.001$, moderate activity ($r = 0.567$, $p < 0.001$, and hard activity ($r = 0.544$, $p < 0.001$ (Table 3).

### 3.7. Gender

Women had significantly greater WOMAC scores ($p = 0.046$) than men with no significant differences in pain scores ($p = 0.163$), ROM ($p = 0.930$), BMI ($p = 0.694$), and distance traveled during the 6-MWT ($p = 0.467$).

## 4. Discussion

The results of this study demonstrate that increased functionality was associated with lower WOMAC and lower pain scores, which is to be expected since when people have less pain it is easier for them to conduct activities of daily living. The same was also true about the 6-MWT, as individuals with lower WOMAC and pain scores were able to walk longer distances. Additionally, participants who had a greater ROM were able to walk a longer distance with the 6-MWT, and participants who were able to walk longer distances with the 6-MWT, on average, participated in more very hard activities. Although there are numerous studies [24–30] which have performed one or two tests in this population, the authors are not aware of any studies that have examined WOMAC pain scores, ROM, and 6-MWT simultaneously. These findings confirm that it is most likely that once people suffer from pain due to OA, their overall functionality is also compromised. Older age was associated with a lower BMI, WOMAC scores, and shorter distance traveled from the 6-MWT, while increases in BMI were associated with increases in WOMAC scores and TEE. Women had greater WOMAC scores than men, indicating that gender may play an additional role in the progression and manifestation of OA. Additionally, this may explain our distribution of males and females included in this study, as the prevalence of OA in the knee is higher in women [31]. These findings provide insight into the functional capacity in overweight and obese individuals with mild-to-moderate OA, which is important for maintenance of knee joint function, as well as targets for possible therapies to prevent progression of OA in this population. These results indicate that these individuals may want to quickly complete tasks in order to have decreased pain. The authors were surprised to find that these individuals also participated in more very hard activities, an unexpected finding that may be due to the short duration of these types of activities, allowing individuals to get a given task finished faster, possibly contributing to less pain.

In this study the WOMAC questionnaire was used to assess functionality and pain. The participants who had higher BMI were found to have more pain, stiffness, and loss of physical function. Oyeyemi et al. [24] observed a similar trend with regard to BMI and functional limitations, where obese participants with knee OA had higher WOMAC scores than normal and overweight counterparts. Contrary to our expectations, findings from our study also showed that the older participants had a lower BMI and WOMAC scores. OA is an age-related disorder, where aging can increase wear and tear of joints, increasing pain and disability [25]. Perceived pain in older individuals due to musculoskeletal conditions is very common and often underreported. Another possible explanation for lower WOMAC scores observed in the older participants in this study may possibly be due to successful pain management as well as improvements in overall quality of life [26]. ROM was inversely related to WOMAC scores, indicating that in individuals with mild-to-moderate knee OA, ROM can be a good indication of preserved functionality. In a study by Kauppila et al. [26] there was no significant association between ROM and self-reported disability in individuals with severe knee OA. These contrasting findings may have been due to the severity of knee OA within the population studied, whereas in our study the individuals did not have as severe knee OA. Individuals who were able to travel greater distances from the 6-MWT had significantly lower WOMAC scores. Our results are similar to those of Sutbeyaz et al. [28] who observed a significant negative correlation between the 6-MWT and WOMAC scores in obese individuals with mild to severe knee OA. In regard to gender, women had greater WOMAC scores than men, which is consistent with previous studies indicating that women with a similar degree of knee OA have greater perceived knee pain in comparison to men [29,30].

The participants in this study who had a greater ROM had a lower WOMAC score, and the participants with greater ROM were able to go a longer distance with the 6-MWT. Participants who were able to walk longer distances with the 6-MWT also participated in more very hard activities throughout their days. The older individuals in this study did not travel as far a distance with the 6-MWT than the middle-aged individuals. A study by Nejati et al. [32] found that adding anaerobic exercises to non-invasive therapies for knee OA decreased pain and improved knee function after three months. A meta-analysis performed by Tanaka et al. [33] examining different exercise therapies in patients who have knee OA found that both muscle strengthening and aerobic exercises were effective in reducing pain, with non-weight bearing strengthening exercises being the most effective. While these studies have identified possible treatments useful for improving both quality of life and the aging process, prevention of the disease is still poorly understood.

Several longitudinal and cross-sectional studies from different countries have recognized the strong association between OA, obesity and reduced functionality [34–37]. The Rotterdam Study, which followed 3585 participants from the Netherlands for over 6 years, observed that a BMI > 27 kg/m$^2$ was associated with a 3.3-fold increased risk and progression of knee OA [34]. Similarly in the Chingford Study, 715 women from the London area were followed for 4 years and women who were in the top tertile of body weight (BMI > 26.4 kg/m$^2$) had an increased risk of knee OA [35]. The China Health and Retirement Longitudinal Study, which was a population based survey that examined women over the age of 45 years from 3 different provinces in China, observed that the prevalence of knee OA was higher in China than that of Americans (the Framingham Study) as well as Europeans (Epidemiological Study of Rheumatic Diseases in Greece), indicating that in addition to obesity there may be genetic and other lifestyle factors which may play an important role in the etiology of knee OA [36].

Participants who had greater TEE also had a higher BMI, and participated in more moderate and hard activities throughout their days in this study. This is of particular importance within this population because less than one in seven men and one in 12 women who have OA of the knee get enough physical activity [37]. A study by Christensen et al. [38] showed that 10% weight loss in obese individuals with knee OA resulted in improvement in functionality by 28%. Thus, increases in TEE may be an optimal component of knee OA management in overweight and obese individuals. As obese individuals with knee OA reduce body weight it may contribute to a reduction in pain and distress associated with movement. A systematic review and meta-analysis from the same group [39] observed that obese adults with knee OA who lost 5% of their body weight had a reduction in joint pain, and when there was a loss of at least 10% of their body weight they had further improvements in joint pain.

Limitations of this study include the calculation of TEE from the Five-City Project questionnaire which is a subjective assessment of physical activity. Many physical activity questionnaires are known to overestimate TEE, particularly in overweight and obese individuals [40,41]. Administration of questionnaires, such as the WOMAC and physical activity recall were subjective measures which, with all self-reports, may have some bias with how it is reported which may have influenced some of our results. Participants in this study were also not homogeneous with regards to gender, with more women being eligible for participation than men. The greater number of female participants may be due to the higher prevalence of OA in women, as well as more women being interested in the study.

**Table 3.** Pearson product-moment correlations between dependent variables ($n = 83$).

| Variables | Age (years) | Height (cm) | Weight (kg) | BMI (kg/m²) | ROM (°) | 6-MWT (m) | MOD (h) | HARD (h) | VHARD (h) | TEE (kcal) | WOMAC | PAIN |
|---|---|---|---|---|---|---|---|---|---|---|---|---|
| Age (years) | 1 | −0.007 | −0.299 [a] | −0.349 [a] | 0.006 | −0.124 | 0.002 | −0.071 | −0.145 | −0.2 | −0.247 [a] | −0.378 |
| Height (cm) | −0.007 | 1 | 0.45 | −0.004 | 0.067 | 0.006 | −0.193 | 0.131 | −0.076 | 0.22 | −0.184 | −0.113 |
| Weight (kg) | −0.299 [a] | 0.45 | 1 | 0.888 | −0.045 | −0.136 | −0.125 | 0.045 | −0.148 | 0.476 [f,g] | 0.145 | 0.149 |
| BMI (kg/m²) | −0.349 [a] | −0.004 | 0.888 | 1 | −0.072 | −0.151 | −0.04 | −0.009 | −0.135 | 0.430 [b] | 0.268 [b] | 0.237 |
| ROM (°) | 0.006 | 0.067 | −0.045 | −0.072 | 1 | 0.561 [c] | 0.063 | 0.139 | 0.2 | 0.159 | −0.338 [d] | −0.222 d [e] |
| 6-MWT | −0.124 | 0.006 | −0.136 | −0.151 | 0.561 [c] | 1 | 0.108 | 0.096 | 0.238 [e] | 0.061 | −0.413 [e] | −0.283 |
| MOD (h) | 0.002 | −0.193 | −0.125 | −0.04 | 0.063 | 0.108 | 1 | 0.236 | 0.055 | 0.567 [g] | 0.03 | 0.09 |
| HARD (h) | −0.071 | 0.131 | 0.045 | −0.009 | 0.139 | 0.096 | 0.236 | 1 | 0.148 | 0.544 [g] | 0.058 | 0.114 |
| VHARD (h) | −0.145 | −0.076 | −0.148 | −0.135 | 0.2 | 0.238 [e] | 0.055 | 0.148 | 1 | 0.078 | −0.109 | −0.014 |
| TEE (kcal) | −0.2 | 0.22 | 0.476 [f,g] | 0.430 [b] | 0.159 | 0.061 | 0.567 [g] | 0.544 [g] | 0.078 | 1 | 0.096 | 0.174 |
| WOMAC | −0.247 [a] | −0.184 | 0.145 | 0.268 [b] | −0.338 [d] | −0.413 [e] | 0.03 | 0.058 | −0.109 | 0.096 | 1 | 0.845 |
| PAIN | −0.378 | −0.113 | 0.149 | 0.237 | −0.222 [d] | −0.283 | 0.09 | 0.114 | −0.014 | 0.174 | 0.845 | 1 |

[a] Significant (−) correlations were found between age and weight, BMI, and total WOMAC, an indicator that as age increases, body weight and knee functionality decline; [b] Significant (+) correlations were found between BMI and TEE, WOMAC, indicating that higher BMI scores are associated with increased TEE and a decline in functionality; Significant (+) [c] and (−) [d] correlations were found between ROM and 6-MWT and with ROM and WOMAC pain scores, respectively. Increased ROM along with a longer 6-MWT was expected as well as a decrease in WOMAC since pain was lower as well. [e] 6-MWT was significantly (−) correlated with WOMAC and pain (pain not significant) while (+) correlating with very hard activity, suggesting lower pain/higher functionality with longer 6-MWT. [g] Significant (+) associations were found between TEE and weight, moderate, and hard activity.

## 5. Conclusions

The results from this study indicate that overweight and obese individuals with knee OA had a greater ROM and TEE from physical activity, less pain and stiffness, and walked longer distances on average than those who had lower ROM and higher pain, which was in agreement with our hypothesis. Further studies are needed to establish the relationship between pain and which types of physical activity will preserve functionality in this population.

**Author Contributions:** N.S.A. wrote the manuscript. N.S.A., B.H.A., and L.B.P. designed the study. L.O., M.L.E., and Z.E.-Z. collected data, performed experiments and revised the manuscript. N.S.A., L.O., B.H.A., L.B.P., S.A.J., K.S.G., and E.M.F. contributed to the interpretation of data and the discussion of the paper. B.H.A. had primary responsibility for final content and overseeing all aspects of this study.

**Funding:** This research received no external funding.

**Acknowledgments:** We would like to acknowledge partial support from the Margaret A. Sitton Professorship that enabled us to conduct this study. We would like to acknowledge Payton for the power calculation and in part helping with the analysis of the data. We also would like to thank the participants for their involvement in the study.

## References

1.  Xing, D.; Xu, Y.; Liu, Q.; Ke, Y.; Wang, B.; Li, Z.; Lin, J. Osteoarthritis and all-cause mortality in worldwide populations: Grading the evidence from a meta-analysis. *Sci. Rep.* **2016**, *6*, 24393. [CrossRef] [PubMed]

2.  Word Health Organization. *Priority Medicines for Europe and the World 2013 Update. vol. 6.12 Osteoarthritis-Priority Diseases and Reasons for Inclusion*; Word Health Organization: Geneva, Switzerland, 2013.

3.  Woolf, A.D.; Pfleger, B. Burden of major musculoskeletal conditions. *Bull. World Health Organ.* **2003**, *81*, 646–656. [PubMed]

4.  Bhatia, D.; Bejarano, T.; Novo, M. Current interventions in the management of knee osteoarthritis. *J. Pharm. Bioallied Sci.* **2013**, *5*, 30–38. [CrossRef] [PubMed]

5.  Li, G.; Yin, J.; Gao, J.; Cheng, T.S.; Pavlos, N.J.; Zhang, C.; Zheng, M.H. Subchondral bone in osteoarthritis: Insight into risk factors and microstructural changes. *Arthritis Res. Ther.* **2013**, *15*, 223. [CrossRef] [PubMed]

6.  Henrotin, Y.; Pesesse, L.; Sanchez, C. Subchondral bone and osteoarthritis: Biological and cellular aspects. *Osteoporos Int.* **2012**, *23* (Suppl. 8), S847–S851. [CrossRef] [PubMed]

7.  Cisternas, M.G.; Murphy, L.; Sacks, J.J.; Solomon, D.H.; Pasta, D.J.; Helmick, C.G. Alternative Methods for Defining Osteoarthritis and the Impact on Estimating Prevalence in a US Population-Based Survey. *Arthritis Care Res.* **2016**, *68*, 574–580. [CrossRef] [PubMed]

8.  Bitton, R. The economic burden of osteoarthritis. *Am. J. Manag. Care* **2009**, *15*, S230–S235. [PubMed]

9.  Coggon, D.; Reading, I.; Croft, P.; McLaren, M.; Barrett, D.; Cooper, C. Knee osteoarthritis and obesity. *Int. J. Obes. Relat. Metab. Disord.* **2001**, *25*, 622–627. [CrossRef] [PubMed]

10. King, L.K.; March, L. Anandacoomarasamy A: Obesity & osteoarthritis. *Indian J. Med. Res.* **2013**, *138*, 185–193. [PubMed]

11. Berry, P.A.; Wluka, A.E.; Davies-Tuck, M.L.; Wang, Y.; Strauss, B.J.; Dixon, J.B.; Proietto, J.; Jones, G.; Cicuttini, F.M. The relationship between body composition and structural changes at the knee. *Rheumatology* **2010**, *49*, 2362–2369. [CrossRef] [PubMed]

12. Sowers, M.R.; Karvonen-Gutierrez, C.A. The evolving role of obesity in knee osteoarthritis. *Curr. Opin. Rheumatol.* **2010**, *22*, 533–537. [CrossRef] [PubMed]

13. Arden, N.; Nevitt, M.C. Osteoarthritis: Epidemiology. *Best Pract. Res. Clin. Rheumatol.* **2006**, *20*, 3–25. [CrossRef] [PubMed]

14. Loeser, R.F. Aging processes and the development of osteoarthritis. *Curr. Opin. Rheumatol.* **2013**, *25*, 108–113. [CrossRef] [PubMed]

15. Conley, S.; Rosenberg, A.; Crowninshield, R. The female knee: Anatomic variations. *J. Am. Acad. Orthop. Surg.* **2007**, *15* (Suppl. 1), S31–S36. [CrossRef] [PubMed]

16. Srikanth, V.K.; Fryer, J.L.; Zhai, G.; Winzenberg, T.M.; Hosmer, D.; Jones, G. A meta-analysis of sex differences prevalence, incidence and severity of osteoarthritis. *Osteoarthr. Cartil.* **2005**, *13*, 769–781. [CrossRef] [PubMed]

17. Steultjens, M.P.; Dekker, J.; van Baar, M.E.; Oostendorp, R.A.; Bijlsma, J.W. Range of joint motion and disability in patients with osteoarthritis of the knee or hip. *Rheumatology* **2000**, *39*, 955–961. [CrossRef] [PubMed]

18. Angst, F.; Aeschlimann, A.; Steiner, W.; Stucki, G. Responsiveness of the WOMAC osteoarthritis index as compared with the SF-36 in patients with osteoarthritis of the legs undergoing a comprehensive rehabilitation intervention. *Ann. Rheum. Dis.* **2001**, *60*, 834–840. [PubMed]

19. ATS Committee on Proficiency Standards for Clinical Pulmonary Function Laboratories. ATS statement: Guidelines for the six-minute walk test. *Am. J. Respir. Crit. Care Med.* **2002**, *166*, 111–117.

20. Sallis, J.F.; Haskell, W.L.; Wood, P.D.; Fortmann, S.P.; Rogers, T.; Blair, S.N.; Paffenbarger, R.S. Physical activity assessment methodology in the Five-City Project. *Am. J. Epidemiol.* **1985**, *121*, 91–106. [CrossRef] [PubMed]

21. Bellamy, N.; Buchanan, W.W.; Goldsmith, C.H.; Campbell, J.; Stitt, L.W. Validation study of WOMAC: A health status instrument for measuring clinically important patient relevant outcomes to antirheumatic drug therapy in patients with osteoarthritis of the hip or knee. *J. Rheumatol.* **1988**, *15*, 1833–1840. [PubMed]

22. Guyatt, G.H.; Sullivan, M.J.; Thompson, P.J.; Fallen, E.L.; Pugsley, S.O.; Taylor, D.W.; Berman, L.B. The 6-minute walk: A new measure of exercise capacity in patients with chronic heart failure. *Can. Med. Assoc. J.* **1985**, *132*, 919–923. [PubMed]

23. Cohen, J. *Statistical Power Analysis for the Behavioral Sciences*; Lawrence Erlbaum Associates: Hillsdale, NJ, USA, 1988.

24. Oyeyemi, A.L. Body mass index, pain and function in individuals with knee osteoarthritis. *Niger. Med. J.* **2013**, *54*, 230–235. [CrossRef] [PubMed]

25. Shane Anderson, A.; Loeser, R.F. Why is osteoarthritis an age-related disease? *Best Pract. Res. Clin. Rheumatol.* **2010**, *24*, 15–26. [CrossRef] [PubMed]

26. Fitzcharles, M.A.; Lussier, D.; Shir, Y. Management of chronic arthritis pain in the elderly. *Drugs Aging* **2010**, *27*, 471–490. [CrossRef] [PubMed]

27. Kauppila, A.M.; Kyllonen, E.; Mikkonen, P.; Ohtonen, P.; Laine, V.; Siira, P.; Niinimaki, J.; Arokoski, J.P. Disability in end-stage knee osteoarthritis. *Disabil. Rehabil.* **2009**, *31*, 370–380. [CrossRef] [PubMed]

28. Sutbeyaz, S.T.; Sezer, N.; Koseoglu, B.F.; Ibrahimoglu, F.; Tekin, D. Influence of knee osteoarthritis on exercise capacity and quality of life in obese adults. *Obesity* **2007**, *15*, 2071–2076. [CrossRef] [PubMed]

29. Glass, N.; Segal, N.A.; Sluka, K.A.; Torner, J.C.; Nevitt, M.C.; Felson, D.T.; Bradley, L.A.; Neogi, T.; Lewis, C.E.; Frey-Law, L.A. Examining sex differences in knee pain: The multicenter osteoarthritis study. *Osteoarthr. Cartil.* **2014**, *22*, 1100–1106. [CrossRef] [PubMed]

30. Alves, J.C.; Bassitt, D.P. Quality of life and functional capacity of elderly women with knee osteoarthritis. *Einstein* **2013**, *11*, 209–215. [CrossRef] [PubMed]

31. Zhang, Y.; Jordan, J.M. Epidemiology of osteoarthritis. *Clin. Geriatr. Med.* **2010**, *26*, 355–369. [CrossRef] [PubMed]

32. Nejati, P.; Farzinmehr, A.; Moradi-Lakeh, M. The effect of exercise therapy on knee osteoarthritis: A randomized clinical trial. *Med. J. Islam. Repub. Iran* **2015**, *29*, 186. [PubMed]

33. Tanaka, R.; Ozawa, J.; Kito, N.; Moriyama, H. Effects of exercise therapy on walking ability in individuals with knee osteoarthritis: A systematic review and meta-analysis of randomised controlled trials. *Clin. Rehabil.* **2016**, *30*, 36–52. [CrossRef] [PubMed]

34. Reijman, M.; Pols, H.A.; Bergink, A.P.; Hazes, J.M.; Belo, J.N.; Lievense, A.M.; Bierma-Zeinstra, S.M. Body mass index associated with onset and progression of osteoarthritis of the knee but not of the hip: The Rotterdam Study. *Ann. Rheum. Dis.* **2007**, *66*, 158–162. [CrossRef] [PubMed]

35. Hart, D.J.; Doyle, D.V.; Spector, T.D. Incidence and risk factors for radiographic knee osteoarthritis in middle-aged women: The Chingford Study. *Arthritis Rheum.* **1999**, *42*, 17–24. [CrossRef]

36. Tang, X.; Wang, S.; Zhan, S.; Niu, J.; Tao, K.; Zhang, Y.; Lin, J. The Prevalence of Symptomatic Knee Osteoarthritis in China: Results From the China Health and Retirement Longitudinal Study. *Arthritis Rheumatol.* **2016**, *68*, 648–653. [CrossRef] [PubMed]

37. Dunlop, D.D.; Song, J.; Semanik, P.A.; Chang, R.W.; Sharma, L.; Bathon, J.M.; Eaton, C.B.; Hochberg, M.C.; Jackson, R.D.; Kwoh, C.K.; et al. Objective physical activity measurement in the osteoarthritis initiative: Are guidelines being met? *Arthritis Rheum.* **2011**, *63*, 3372–3382. [CrossRef] [PubMed]

38. Christensen, R.; Astrup, A.; Bliddal, H. Weight loss: The treatment of choice for knee osteoarthritis? A randomized trial. *Osteoarthr. Cartil.* **2005**, *13*, 20–27. [CrossRef] [PubMed]

39. Christensen, R.; Bartels, E.M.; Astrup, A.; Bliddal, H. Effect of weight reduction in obese patients diagnosed with knee osteoarthritis: A systematic review and meta-analysis. *Ann. Rheum. Dis.* **2007**, *66*, 433–439. [CrossRef] [PubMed]

40. Prince, S.A.; Adamo, K.B.; Hamel, M.E.; Hardt, J.; Connor Gorber, S.; Tremblay, M. A comparison of direct versus self-report measures for assessing physical activity in adults: A systematic review. *Int. J. Behav. Nutr. Phys. Act.* **2008**, *5*, 56. [CrossRef] [PubMed]

41. Lagerros, Y.T.; Mucci, L.A.; Bellocco, R.; Nyrén, O.; Bälter, O.; Bälter, K.A. Validity and reliability of self-reported total energy expenditure using a novel instrument. *Eur. J. Epidemiol.* **2006**, *21*, 227–236. [CrossRef] [PubMed]

# 5

# Rationale and Protocol for a Randomized Controlled Trial Comparing Fast versus Slow Weight Loss in Postmenopausal Women with Obesity—The TEMPO Diet Trial

Radhika V. Seimon [1] (iD), Alice A. Gibson [1] (iD), Claudia Harper [1] (iD), Shelley E. Keating [2] (iD), Nathan A. Johnson [1,3], Felipe Q. da Luz [1,4] (iD), Hamish A. Fernando [1], Michael R. Skilton [1] (iD), Tania P. Markovic [1,5], Ian D. Caterson [1,5] (iD), Phillipa Hay [6] (iD), Nuala M. Byrne [7] and Amanda Sainsbury [1,4,*] (iD)

[1]   Faculty of Medicine and Health, Charles Perkins Centre, The University of Sydney, the Boden Institute of Obesity, Nutrition, Exercise & Eating Disorders, Camperdown, NSW 2006, Australia; radhika.seimon@sydney.edu.au (R.V.S.); alice.gibson@sydney.edu.au (A.A.G.); claudia.harper@sydney.edu.au (C.H.); nathan.johnson@sydney.edu.au (N.A.J.); felipe.quintodaluz@sydney.edu.au (F.Q.d.L.); hamish.fernando@sydney.edu.au (H.A.F.); michael.skilton@sydney.edu.au (M.R.S.); tania.markovic@sydney.edu.au (T.P.M.); ian.caterson@sydney.edu.au (I.D.C.)
[2]   School of Human Movement and Nutrition Sciences, Centre for Research on Exercise, Physical Activity and Health, The University of Queensland, Brisbane, QLD 4072, Australia; s.keating@uq.edu.au
[3]   Faculty of Health Sciences, The University of Sydney, Lidcombe, NSW 2141, Australia
[4]   Faculty of Science, School of Psychology, The University of Sydney, Camperdown, NSW 2006, Australia
[5]   Metabolism & Obesity Services, Royal Prince Alfred Hospital, Camperdown, NSW 2050, Australia
[6]   School of Medicine, Western Sydney University, Translational Health Research Institute (THRI), Locked Bag 1797, Penrith, NSW 2751, Australia; P.Hay@westernsydney.edu.au
[7]   School of Health Sciences, College of Health and Medicine, University of Tasmania, Launceston, TAS 7250, Australia; nuala.byrne@utas.edu.au
*    Correspondence: amanda.salis@sydney.edu.au

**Abstract:** Very low energy diets (VLEDs), commonly achieved by replacing all food with meal replacement products and which result in fast weight loss, are the most effective dietary obesity treatment available. VLEDs are also cheaper to administer than conventional, food-based diets, which result in slow weight loss. Despite being effective and affordable, these diets are underutilized by healthcare professionals, possibly due to concerns about potential adverse effects on body composition and eating disorder behaviors. This paper describes the rationale and detailed protocol for the TEMPO Diet Trial (**T**ype of **E**nergy **M**anipulation for **P**romoting optimal metabolic health and body composition in **O**besity), in a randomized controlled trial comparing the long-term (3-year) effects of fast versus slow weight loss. One hundred and one post-menopausal women aged 45–65 years with a body mass index of 30–40 kg/m$^2$ were randomized to either: (1) 16 weeks of fast weight loss, achieved by a total meal replacement diet, followed by slow weight loss (as for the SLOW intervention) for the remaining time up until 52 weeks ("FAST" intervention), or (2) 52 weeks of slow weight loss, achieved by a conventional, food-based diet ("SLOW" intervention). Parameters of body composition, cardiometabolic health, eating disorder behaviors and psychology, and adaptive responses to energy restriction were measured throughout the 3-year trial.

**Keywords:** weight loss; diet-reducing; obesity; clinical protocol; rationale

## 1. Introduction

The worldwide prevalence of obesity is increasing at an alarming rate [1]. Obesity is associated with a number of complications including type 2 diabetes, cardiovascular disease as well as many cancers [2], and is responsible for significant health care costs [1,3]. In Australia, in 2008 alone, overweight and obesity cost Australian society and government AU$56.6 billion in direct and indirect costs [4], while in the USA the direct medical costs of obesity were estimated at US$190 billion in 2012 [5], with the annual costs of treating obesity-related diseases in the USA estimated to increase by an additional US$48–$66 billion by 2030 [6]. However, if obesity were effectively treated, the costs of obesity-related health complications would be significantly reduced [4]. Thus, implementing effective obesity treatments is essential to reducing obesity-related comorbidities and the associated costs.

Management strategies for weight reduction include lifestyle interventions (i.e., changes in diet, physical activity and behavior), pharmacological treatment [7] and surgery [8,9]. However, lifestyle interventions are considered the first-line treatment for overweight and obesity, and are also an important component of pharmacological and surgical treatments [10]. Recent studies have noted that weight loss of as little as 3–5% of initial body weight can induce clinically meaningful reductions in some cardiovascular risk factors, diabetes and osteoarthritis, with larger weight losses producing even greater health benefits [10–13]. Although weight loss can usually be achieved through lifestyle interventions, the overwhelming majority of people regain the weight lost over the long-term (several years). A major reason for this weight regain is that the body responds to energy restriction and weight loss with a series of adaptive responses such as an increased drive to eat, a decrease in physical activity, and a decrease in energy expenditure [14,15]. In addition, energy restriction and weight loss induce adaptive responses in neuroendocrine status that may have adverse consequences on body composition, such as loss of bone mineral density (BMD) and lean mass, as well as muscle strength (which together potentially increase the risk of osteoporosis, sarcopenia and frailty), and promote regain of visceral adipose tissue (VAT), in turn increasing the risk of cardiometabolic diseases such as type 2 diabetes and cardiovascular disease [15].

As mentioned, greater weight losses in people with overweight or obesity are usually associated with greater health benefits. Although a number of dietary approaches have been advocated for the treatment of obesity [16,17], the dietary interventions that induce the greatest and longest-lasting weight losses are very low energy diets (VLEDs) [18]. These, by definition, involve restricting dietary energy intake to <3350 kJ (<800 kcal) per day [19]. VLEDs are most commonly administered as total meal replacement diets, which involve replacing all, or almost all, foods with nutritionally replete meal replacement products such as shakes, soups, bars, or desserts. The short-term success of VLEDs is high, resulting in fast and substantial weight losses of ~1.5–2.5 kg per week, typically over periods of 8–16 weeks [20], while reducing hunger and increasing satiety [21]. An individual commencing a VLED has an ~80% chance of losing ≥12.5% of their initial body weight, compared to ~50% of people commencing conventional, food-based diets that involve moderately restricting dietary energy intake by ~2000 kJ (500 kcal) per day, inducing slow weight loss [22]. The long-term success of VLEDs may also be greater than conventional, food-based diets, because greater initial weight loss has been shown to be predictive of long-term success in weight maintenance [23,24]. This is in keeping with recent evidence showing that there is no faster weight regain in response to fast than to slow weight loss [22,25,26]. Moreover, at 1 and 5 years after commencement of a VLED, ~60% and ~30% of people weigh ≥10% less than their initial body weight, respectively [18,27]. In addition, a meta-analysis showed that weight loss at 4–5 years after a VLED or a conventional, food-based diet was 6.6% versus 2.1%, respectively [18]. Besides achieving greater long-term weight loss, VLEDs are approximately three times cheaper to administer than conventional, food-based diets, in terms of the cost of dietetics support [28]. In terms of the cost to consumers, total meal replacement products—when used in place of all meals and snacks—are cheaper than the average per capita food expenditure [29].

Despite being an effective and affordable option for the dietary treatment of obesity, VLEDs are underutilized by healthcare professionals [28,30]. A 2002 survey of dietitians in Australia revealed that only 3.2% of respondents reported prescribing a VLED or fast weight loss to manage overweight or obesity in their clients [30]. This was corroborated in a 2008 survey, which revealed that only 1.5% of dietitians in Australia recommended VLEDs to their clients for weight loss [28]. Part of the reason for this underutilization of VLEDs may be due to concerns regarding adverse psychological outcomes, particularly with regards to inducing or exacerbating binge eating disorders, although these concerns may be unfounded [31]. Other safety concerns are the possibility that fast weight loss may have adverse effects on body composition. Indeed, the greater degree of energy restriction used to achieve fast weight loss could conceivably induce stronger adaptive responses than those seen during slow weight loss with a conventional food-based diet, and this may adversely affect body composition (BMD, lean mass/function, and fat mass/distribution) and cardiometabolic risk factors relative to slow weight loss. A systematic review comparing VLEDs and low energy diets (LEDs), which may respectively be defined as providing <3400 kJ (<800 kcal) per day as mentioned above [19], and between 3400–5000 kJ (800–1200 kcal) per day [32,33], showed that larger energy deficits induce greater losses of fat free mass in adults with overweight and obesity [34]. However, the studies included in that systematic review differed in total weight loss, duration of the intervention, and did not include studies where participants were randomly assigned to a VLED or LED. More recent studies have similarly shown significantly greater losses of lean body mass after fast weight loss (of at least 5% of initial body weight in 5 weeks) compared to after slow weight loss (of at least 5% of initial body weight in 15 weeks) in postmenopausal women [35] and in men and women [36] with overweight or obesity. Short-term outcomes of faster versus slower weight loss have also been reported in elite athletes, where fast weight loss of ~1.4% of body weight per week over 5.3 ± 0.9 weeks was associated with greater loss of lean mass and inferior performance on upper body strength tests compared to slower weight loss of ~0.7% of body weight per week over 8.5 ± 2.2 weeks [37]. However, responses to fast or slow weight loss could conceivably be different between elite athletes and people with overweight and obesity. To our knowledge, no study has directly compared the long-term effects of fast weight loss (achieved via VLED in a total meal replacement diet involving severe energy restriction) in comparison to slow weight loss (achieved via a conventional food-based diet involving moderate energy restriction) on body composition in people with obesity.

Therefore, the aim of the current work is to make a head-to-head comparison of the long-term (3-year) effects of fast versus slow weight loss, notably with respect to body composition, but also on eating behavior. This is addressed in the randomized controlled TEMPO Diet Trial (**T**ype of **E**nergy **M**anipulation for **P**romoting optimum metabolic health and body composition in **O**besity), the protocol for which is described here.

## 2. Materials and Methods

### 2.1. Ethics and Participants

The TEMPO Diet Trial is a randomized controlled trial designed to assess the long-term effects of fast versus slow weight loss on body composition and cardiometabolic health in postmenopausal women aged 45–65 years and with a BMI of 30–40 kg/m$^2$. The standardized inclusion and exclusion criteria for the TEMPO Diet Trial are listed in Table 1. Our target sample size of 100 participants was determined based on power calculations with body composition as the primary outcome, and allowing for up to 20% attrition as seen in previously-published weight loss interventions [38–40]. Multiple strategies were used to fully recruit participants into the trial ($n$ = 101) from March 2013 to July 2016. Recruitment strategies included word of mouth, free publicity on radio and TV, printed advertorials, internet-based advertisements, clinical trial databases and intranets, flyer distribution at community events, hospitals, the local tertiary education campus, local health service centers and residential mailboxes, as well as referrals from healthcare professionals. Full details of the recruitment process and recruitment strategies for the trial have been published previously [41].

**Table 1.** Inclusion and exclusion criteria for the TEMPO Diet Trial.

| Inclusion Criteria |
|---|
| Female, due to the estimated lifetime risk of osteoporotic fractures being 3-fold higher in women than in men (40% versus 13%) [42] |
| 45–65 years of age |
| Postmenopausal for $\geq$5 years (calculated from date of last menses), to circumvent known effects of female sex hormone cycles and the menopausal transition on parameters under investigation |
| Body mass index (BMI) 30–40 kg/m$^2$ |
| Weight stable ($\pm$2 kg) for $\geq$past 6 months |
| English-speaking |
| Living in the Sydney metropolitan area (defined by the City of Sydney Statistical Division [43,44]) and able to attend all in-person appointments at the University of Sydney Camperdown campus |
| Sedentary (defined as <3 h of structured physical activity per week) |
| Consider themselves capable of completing activities required for the trial (e.g., keeping a food, activity, and sleep diary, wearing accelerometers for seven days at a time, etc.) |

| Exclusion Criteria |
|---|
| Not ambulatory, or having restrictions to physical movement that would impede completion of trial activities |
| Osteoporosis |
| Extreme anemia that could be exacerbated by very low energy/total meal replacement diet |
| Hyperthyroidism or hypothyroidism |
| Diabetes mellitus (defined by fasting blood glucose level $\geq$7.0 mmol/L and glycated hemoglobin (HbA$_{1c}$) $\geq$6.5%) [45] |
| Cardiovascular disease |
| Gastrointestinal disease |
| Previous gastric or other surgery that may affect appetite |
| Any loose metal in the body (e.g., pacemaker or bullet) that is contraindicated for magnetic resonance imaging (MRI) for safety reasons, or which may result in artefacts in medical imaging |
| Planning to undertake any major surgery in the next three years |
| Tobacco use |
| Alcohol or drug dependency |
| Taking medication that affects heart rate, body composition or bone mass (e.g., beta-blockers, glucocorticoids) |
| Having taken anti-resorptive therapy within the last three years |
| Having taken medication that affects appetite, metabolism, or weight within the past 6 months |
| Any of the following contraindications for following a very low energy/total meal replacement diet: lactose intolerance; following a strict vegan diet; or unwillingness to be randomized to one of the two diets |
| Donated whole blood within three months prior to commencement on the trial |
| Hepatic or renal impairments (which can be contraindications for following a very low energy/total meal replacement diet) |

Ethical approval was obtained from the Sydney Local Health District, Royal Prince Alfred Hospital Human Research Ethics Committee. The trial was prospectively registered with the Australian New Zealand Clinical Trials Registry (ANZCTR Reference Number 12612000651886). It is being conducted at the Charles Perkins Centre Royal Prince Alfred Clinic on the University of Sydney campus in Camperdown, NSW, Australia, with Magnetic Resonance Imaging (MRI) scans being performed at I-Med Radiology, Camperdown, NSW, Australia.

## 2.2. Interventions

Eligible participants were randomized to either a "FAST" or "SLOW" weight loss intervention. The FAST intervention involved a total meal replacement diet (KicStart[TM] meal replacement products [shakes and soups] from Prima Health Solutions Pty Ltd., Brookvale, NSW, Australia) involving severe energy restriction (target range for energy restriction was 65–75% relative to estimated energy expenditure) for 16 weeks, or until a BMI of no lower than 20 kg/m$^2$ was reached, whichever came first, followed by slow weight loss (as for the SLOW intervention) for the remaining time up until 52 weeks (FAST intervention). The SLOW intervention involved a food-based, moderately energy-restricted diet (target range for energy restriction was 25–35% relative to estimated energy expenditure) for a total of 52 weeks. As such, we aimed for a minimum difference in energy restriction between women in the FAST versus SLOW interventions of 30% of estimated energy expenditure. The SLOW intervention was based on the Australian Guide to Healthy Eating (AGHE) [46], which provides recommendations as to the average number of standard serves of the five core food groups (vegetables, fruits, grains and cereals, meat and meat alternatives, reduced fat dairy) an individual should consume in order to meet their nutritional requirements, based on age and sex. In order to simplify adherence to the SLOW intervention in the TEMPO Diet Trial we defined six food groups. The meat and meat alternative and reduced fat dairy core food groups were collapsed into a 'proteins' group, and starchy vegetables were incorporated into the grains and cereals group to form a 'carbohydrates' group while also having a vegetables, fruits, fats, and discretionary foods group. For the FAST intervention, prescribed daily carbohydrate intake was less than 100 g. A protein intake of 1.0 g per kg of actual body weight per day was prescribed for both interventions. As it is not possible to achieve a protein intake of 1.0 g per kg using meal replacement products alone, without increasing energy and carbohydrate intake above target levels for the FAST intervention, the total meal replacement diet (KicStart[TM]) was supplemented with a whey protein isolate (Beneprotein®, Nestlé HealthCare Nutrition Inc, Florham Park, NJ, USA). The development process and rationale behind the dietary interventions for the TEMPO Diet Trial, as well as full details of the dietary interventions, have been published previously [47].

## 2.3. Study Protocol

Two weeks prior to commencement of the dietary interventions (−2 weeks), eligible prospective participants attended our clinical research facility for interim measurement of weight, and for administration of several questionnaires and an interview related to the outcomes shown at −2 weeks in Table 2. They were instructed to maintain a steady weight (±1 kg) until 0 weeks, and two more face-to-face appointments were scheduled (one at −1 weeks, and another at 0 weeks). During this period, participants were requested to complete a food, activity and sleep diary for 7 days, to wear a pedometer and activity monitor for 7 days, to weigh themselves every morning at home before breakfast and record the results, to purchase an athletic bra and leggings suitable for use in the trial during the anthropometry and body composition measurements, and to bring all data and materials to the face-to-face appointments at −1 and 0 weeks. This procedure was implemented to not only help reduce variability in outcome measures at 0 weeks by facilitating weight stability, but also to help ensure that participants who continued to −1 weeks and beyond were likely to comply with trial requirements. It should be noted that all prospective participants successfully completed all requested tasks by −1 weeks and proceeded to randomization at that time point as described below, marking their official enrolment into the trial. At −1 weeks participants met with the trial dietitian (A.A.G. or C.H.) for a detailed weight history and counselling on following the diet to which they had been randomized, and certain outcome measures were undertaken or commenced at this time point.

**Table 2.** Outcomes measured at each time point during the TEMPO Diet Trial.

| Time (Months) from Start of Dietary Intervention | ~0 | | | ~0.25 | ~1 | ~4 | | | ~6 | | | ~12 | | ~24 | | ~36 | |
|---|---|---|---|---|---|---|---|---|---|---|---|---|---|---|---|---|---|
| Time (Weeks) from Start of Dietary Intervention | -2 | -1 | 0 | 1 | 4 | 15 | 16 | 17§ | 25 | 26 | 29 | 51 | 52 | 103 | 104 | 155 | 156 |
| **Body Composition** | | | | | | | | | | | | | | | | | |
| Height | | | X | | | | | | | | | | | | | | X |
| Weight (and Body Mass Index) | | X | X | X | X | | X | X | | X | | | X | | X | | X |
| **Bone** | | | | | | | | | | | | | | | | | |
| Bone Mineral Density and Bone Mineral Content | | | | | | | | | | | | | | | | | |
| Hip (DXA) | | | X | | X | | X | | | X | | | X | | X | | X |
| Lumbar Spine (DXA) | | | X | | X | | X | | | X | | | X | | X | | X |
| Markers of Bone Turnover | | | | | | | | | | | | | | | | | |
| Markers of Bone Formation | | | | | | | | | | | | | | | | | |
| N-Terminal Propeptide of Type I Procollagen (P1NP) (Serum) | | | X | | X | | X | | | X | | | X | | X | | X |
| Osteocalcin (Serum) | | | X | | X | | X | | | X | | | X | | X | | X |
| Markers of Bone Resorption | | | | | | | | | | | | | | | | | |
| C-Terminal Telopeptide of Type I Collagen (CTX) (Serum) | | | X | | X | | X | | | X | | | X | | X | | X |
| N-Terminal Telopeptide of Type I Collagen (NTX) (Urine) | | | X | | X | | X | | | X | | | X | | X | | X |
| **Lean Tissues** | | | | | | | | | | | | | | | | | |
| Fat Free Mass (DXA) | | | X | | X | | X | | | X | | | X | | X | | X |
| Fat Free Mass (4-Compartment Model, Using): Bone Mineral Content (DXA) / Body Volume (BodPod) / Total Body Water (Deuterium Dilution) | | | X | | X | | X | | | X | | | X | | X | | X |
| Fat Free Mass (Using): Body Volume (BodPod) / Total Body Water (Deuterium Dilution) | | | X | X | X | | X | X | | X | | | X | | X | | X |
| Thigh Muscle Cross Sectional Area (MRI) | X | | | | | X | | | X | | | X | | | | | |
| Muscle Strength (Hand Dynamometry) | | | X | | X | | X | | | X | | | X | | X | | X |
| **Fat Mass and Distribution** | | | | | | | | | | | | | | | | | |
| Waist Circumference | | X | X | X | X | | X | X | | X | | | X | | X | | X |
| Hip Circumference | | X | X | X | X | | X | X | | X | | | X | | X | | X |
| Ratio of Waist to Hip Circumference | | X | X | X | X | | X | X | | X | | | X | | X | | X |

**Table 2.** *Cont.*

| Time (Months) from Start of Dietary Intervention | ~0 | | | ~0.25 | ~1 | ~4 | | | ~6 | | | ~12 | | ~24 | | ~36 | |
| --- | --- | --- | --- | --- | --- | --- | --- | --- | --- | --- | --- | --- | --- | --- | --- | --- | --- |
| **Time (Weeks) from Start of Dietary Intervention** | −2 | −1 | 0 | 1 | 4 | 15 | 16 | 17§ | 25 | 26 | 29 | 51 | 52 | 103 | 104 | 155 | 156 |
| Fat Mass (DXA) | | | X | | | | X | | | X | | | X | | X | | X |
| Fat Mass (4-Compartment Model) | | | X | | | | X | | | X | | | X | | X | | X |
| Fat Mass (Body Volume and Total Body Water) | | | X | X | | | X | X | | X | | | X | | X | | X |
| Abdominal Fat (MRI) | | X | | | | X | | | X | | | X | | X | | X | |
| Intrahepatic Lipid ($^1$H-MRS) | | X | | | | X | | | X | | | X | | X | | X | |
| Thigh Fat (MRI) | | X | | | | X | | | X | | | X | | X | | X | |
| **Cardiometabolic Health (in Addition to Waist Circumference)** | | | | | | | | | | | | | | | | | |
| Blood Pressure | | | X | | | | X | | | X | | | X | | X | | X |
| **Circulating Markers of Cardiometabolic Health** | | | | | | | | | | | | | | | | | |
| Glucose (Serum) | | | X | | | | X | | | X | | | X | | X | | X |
| Glycosylated Hemoglobin (Whole Venous Blood) | | | X | | | | X | | | X | | | X | | X | | X |
| Insulin (Serum) | | | X | | | | X | | | X | | | X | | X | | X |
| Triglycerides (Serum) | | | X | | | | X | | | X | | | X | | X | | X |
| Cholesterols (Serum) | | | X | | | | X | | | X | | | X | | X | | X |
| **Vascular Function and Structure** | | | | | | | | | | | | | | | | | |
| Flow Mediated Dilatation (FMD) | | | X | | | | X | | | X | | | X | | X | | X |
| Carotid Intima Media Thickness (cIMT) | | | X | | | | X | | | X | | | X | | X | | X |
| **Eating Disorder Behaviors/Psychology** | | | | | | | | | | | | | | | | | |
| Eating Disorders Examination | X | | | | | | | | | | X | X | | X | | X | |
| Eating Disorders Examination Questionnaire † | X | | | | X | | | | | | X | X | | X | | X | |
| Loss of Control over Eating Scale † | X | | | | X | | | | | | X | X | | X | | X | |
| Three Factor Eating Questionnaire | X | | | | | | | | | | X | X | | X | | X | |
| Dutch Eating Behavior Questionnaire | X | | | | | | | | | | X | X | | X | | X | |
| **Mini International Neuropsychiatric Interview (MINI)** | | | | | | | | | | | | | | | | | |
| All Questions | X | | | | | | | | | | | | | | | | |
| Lifetime History of Eating Disorder Questions | X | | | | | | | | | | | | | | | | |
| Eating Disorder Questions Only | | | | | | | | | | | X | X | | X | | X | |
| **General Mental Health** | | | | | | | | | | | | | | | | | |
| Rosenberg Self-Esteem Scale | X | | | | | | | | | | X | X | | X | | X | |
| 36-Item Short Form Survey (SF-36) | X | | | | | | | | | | X | X | | X | | X | |
| Depression, Anxiety and Stress Scale (DASS-21) | X | | | X | X | | X | | | X | X | X | X | X | X | X | X |

**Table 2.** *Cont.*

| Time (Months) from Start of Dietary Intervention | ~0 | | | ~0.25 | ~1 | | ~4 | | | | ~6 | | ~12 | | ~24 | | ~36 | |
|---|---|---|---|---|---|---|---|---|---|---|---|---|---|---|---|---|---|---|
| Time (Weeks) from Start of Dietary Intervention | -2 | -1 | 0 | 1 | 4 | 15 | 16 | 17§ | 25 | 26 | 29 | 51 | 52 | 103 | 104 | 155 | 156 |
| **Mindfulness and Personality** | | | | | | | | | | | | | | | | | |
| Langer Mindfulness Scale | X | | | | | | | | | | | | | | | | |
| Five Facet Mindfulness Questionnaire | X | | | | | | | | | | | | | | | | |
| Big Five Inventory | | | X | | | | | | | | | | | | | | |
| **Adaptive Responses to Energy Restriction** | | | | | | | | | | | | | | | | | |
| Energy Intake, and Factors Influencing it | | | | | | | | | | | | | | | | | |
| Food Diary | | | X | X⌘ | X⌘ | | X | X | | X | | | X | | X | | X |
| Drive to Eat | | | | | | | | | | | | | | | | | |
| General Food Craving Questionnaire—State | X | | | | | | | | | | | X | | X | | X | |
| Eating Self-Efficacy Scale | | | X | | X | | X | | | X | | | X | | X | | X |
| Subjective Drive to Eat (Visual Analogue Scales)—Fasting and Postprandial | | | X | X | X | | X | X | | X | | | X | | X | | X |
| Appetite-Regulating Hormones | | | | | | | | | | | | | | | | | |
| Ghrelin (Plasma)—Fasting and Postprandial | | | X | X | X | | X | X | | X | | | X | | X | | X |
| Peptide YY (Plasma)—Fasting and Postprandial | | | X | X | X | | X | X | | X | | | X | | X | | X |
| Leptin (Plasma) | | | X | X | X | | X | X | | X | | | X | | X | | X |
| Ketones | | | | | | | | | | | | | | | | | |
| β-Hydroxybutyrate (Whole Venous Blood) | | | X | X | X | | X | X | | X | | | X | | X | | X |
| Acetoacetic Acid (Urine) | | | X | X | X | | X | X | | X | | | X | | X | | X |
| **Physical Activity** | | | | | | | | | | | | | | | | | |
| Self-Efficacy to Regulate Exercise | | | X | X | X | | X | | | X | | | X | | X | | X |
| Pedometer Step Count | | | X | X | X | | X | X | | X | | | X | | X | | X |
| Physical Activity Diary | | | X | X | X | | X | X | | X | | | X | | X | | X |
| Accelerometry | | | X | X | X | | X | X | | X | | | X | | X | | X |
| Sleep (in Addition to Accelerometry) | | | | | | | | | | | | | | | | | |
| Sleep Diary | | | X | X | X | | X | | | X | | | X | | X | | X |
| Epsworth Sleepiness Scale | | | X | X | X | | X | | | X | | | X | | X | | X |
| Pittsburgh Sleep Quality Index | | | X | X | X | | X | | | X | | | X | | X | | X |
| **Energy Expenditure** | | | | | | | | | | | | | | | | | |
| Resting Energy Expenditure (Indirect Calorimetry) | | | X | X | X | | X | X | | X | | | X | | X | | X |
| Body Temperature | | | X | X | X | | X | X | | X | | | X | | X | | X |

**Table 2.** *Cont.*

| Time (Months) from Start of Dietary Intervention | ~0 | | | ~0.25 | ~1 | ~4 | | | | ~6 | | ~12 | | ~24 | | ~36 | |
|---|---|---|---|---|---|---|---|---|---|---|---|---|---|---|---|---|---|
| **Time (Weeks) from Start of Dietary Intervention** | -2 | -1 | 0 | 1 | 4 | 15 | 16 | 17§ | 25 | 26 | 29 | 51 | 52 | 103 | 104 | 155 | 156 |
| **Neuroendocrine Status** | | | | | | | | | | | | | | | | | |
| *Hypothalamo-Pituitary-Adrenal Axis* | | | | | | | | | | | | | | | | | |
| Cortisol (Serum) | | | X | | | | X | X | | X | | | X | | X | | X |
| Adrenocorticotropic Hormone (Plasma) | | | | | | | X | X | | X | | | X | | X | | X |
| *Hypothalamo-Pituitary-Thyroid Axis* | | | | | | | | | | | | | | | | | |
| Free Triiodothyronine or 3,3′,5-Triiodothyronine (T3) (Serum) | | | X | | | | X | X | | X | | | X | | X | | X |
| Reverse T3 (Serum) | | | X | | | | X | X | | X | | | X | | X | | X |
| Free Thyroxine or 3,5,3′,5′-Tetraiodothyronine (T4) (Serum) | | | X | | | | X | X | | X | | | X | | X | | X |
| Thyroid Stimulating Hormone (Serum) | | | X | | | | X | X | | X | | | X | | X | | X |
| *Hypothalamo-Pituitary-Gonadotropic Axis* | | | | | | | | | | | | | | | | | |
| Estradiol (Serum) | | | X | | | | X | X | | X | | | X | | X | | X |
| Sex Hormone Binding Globulin (Serum) | | | X | | | | X | X | | X | | | X | | X | | X |
| *Hypothalamo-Pituitary-Somatotropic Axis* | | | | | | | | | | | | | | | | | |
| Insulin-Like Growth Factor-1 (Serum) | | | X | | | | X | X | | X | | | X | | X | | X |
| Insulin-Like Growth Factor Binding Proteins (Serum) | | | X | | | | X | X | | X | | | X | | X | | X |
| **Miscellaneous** | | | | | | | | | | | | | | | | | |
| Energy Homeostasis Questionnaire | X | | | | | | | | | | | | | | | | |
| **General** | | | | | | | | | | | | | | | | | |
| Preferred Intervention | | | X | | | | | | | | | | | | | | |
| Diet Side Effect Questionnaire | | | | X | X | | | | | | | | | | | | |

§ Only measured in participants in the FAST intervention. ⌘ While food diary data was collected at 8–9 time points, the food diaries served the dual purpose of providing data for analysis, as well as assisting with adherence to the prescribed dietary intervention. † The Eating Disorders Examination Questionnaire and the Loss of Control Over Eating Scale were additionally collected at 8, 12 and 20 weeks. All samples of blood and urine are collected in the fasting state unless otherwise stated, and except for the urine sample taken after deuterium administration for determination of total body water. All pedometer and accelerometer measures, as well as food, activity, and sleep diaries, were commenced a week prior to the measurement time point. DXA, Dual-energy X-ray absorptiometry; $^{1}$H-MRS, proton magnetic resonance spectroscopy; MRI, magnetic resonance imaging.

Table 2 lists the schedule of all outcome measures for the trial. In brief, there are 8–9 major time points over the 3-year trial (0, 0.25, 1, 4, (and 4.25 for those in the FAST intervention), 6, 12, 24, and 36 months relative to commencement of the dietary interventions), with measurements undertaken during 1–3 face-to-face appointments at our clinical research facility, ideally scheduled at $\pm 2$ weeks of these major time points as shown in Table 2. We undertook measurements over 1–3 face-to-face appointments at each major time point because the measurements took up to 13 h to complete (which would have been too burdensome for participants if conducted in a single appointment of greater than 7 h in duration), and because some measurements (i.e., those for which participants were given a food, activity and sleep diary to complete for 7 days, and were requested to wear a pedometer and an activity monitor for 7 days) required meeting with participants a week before in order to provide materials and instructions for data collection over the ensuing week. Participants were given medical certificates to enable them to take leave of absence from work for trial appointments (if required), and—while in our clinical research facility—they were given a meal every 3–4 h, or a coffee voucher to use in the adjacent café during breaks from testing. The measurements at 0 and 0.25 months (0 and 1 weeks), as well as those at 4 and 4.25 months (16 and 17 weeks), were always done exactly 1 week apart. The measurements at 1 month were done within $\pm 2$ days from the exact date. The measurements at 4 and 6 months were done within $\pm 1$ week from the exact date. The measurements at 12 months were done within $\pm 2$ weeks from the exact date, while the measurements at 24 and 36 months were done within $\pm 4$ weeks from the exact date.

In addition to attending our clinical research facility for data collection, participants were required to attend 21–22 individual dietary appointments with the trial dietitian (A.A.G. or C.H.). The initial individual dietary appointment at week 0 was scheduled for approximately 90 min, which is also when participants in the FAST intervention received their first meal replacement products (shakes and soups) and protein supplementation as required [47]. Subsequent individual dietary appointments (for review) were scheduled for 30 min approximately every 2 weeks for the first 26 weeks of the intervention (i.e., at 1, 2, 4, 6, 8, 10, 12, 15, 16, 18, 20, 25, and 26 weeks relative to commencement of the dietary interventions, plus an extra appointment at 17 weeks for participants in the FAST intervention during their transition from the FAST to the SLOW intervention), and then approximately every month until 52 weeks (i.e., at 29, 33, 37, 41, 45, 51, and 52 weeks). To increase compliance with individual dietary appointments, participants were able to complete appointments that did not require face-to-face contact (i.e., to collect a food, activity, and sleep diary or to collect meal replacement products and protein) via telephone. After 52 weeks, participants were given the option of attending monthly group support meetings of 60–90 min in duration each, facilitated on a rotating basis by different members of the research team (R.V.S., A.A.G., C.H., F.Q.d.L. and A.S.), sometimes in association with a guest facilitator.

### 2.4. Randomization

At −1 weeks, participants were randomized (and enrolled) into the trial using stratified permuted block randomization [48]. Specifically, they were stratified by BMI (30–34.9 kg/m$^2$; 35–40 kg/m$^2$) and age (45–54.9 years; 55–65 years). Individuals in each of the 4 stratified groups were then randomized in blocks of 2 and with a 1:1 ratio into the FAST or SLOW intervention. To avoid bias, randomization was undertaken by an investigator (A.S.) who had not had contact with participants before randomization and was not involved in implementation of the 52-week dietary interventions. Researchers undertaking screening (R.V.S., A.A.G., C.H.) and dietary interventions (A.A.G., C.H.) were not aware of the method used for randomization and were not able to predict which intervention a particular participant would be randomized to.

### 2.5. Preparing Participants Before Outcome Measurements

One week prior to each face-to-face appointment at our clinical research facility, detailed instructions were e-mailed to each participant regarding what they needed to do prior to the day of the appointment as well as on the appointment day itself. At all appointments that involved measurement of weight and blood or urine sampling (i.e., at 0, 1, 4, 16 [and 17 for those in the FAST intervention], 26, 52, 104, and 156 weeks as shown in Table 2), participants were asked to attend our clinical research facility after an overnight fast (eight hours or more). They were instructed to drink plenty of fluid the day before so that they would be adequately hydrated on the day. In preparation for urine sample collection, participants were asked to drink a glass of water (250 mL) and to void their bladder once at home before attending our clinical research facility. They were also instructed to minimize physical activity on the morning of the appointment day, to minimize possible confounding of resting energy expenditure measurement.

### 2.6. Outcome Measures

All anthropometry and body composition data were collected with participants lightly-clothed (i.e., in the close-fitting sports bra and leggings that they purchased for use in the trial), without shoes, and with all metal jewelry, accessories, and electronic devices removed.

### 2.6.1. Body Composition

#### Height

Height was measured to the nearest 0.1 cm using a stadiometer (Harpenden Stadiometer, Holtain Ltd., Crymych, UK). Two measurements were taken, and if the difference between the measurements was >0.5 cm, a third measurement was taken. The average of the two measurements (or the average of the two closest measurements if a third measurement was taken) was recorded as the result.

#### Weight (and BMI)

Body weight was measured to the nearest 0.1 kg with a calibrated scale (Tanita BWB-800 digital scale, Wedderburn Pty Ltd., Sydney, Australia). Two measurements were taken, and if the difference between the measurements was >0.5 kg, a third measurement was taken. The average of the two measurements (or the average of the two closest measurements if a third measurement was taken) was recorded as the result. BMI ($kg/m^2$) was calculated by dividing weight (in kg) by height (in m) squared.

#### Bone

#### Bone Mineral Density (BMD) and Bone Mineral Content (BMC)

A dual-energy X-ray absorptiometry (DXA) machine (Discovery W model, Hologic Inc, Bedford, MA, USA) was used to measure BMD ($g/cm^2$) and BMC (g) of the total left hip and anterior posterior lumbar spine (L1-L4). Scans were conducted in accordance with the recommendations outlined in the manufacturer's manual and were assisted by use of the Hologic hip positioning fixture and a large square cushion for the hip and spine scans, respectively. Scans were analyzed using the integrated Hologic APEX Software (version 4, Hologic Inc, Bedford, MA, USA). Regions of interest were manually inspected, with adjustments where necessary. The DXA machine was serviced annually, subject to regular quality assurance testing, and calibrated on each day of use with a Hologic phantom spine.

#### Markers of Bone Turnover

#### Markers of Bone Formation

For the subsequent analysis of serum N-terminal propeptide of type I procollagen (P1NP) and osteocalcin, an intravenous cannula was inserted into a forearm vein and venous blood samples were collected into serum tubes from Becton Dickinson (BD, Australia New Zealand, North Ryde, NSW, Australia) and allowed to clot at room temperature. Serum was obtained by centrifugation of blood samples at 3200 rpm (~$1600 \times g$) for 10 min at 4 °C (Eppendorf Centrifuge 5702, Eppendorf

AG, Hamburg, Germany). Serum aliquots were pipetted into CryoPure® tubes (Sarstedt Australia, Technology Park, SA, Australia) and immediately stored at −80 °C until analysis.

### Markers of Bone Resorption

For the subsequent analysis of C-terminal telopeptide of type I collagen (CTX), venous blood samples were collected into serum tubes and serum was prepared and stored as described above until subsequent analysis. In addition, a fasting urine sample was collected from participants and pipetted into a CryoPure® tube and immediately stored at −80 °C until subsequent analysis of N-terminal telopeptide of type I collagen (NTX).

### Lean Tissues

### Fat Free Mass (FFM, DXA)

A whole-body DXA scan was carried out to quantify FFM (kg) and fat mass (FM) (kg and % of body weight), using the DXA machine as described above. During the scan, participants lay supine on the scanning table with their arms at their sides. Scans were conducted in accordance with the procedure outlined in the manufacturer's manual and were analyzed using the integrated Hologic APEX Software, which was used to define regions of the body (i.e., head, arms, trunk, and legs).

### Fat Free Mass (4-Compartment Model)

The 4-compartment model was used because it is the most accurate way to assess body composition under conditions (such as weight loss) where body composition is changing [49–51]. This gold-standard method can be explained by considering the body to be composed of a variety of "compartments" which include bone, fat, water, and a "residual" compartment that is largely made up of protein (mostly muscle) but which also includes non-bone mineral and glycogen. When estimating body composition, the accuracy of the measurement depends on how many compartments can be measured directly, with each direct measurement reducing the number of assumptions that need to be made. For example, methods that utilize a 2-compartment model, such as bioelectrical impedance, generally separate the body into a fat compartment and a fat free compartment. Because this method directly measures only the fat compartment, not the fat free compartment, a number of assumptions are made for the estimation of FFM, especially regarding its density, which is highly variable depending on the relative proportions of muscle mass, BMC, and total body water (TBW). All of these variables change from one person to the next, and also within the same person under different conditions (e.g., before and after weight loss). Methods that utilize a 3-compartment model, such as DXA, air displacement plethysmography and underwater weighing, are more accurate than methods that draw on a 2-compartment model, but none of these methods control for inter-individual variability (and intra-individual variability over time) in both BMC *and* TBW.

With the 4-compartment model, direct measurements of BMC using DXA, body volume using air displacement plethysmography or underwater weighing, and TBW using the deuterium dilution technique, reduces the number of assumptions that need to be made when calculating body composition, because the masses of most of the components of the fat free compartment are measured rather than assumed. FFM (and FM) using the 4-compartment model can be calculated from the equations below [52]:

$$FFM\ (kg) = body\ weight\ (kg) - FM\ (kg) \tag{1}$$

$$FM\ (kg) = [2.748 \times body\ volume\ (L)] - [0.699 \times TBW\ (kg)] + [1.129 \times BMC\ (kg)] - 2.051 \times body\ weight\ (kg)] \tag{2}$$

### Body Volume (BodPod)

As described above, the 4-compartment model requires body volume to calculate FFM (and FM), and this was measured via air displacement plethysmography using a BOD POD® (COSMED USA

Inc, Concord, CA, USA) following the manufacturer's recommended procedures. In addition to the attire described above for anthropometry and body composition assessment, each participant also wore a Lycra swim cap during body volume measurement. After initial calibration of the BodPod®, participants were weighed on an electronic scale. The resulting body weight, as well as sex, age, and height, were entered into the BodPod® software system (BOD POD version 5.4.3) to estimate (predict) thoracic lung volume. Participants were given a brief description of the procedure before entering the BodPod® chamber for the first of two sequential body volume measurements. If the difference between these two measurements was >0.150 L, a third measurement was taken. The average of the two measurements (or the average of the two closest measurements if a third measurement was taken) was recorded as the result for body volume.

Total Body Water (TBW, Deuterium Dilution)

Stock deuterium oxide (99.9% atom % D, Sigma-Aldrich Co, St Louis, MO, USA) was diluted to a 10% dosing solution ($v/v$) by adding 100 mL of the stock deuterium oxide to 900 mL of tap water. The 10% deuterium oxide dosing solution was then autoclaved and stored at $-4\,°C$. When arriving at the clinical research facility on testing days after an overnight-fast, participants were instructed to first void the bladder (and in doing so also collect a urine sample, the 'pre-dose urine sample'). Participants were then given a dose of 0.5 g per kg of body weight of the 10% deuterium oxide dosing solution in a cup with a straw. The weight of the cup + straw, and the weight of the cup + straw + calculated dose of 10% deuterium oxide, were recorded. Participants were asked to ingest as much of the liquid as they could using the straw provided, and then the weight of the cup + straw was recorded again to account for any leftover 10% deuterium oxide dose remaining in the cup. After a six-hour equilibrium period, during which time participants were given a total of 650 mL of tap water to drink, participants were asked to collect another urine sample (the 'post-dose urine sample'). All urine samples were labelled and stored at $-80\,°C$ before processing for analysis of deuterium content. To this end, 5 mL of each urine sample was passed through 200 mg of charcoal to remove organic matter, and 1 mL of the filtrate was pipetted into clear 2 mL screw-top vials sealed with caps containing a hole with a polytetrafluoroethylene/silicone septum (product numbers SV08CW and AC08WK, respectively, Pacific Laboratory Products, Victoria, Australia). Cavity ring-down spectroscopy was used to determine the abundance of deuterium in the processed urine samples, as well as in the tap water and a sample of the 10% deuterium oxide dosing solution (which was diluted 1 in 100 with tap water to make a 0.1% dilution of the original stock deuterium oxide), using a Picarro L2130-i Isotopic Water Analyzer (Picarro Inc, Santa Clara, CA, USA). TBW was calculated using the following equation [53]:

$$TBW = [(W \times A)/a] \times [(\delta dose - \delta tap)/(\delta post - \delta pre)] \times [1/(1000 \times 1.041)] \qquad (3)$$

W is weight of water used to further dilute the 10% deuterium oxide dosing solution to 0.1% (g)
A is weight of the 10% deuterium oxide dosing solution consumed by the participant (g)
a is weight of the 10% deuterium oxide dosing solution that was further diluted to 0.1% (g)
$\delta dose$ is abundance of deuterium in the 0.1% deuterium oxide solution (ppm)
$\delta tap$ is abundance of deuterium in the tap water used to make the dilutions (ppm)
$\delta post$ is abundance of deuterium in the processed post-dose urine sample (ppm)
$\delta pre$ is abundance of deuterium in the processed pre-dose urine sample (ppm)

Thigh Muscle Cross Sectional Area (MRI)

Thigh muscle cross sectional area was determined using MRI with participants lying in a supine position and having removed any metal accessories. Axial images were acquired with a 3.0T MRI scanner (the Discovery MR750 3.0T model from GE Healthcare, Milwaukee, WI, USA), between the base of the femoral head and mid-patella (repetition time = 700 ms, echo time = 10 ms, flip angle = 111°)

with a slice thickness of 1 cm and an inter-slice gap (i.e., the distance between the surfaces of adjacent slices) of 1 cm. For subsequent analysis the median slice between these two points was segmented manually using specialist analysis software (SliceOMatic Version 5.0 rev-6b, Tomovision Inc, Montreal, QC, Canada). When there was an even number of slices between these two points, the inferior of the two slices was selected for analysis. Total skeletal muscle area (and volume) of the thigh muscles (rectus femoris, vastus lateralis, vastus intermedius, vastus medialis, satorius, biceps femoris short head, biceps femoris long head, semitendinosis, semimembranosis, gracilis, and the adductor group) was defined using the region-growing mode of the software, with thresholds adjusted manually as required. Analysis was undertaken by a trained experimenter blinded to treatment allocation.

## Muscle Strength (Hand Dynamometry)

Handgrip strength was assessed using a commercially-available hydraulic hand dynamometer (Jamar®, Model 5030J1, Patterson Medical, Bolingbrook, IL, USA) in accordance with a standardized protocol [54]. In brief, participants were seated upright in an armed chair, with both feet flat on the ground, their forearm resting on the chair arm with an elbow angle of 90° and their wrist positioned over the edge of the chair arm. Participants were instructed to grip the hand dynamometer by the handle and to squeeze as hard as they could. The investigator provided verbal encouragement, and the peak value was recorded to the nearest 1 kg. Three measurements were alternatively recorded for both the left and the right hand, and the maximum reading of the three measurements was used as the result for each hand. A one-minute interval was timed between subsequent measures of the same hand to avoid fatigue. Participants were asked to identify their dominant hand, which was recorded, and handgrip strength was recorded as dominant and non-dominant handgrip strength.

## Fat Mass and Distribution

## Waist and Hip Circumference (and Ratio of Waist to Hip Circumference)

Waist and hip circumferences were measured to the nearest 0.1 cm using a narrow, flexible, and inelastic steel tape (Lufkin W606PM, Apex Tool Group, NC, USA). Participants were asked to breathe normally and to stand with their weight evenly distributed and their arms crossed across their chest during measurements. Waist circumference was measured directly on the skin, at each of the three most commonly used sites worldwide [55]; at the mid-axillary line (i.e., at the halfway point between the bony landmarks of the lowest rib and the top of the iliac crest); at the narrowest part of the torso, and at the level of the umbilicus. Hip circumference measurement was taken at the point of greatest protuberance of the participant's buttocks when viewed from the side. At each site, two measurements were taken, and if the difference between the measurements was >1 cm, a third measurement was taken. The average of each of the two measurements at each site (or the average of the two closest measurements if a third measurement was taken) was recorded as the result.

## Fat Mass (DXA) and Fat Mass (4-Compartment Model)

As described above with FFM (DXA) and FFM (4-compartment mode).

## Abdominal Fat (MRI)

Abdominal fat volumes, namely visceral adipose tissue (VAT) and subcutaneous adipose tissue (SAT) volumes, were quantified using MRI as described above for the section entitled *Thigh Muscle Cross Sectional Area*. Axial T1-weighted fast field echo images were acquired from diaphragm to pelvis (repetition time = 3.8 ms, echo time = 2.1 ms, flip angle = 12°), with a slice thickness of 10 mm and an inter-slice gap of 10 mm. Images were acquired during suspended end-expiration, with a breath-hold duration of approximately 15–18 s per acquisition. Following the scan, all image slices from the base of the lungs to the pelvic floor were segmented manually. VAT was quantified using the Region Growing mode of the analysis software (SliceOMatic Version 5.0 rev-6b, Tomovision Inc, Montreal, QC, Canada), and SAT was quantified using the Mathematical Morphology mode of the software, with thresholds adjusted manually as required. The software was used to automatically calculate the surface area of VAT and SAT on each slice by multiplying the number of pixels tagged by the surface area of one pixel. The inter-slice volume (i.e., the volume of the inter-slice gap) was extrapolated using a cone formula that considered the surface area of the superior and inferior surfaces of the inter-slice gap, as well as the thickness of the inter-slice gap. The total volume of each of the inter-slice gaps was then summed to the total volume of each of the slices (surface area × slice thickness) to calculate the total abdominal volumes of VAT and SAT.

### Intrahepatic Lipid ($^1$H-MRS)

Intrahepatic lipid was measured by proton magnetic resonance spectroscopy ($^1$H-MRS) using a 3.0T MRI scanner (Discovery MR750 3.0T from GE Healthcare, Milwaukee, WI, USA) and analyzed by an assessor blinded to intervention group. Intrahepatic lipid was analyzed by image-guided, localized $^1$H-MRS with a voxel of 30 mm × 30 mm × 20 mm using the whole-body (Q body) coil and a 32-channel torso array coil (NeoCoil), with volumes of interest centered in the right lobe of the liver. Participants lay supine, with spectra acquired during respiratory gating. Spectra were acquired using the PRESS (point resolved spectroscopy) technique (TR = 3000–6000 ms dependent on participant respiration rate, TE = 35 ms, 32 measurements, 4092 sample points). Placement of the voxel in the liver was kept as consistent as possible between measures within each participant, by noting (via image capture) the location of the voxel at the first measurement time point (i.e., at −1 weeks), and replicating this placement as closely as possible in subsequent measurement time points in the same participant. Variation was further minimized by the use of a large voxel, and we have previously shown that the coefficient of variation for this technique is approximately 7% [56]. Fully automated high-order shimming was performed on the volume of interest to ensure maximum field homogeneity. The in vivo water signal was used as the internal standard. Spectral data were post-processed by magnetic resonance user interface software (jMRUI version 5.2, EU Project). Hepatic water signal amplitudes were measured from the acquired non-water suppressed spectra using HLSSVD (Hankel Lanczos Squared Singular Values Decomposition). For hepatic lipid concentration and composition, a five-resonance model was employed [56]. Resonances were fitted for water (4.7 ppm) and fatty acid functional groups: diallylic (2.8–3.1 ppm), other lipids (2.0–2.4 ppm), methylene (1.2–1.4 ppm), and methyl (0.8–1.0 ppm). The signal amplitude was obtained in absolute units for each resonance using AMARES fitting (Advanced Method for Accurate, Robust, and Efficient Spectral), a nonlinear least squares quantitation algorithm, as previously described [57]. Peak amplitudes were determined using prior knowledge that we have detailed previously [56]. The resonances were fitted assuming a Gaussian line shape for all lipid resonances. The zero-order and first-order phase corrections were manually estimated.

### Thigh Fat (MRI)

The MRI scans of the thigh that were described under the section entitled *Thigh Muscle Cross Sectional Area* (above) were used to quantify three types of thigh fat using specialist analysis software (SliceOMatic Version 5.0 rev-6b, Tomovision Inc, Montreal, QC, Canada): SAT of the thigh, subfascial adipose tissue, and intermuscular adipose tissue. SAT of the thigh was identified using the Mathematical Morphology mode of the software as described above for SAT under the heading of *Abdominal Fat*, while the two other adipose tissue compartments—subfascial adipose tissue and intermuscular adipose tissue—were defined using the Region Growing mode of the analysis software, with thresholds adjusted manually as required.

### 2.6.2. Cardiometabolic Health (in Addition to Waist Circumference)

### Blood Pressure

Blood pressure was measured using an automated device from Welch Allyn Medical Products (Skaneateles Falls, NY, USA). Participants rested in a sitting position for two minutes before two measurements were recorded for both the left and right arms. The average of the two recordings was used as the result for each arm.

## Circulating Markers of Cardiometabolic Health

Venous blood was collected and serum prepared and stored as described above for the section entitled *Markers of Bone Turnover*, for subsequent analysis of glucose, insulin, triglycerides, and cholesterols. Whole venous blood was collected directly into a CryoPure® tube and frozen at $-80\,°C$ until subsequent analysis of glycosylated haemoglobin.

## Vascular Function and Structure

## Flow Mediated Dilatation (FMD)

Ultrasound assessment of brachial artery FMD was performed on the right arm in a slightly darkened, temperature-controlled room using an EPIQ 7 Ultrasound System with an L12-3 linear array transducer (Philips, Bothell, WA, USA). Simultaneous electrocardiogram (ECG) recordings were made throughout. The brachial artery was scanned in longitudinal sections 2–10 cm above the antecubital fossa. Ultrasound images were recorded for 30 s at rest, and arterial flow velocity was measured with a pulsed Doppler signal. Increased blood flow was induced by inflation of a blood pressure cuff placed around the forearm, to a suprasystolic pressure of at least 50 mmHg above resting systolic blood pressure. This occlusion was maintained for 5 min, and then the cuff was deflated. Within the first 15 s after the pressure from the cuff was released, a pulsed Doppler velocity signal was acquired to assess the post-occlusive hyperemia. B-mode ultrasound was recorded from 30 s to 2 min post-occlusion, and saved in the DICOM format (Digital Imaging and Communications in Medicine). Brachial artery diameter was subsequently measured offline by a reader blinded to participant characteristics and time point, using semi-automated software (Brachial Analyzer for Research, Medical Imaging Applications LLC, Coralville, IA, USA). Dilatation at 50–70 s after cuff release (FMD60), and the maximum percentage increase in brachial artery diameter in response to hyperemia (%FMD), was recorded.

## Carotid Intima Media Thickness (cIMT)

cIMT is a validated non-invasive marker of subclinical atherosclerosis in adults [58]. The procedure was conducted in the same slightly darkened room as FMD, immediately before the FMD measures, with the participant resting in a supine position with their neck slightly hyperextended and rotated 45°. B-mode ultrasound images were acquired using the EPIQ 7 Ultrasound System with a L12-3 linear array transducer as described above. Both the left and the right common carotid arteries were visualized just proximal to the bulb, in the longitudinal plane and at three distinct angles each (a total of six angles; 90°, 120°, 150°, 210°, 240°, and 270°), identified using a Meijer's Arc. Two 10-s loops were acquired for each angle (12 loops in total per time point for each participant). B-mode images were saved in the DICOM format and imported into a semi-automated program for analysis of cIMT (Carotid Analyzer for Research, Medical Imaging Applications LLC, Coralville, IA, USA). The best quality loop from each angle was analyzed, with the region of interest placed 5–10 mm proximal to the start of the carotid bulb. Mean cIMT, maximum cIMT, and diameter were measured. The mean of the mean cIMT measures from all 6 angles was calculated, as was the mean of the maximum cIMT from all 6 angles.

## 2.6.3. Eating Disorder Behaviors/Psychology

## Eating Disorders Examination (EDE)

The EDE-v16 is an investigator-led interview that is considered the gold standard instrument for the assessment of eating disorders [59]. It is used to assess eating disorder behaviors (i.e., binge eating, purging, very strict dieting) and eating disorder psychopathology, namely restraint, eating concern, weight, and shape overvaluation. It has robust psychometric qualities. A global score can be derived of dietary restraint, eating and weight/shape cognitions.

### Eating Disorders Examination Questionnaire (EDE-Q)

The EDE-Q-v6 modified, is the self-reported questionnaire based on the gold standard EDE for the assessment of eating disorder behaviors and psychopathology [60,61]. In order to exemplify the concepts in the EDE-Q (e.g., objective binge eating) to participants, an initial explanatory text was presented before participants answered the EDE-Q. This initial explanatory text was published in another study [62]. Additionally, we added a question regarding subjective binge eating, as per a previous publication [63]: "Have you had other episodes of eating in which you have had a sense of having lost control and eaten more than you would like, but *have not eaten a very large amount* of food given the situation? Over the past 28 days how many *days* approximately would this have happened?" We also replaced the words "16 ounce" with "450 g" due to this questionnaire being administered in Australia where the metric (rather than the imperial) system is used. Questions regarding weight, height, and menstrual periods were removed because weight and height are available from laboratory measurements, and because all participants in the TEMPO Diet Trial are postmenopausal women.

### Loss of Control over Eating Scale (LOCES)

The experience of loss of control over eating constitutes a clinically significant feature of eating disorders. However, this feature is assessed only in a dichotomous "yes or no" manner in the EDE and EDE-Q, and this may lead to imprecise assessments. Therefore, the LOCES was used in the current trial to complement assessments from the EDE and EDE-Q. The LOCES is a scale used to assess this essential feature of eating disorders, namely the experience of loss of control over eating [64] in both clinical and non-clinical samples [65].

### Three Factor Eating Questionnaire (TFEQ)

The TFEQ is a self-report 51-item questionnaire used to assess three aspects of eating behavior, namely "cognitive restraint of eating", "disinhibition" and "hunger" [66,67]. Two items (item 1 and 4) on the questionnaire were modified: (1) "When I smell a sizzling steak or a juicy piece of meat, I find it very difficult to keep from eating, even if I have just finished a meal" was changed to "When I smell a sizzling steak *or some delicious savory food*, I find it very difficult to keep from eating, even if I have just finished a meal", to make the question appropriate for vegetarians; (4) "When I have eaten my quota of calories, I am usually good about not eating anymore" was changed to "When I have eaten my quota of calories / *kilojoules*, I am usually good about not eating anymore" [68], because an increasing number of individuals in Australia count kilojoules (metric) instead of calories (imperial).

### Dutch Eating Behaviour Questionnaire (DEBQ)

The DEBQ is a self-report 31-item questionnaire that contains three scales that assess three different types of eating behavior, namely "restrained eating", "emotional eating" and "external eating" [69,70].

### Mini International Neuropsychiatric Interview (MINI)

### All Questions

The MINI (version 7.0.0) [71] is a structured interview used to assess the occurrence of psychiatric disorders in accordance with the criteria of the Diagnostic and Statistical Manual of Mental Disorders fifth edition (DSM-5) [64]. In the current trial, the complete MINI (i.e., all questions) was only administered once, at −2 weeks.

### Lifetime History of Eating Disorder Questions

Questions from the MINI (version 7.0.0) that assess binge eating disorder, bulimia nervosa and anorexia nervosa were adapted to assess the lifetime occurrence of these eating disorders (that is, whether a participant had any of these disorders at any time in the past), using the DSM-5 criteria.

### Eating Disorder Questions Only

At all other time points (besides the −2-week time point) where the MINI was administered (i.e., at 29, 51, 103, and 154 weeks as shown in Table 2), only the sections of the MINI (version 7.0.0) that assess binge eating disorder and bulimia nervosa was used.

### General Mental Health

### Rosenberg Self-Esteem Scale

This instrument assesses self-worth by measuring both negative and positive feelings regarding the self. This scale contains 10 items that are answered in a 4-point Likert scale that ranges from "Strongly agree" to "Strongly disagree" [72].

### 36-Item Short Form Survey (SF-36)

The SF-36 is a self-report survey used to assess health status regarding pain, mental health, vitality, general health perception, and limitations in usual activities because of physical or emotional problems [73].

### Depression, Anxiety and Stress Scale (DASS-21)

The DASS-21 is a self-report scale with 21 items used to assess symptoms of depression, anxiety and psychological stress in both clinical and non-clinical samples [74–76].

### Mindfulness and Personality

### Langer Mindfulness Scale (LMS)

The LMS is a 14-item questionnaire that assesses three sub facets of mindfulness: (1) novelty seeking (i.e., having an open and curious orientation to the environment), (2) novelty producing (i.e., an individual's tendency to create new categories rather than relying on those previously formed) and (3) engagement (i.e., the ability to attend to changes in the environment) [77]. Participants are asked to answer the items on a 7-point Likert scale ranging from "Disagree" to "Agree". The LMS has adequate internal consistency and temporal stability, and correlates appropriately with other instruments assessing theoretically-related constructs [78].

### Five Facet Mindfulness Questionnaire

This 39-item self-report questionnaire was used to assess five different facets of mindfulness, namely observing, describing, acting with awareness, non-judging of inner experience, and non-reactivity to inner experience [79].

### Big Five Inventory

This is used to measure five different dimensions of personality and each of these five different dimensions of personality is subdivided into six personality facets [80–82].

### 2.6.4. Adaptive Responses to Energy Restriction

### Energy Intake, and Factors Influencing it

### Food Diary

Participants were provided with detailed written and verbal instructions prior to completing 7-day estimated food diaries which were reviewed for completeness by a dietitian [83]. These food diaries were used for data collection, as well as to aid in administration of the weight loss interventions. The food diary that was collected from −1 to 0 weeks was used to tailor dietary counselling to each individual participant. At all other time points, the food diary was used to monitor adherence (i.e., servings of food groups, number of meal replacement products consumed per day, etc.), and to provide individualized feedback to participants about their progress. Food diaries were coded and analyzed for nutrient composition and food group serves by trained dietitians, using a standardized protocol and FoodWorks Professional version 8 (Xyris Software, Brisbane, QLD, Australia).

## Drive to Eat

### General Food Craving Questionnaire—State (G-FCQ-S)

The G-FCQ-S assesses state-dependent cravings for tasty foods in general. That is, it assesses whether general food cravings are experienced in response to specific, momentary situations or psychological and physiological states [84].

### Eating Self-Efficacy Scale (ESES)

The ESES is a 25-item scale that rates the likelihood of having difficulty controlling overeating across two factors; one concerned with eating when experiencing negative affect; and the other with eating during socially acceptable circumstances [85,86]. Two items (item 1 and 10) on the questionnaire were modified: (1) "Overeating after work or school" was changed to "Overeating after work or school *(or after your day's activities, if you do not go to work or school)*", as the original version may not be applicable to participants that are not working or at school; (10) "Overeating with family members" was changed to "Overeating with family members *(or with other people, if you do not eat with family members)*", as the original version may not be applicable to participants that do not (regularly) eat with family members.

### Subjective Drive to Eat (Visual Analogue Scales)—Fasting and Postprandial

Subjective appetite perceptions were measured at −20, 0, 15, 30, 45, 60, 90, 120 and 180 min in relation to completion of a standardized breakfast using an Electronic Appetite Rating System (EARS) that has been validated against the pen-and-paper version [87]. The breakfast consisted of a wholemeal English muffin (Tip Top, Enfield, NSW, Australia), 2 eggs (~60 g each, cooked by scrambling in a non-stick pan), 15 g of olive oil spread (Coles Supermarkets Australia Pty Ltd., Hawthorn East, Victoria, Australia), which was used to spread on the muffin and to scramble the eggs, 200 mL orange juice (Just Juice, Docklands, Victoria, Australia) and 300 mL tap water. The meal amounted to ~700 g and ~1900 kJ (~450 kcal). Participants were asked to complete the meal within 10 min, and to rate perceptions of hunger, fullness, how much food they felt they could eat (prospective consumption), desire to eat, and satisfaction, using the EARS tool. Participants move the cursor along a horizontal 100 mm visual analogue scale, anchored at each end with the statements "Not at all" or "None at all" (0 mm) and "Extremely" or "A large amount" (100 mm), to a point on the horizontal line that reflects the intensity of their current state. Gastrointestinal and other symptoms, namely nausea, bloating, irritability, and alertness, were also assessed.

### Appetite-Regulating Hormones—Postprandial and/or Fasting

The venous cannula that was inserted for collection of fasting blood samples (for determination of serum markers of bone turnover and cardiometabolic health) was used to collect blood for plasma preparation and determination of appetite-regulating hormones. Venous blood sample collections were commenced at −18, 32, 62, 122, and 182 min relative to completion of the above-mentioned standardized breakfast (i.e., immediately after measurement of subjective drive to eat, which took approximately 1 min). The blood was collected into ice-cold EDTA-treated tubes (BD, Australia New Zealand, North Ryde, NSW, Australia) containing inhibitors to prevent degradation of hormones. The inhibitors consisted of 1 mg Prefabloc® (Roche Diagnostics, Castle Hill, NSW, Australia), 10 μL dipeptidyl peptidase-IV inhibitor (Merck Millipore, Burlington, MA, USA), and 10 μL protease inhibitor cocktail (Sigma-Aldrich, St Louis, Missouri, USA) per 1 mL whole blood. Immediately after collection, samples were plunged up to the neck into wet ice, and were centrifuged as described above in the section entitled *Markers of Bone Turnover*. Immediately after centrifugation, aliquots of plasma were stored at −80 °C until subsequent analysis of ghrelin and peptide YY (in fasting and postprandial plasma samples) and leptin (in fasting plasma samples only).

## Ketones

### β-Hydroxybutyrate (Whole Venous Blood)

Fasting venous blood from the cannula was used to measure concentrations of circulating ketones (β-hydroxybutyrate) using β-ketone test strips and a ketone monitor (FreeStyle Optium, Abbott Diabetes Care Ltd., Witney, Oxon, UK), as per the manufacturer's protocol.

### Acetoacetic Acid (Urine)

Urinary acetoacetic acid concentrations were estimated using over-the-counter reagent strips (Ketostix®, Bayer Vital GmbH, Leverkusen, Germany), which determine the presence of acetoacetic acid upon reaction with nitroprusside salt. The end of the strip was dipped into a fasting urine sample collected from the participant soon after they arrived at our clinical research facility. The colour of the reagent strip was then compared to the color chart provided with the product, at 15 s after contact with urine.

## Physical Activity

### Self-Efficacy to Regulate Exercise

This scale describes eighteen situations that can make it difficult to maintain an exercise routine, and assesses an individual's confidence in their ability to perform their exercise routine regularly (three or more times a week) during these situations [85]. For each item, participants indicate their confidence to execute the behavior on a 100-point percentage scale comprised of 10-point increments, ranging from "Cannot do at all" (0%) to "highly certain can do" (100%).

### Pedometer Step Count and Physical Activity Diary

Participants were given a calibrated pedometer (Omron Walking Stle HJ-203, Omron Healthcare Co Ltd., Kyoto, Japan) to be worn in a pocket or bra, and were advised to gradually increase daily step counts to a total of 8000–12,000 steps per day, including 30–60 min per day of moderate to vigorous physical activity. This recommendation was based on achieving 200–300 min per week of physical activity, as recommended in the 2009 American College of Sports Physicians physical activity guidelines for weight loss and prevention of weight regain in adults [88]. Participants were asked to record the number of steps displayed on their pedometer in a daily physical activity diary for 7 days. This was done in their food diary, which contained spaces for recording physical activity (and sleep). This diary was thus referred to as the food, activity, and sleep diary.

### Accelerometry

Intensity and duration of daily physical activities, as well as sleep, were measured using an accelerometer (SenseWear Pro Armband®, BodyMedia Inc, Pittsburgh, PA, USA) [89]. Participants were asked to wear the accelerometer continuously for 7 days, on the back of the upper tricep muscle of the left arm, except when showering or for water-based activities (e.g., swimming) as the device is not water proof. Participants were asked to record the time and reasons for taking off the accelerometer in their food, activity, and sleep diary.

Sleep (in Addition to Accelerometry)

Sleep Diary

Participants were asked to record in their food, activity and sleep diary, for seven days, what time they woke up in the morning (which may be different from the time they actually got out of bed), what time they tried to go to sleep the previous night (which may be different from the time they got into bed), and approximately how long (in minutes) it took them to fall asleep the previous night.

Epsworth Sleepiness Scale (ESS)

The ESS consists of eight self-report items, each scored from 0–3, that measure a person's habitual "likelihood of dozing or falling asleep" in common situations of daily living [90,91]. No specific time frame is specified. The ESS score represents the sum of individual items, and ranges from 0–24. Values >10 are considered to indicate significant sleepiness.

Pittsburgh Sleep Quality Index (PSQI)

The PSQI is a 19-item self-report questionnaire for evaluating subjective sleep quality over the previous month, combined into seven clinically-derived component scores, each weighted equally from 0–3 [92]. The seven component scores are added to obtain a global score ranging from 0–21, with higher scores indicating worse sleep quality.

Energy Expenditure

Resting Energy Expenditure (REE, Indirect Calorimetry)

REE was measured via indirect calorimetry using a ventilated hood system (TrueOne2400, ParvoMedics, Inc, Sandy, UT, USA) after an overnight fast. REE was measured with participants lying in a comfortable supine position, with their head on a pillow and a transparent ventilated hood placed over their head. Plastic sheeting attached to the hood was tucked around the participant to form a seal between the air inside and outside the hood. Participants lay in a quiet room with an ambient temperature of ~23–25 °C. The ventilated hood system was calibrated before each measurement using standardized gases and rates of airflow, according to the manufacturer's manual. Volumes of oxygen inspired and carbon dioxide expired were recorded continuously for 45 min, and the first 10 min of data were disregarded, as during this time the participant is considered to be adapting to the hood. REE (kJ/day) was calculated using the modified Weir equation, as previously published [93].

Body Temperature

Body temperature was measured over seven days using the same accelerometer used to measure physical activity and sleep, as described above. Body temperature was measured as it provides an indication of energy expenditure in a variety of mammalian species, including humans [94].

Neuroendocrine Status

As the hypothalamo-pituitary-adrenal, -thyroid, -gonadotropic, and -somatotropic axes are influenced by weight loss and are known to influence body composition if sustained for several weeks [15], serial measurements of hormones within these axes will demonstrate whether there is any differential effect of the FAST versus SLOW intervention on the concentrations of hormones that could adversely affect body composition, as well as the duration of any such changes. A suite of hormones will be measured to allow a more accurate assessment of whether the activity of each axis has been differentially altered by either intervention. Venous blood samples were collected either into serum tubes (BD, Australia New Zealand, North Ryde, NSW, Australia) and allowed to clot at room temperature, or collected into ice-cold EDTA-treated tubes (BD) and immediately plunged up to the neck into wet ice. Serum and plasma were obtained by centrifugation of blood samples as described above in the section entitled *Markers of Bone Turnover*, and aliquots were pipetted into

CryoPure® tubes and immediately stored at −80 °C until analysis. Serum and plasma samples were used for analysis of cortisol and adrenocorticotropic hormone, respectively, as indices of activity of the hypothalamo-pituitary-adrenal axis. Serum samples were used for analysis of free triiodothyronine or 3,3′,5-triiodothyronine (T3), reverse T3, free thyroxine or 3,5,3′,5′-tetraiodothyronine (T4), and thyroid stimulating hormone (TSH), as indices of activity of the hypothalamo-pituitary-thyroid axis; estradiol and sex hormone binding globulin, as indices of activity of the hypothalamo-pituitary-gonadotropic axis; and insulin-like growth factor-1 and insulin-like growth factor binding proteins, as indices of activity of the hypothalamo-pituitary-somatotropic axis.

Miscellaneous

Energy Homeostasis Questionnaire

This was a custom-built, experimental questionnaire in which we aimed to determine whether an individual's propensity to lose weight or keep it off, or to mount adaptive physiological responses to energy restriction or energy excess, could be predicted by self-report of traits such as hunger, energy levels or body temperature after periods of relatively reduced or increased energy intake.

2.6.5. General

Preferred Intervention

We asked participants to select 1 of 3 statements that best reflected how they felt when they found out which of the two interventions they had been randomized to. The statements were "I was disappointed", "I was pleased", and "I would have been pleased to have been randomized to either of the two diets", with the different options listed in random order for each participant. This was asked in order to ascertain whether being randomized to the preferred intervention had any effect on the amount of weight that a participant lost on that intervention.

Diet Side Effect Questionnaire

The aim of this custom-built questionnaire was to capture and quantitate any side effects from the FAST intervention.

*2.7. Statistical Analyses*

Data analysis will be conducted using intention to treat principles. Exploratory analyses will be performed using appropriate statistical methods, such as the generalized linear mixed-model, as deemed appropriate.

## 3. Discussion

The observed reticence of healthcare professionals to prescribe dietary obesity treatments that induce fast weight loss [28,30] suggests an underlying assumption that fast weight loss is less advisable than slow weight loss. Potential concerns about the safety of fast weight loss—notably for musculoskeletal integrity but also for eating disorder behaviors—may contribute to the low utilization of fast weight loss by healthcare professionals. Given the short- and longer-term effectiveness of VLEDs as a dietary obesity treatment [18,20,22–24,27], it is necessary to know whether any concerns about their safety are founded, as the escalating obesity epidemic mandates use of all safe and effective obesity treatment options.

## 4. Conclusions

To our knowledge, the TEMPO Diet Trial will be the first randomized controlled trial to compare the long-term effects of fast weight loss (achieved via VLED in a total meal replacement diet involving severe energy restriction) to slow weight loss (achieved via a conventional food-based diet involving moderate energy restriction) on gold-standard measures of musculoskeletal integrity and eating disorder behaviors. This work has the potential to advance the treatment of obesity by providing information about the safety or otherwise of dietary obesity treatments that induce fast versus slow weight loss.

**Author Contributions:** Conceptualization, I.D.C., N.M.B. and A.S.; Methodology, R.V.S., A.A.G., C.H., S.E.K., N.A.J., F.Q.d.L., H.A.F., M.R.S., T.P.M., I.D.C., P.H., N.M.B. and A.S.; Writing—Original Draft Preparation, R.V.S. and A.S.; Writing—Review & Editing, R.V.S., A.A.G., C.H., S.E.K., N.A.J., F.Q.d.L., H.A.F., M.R.S., T.P.M., I.D.C., P.H., N.M.B. and A.S.; Supervision, R.V.S., A.A.G., S.E.K., N.A.J., M.R.S., T.P.M., I.D.C., P.H. and A.S.; Project Administration, R.V.S. and A.S.; Funding Acquisition, I.D.C., N.M.B. and A.S.

**Funding:** This work was supported by the National Health and Medical Research Council (NHMRC) of Australia via an Early Career Research Fellowship to R.V.S. (1072771) and S.E.K. (1122190), as well as a Project Grant (1026005) to A.S., N.M.B. and I.D.C., and Senior Research Fellowships (1042555 and 1135897) to A.S. The University of Sydney and the Endocrine Society of Australia additionally supported this work via a Sydney Outstanding Academic Researcher (SOAR) Fellowship to A.S., and a Postdoctoral Research Award to R.V.S., respectively. The Australian Government's Department of Education & Training also supported this research via an Australian Postgraduate Award to A.A.G., and an International Postgraduate Research Scholarship to H.A.F. F.Q.d.L. was supported by the CAPES Foundation, Ministry of Education of Brazil, via a postgraduate scholarship. MRS is supported by a Future Leader fellowship from the National Heart Foundation of Australia (100419).

**Conflicts of Interest:** A.A.G. has received payment from the Pharmacy Guild of Australia and from Nestlé Health Science for oral presentations at conferences. M.R.S. receives in-kind support (investigational product) from Swisse Wellness Pty Ltd. T.P.M. is on the NovoNordisk Obesity Advisory Board and the Nestlé Health Science Optifast® VLCD™ Advisory Board, has received funds for performing clinical trials from Pfizer, NovoNordisk, SFI, the Australian Egg Corporation, and has given talks on obesity for NovoNordisk. I.D.C. is president of the World Obesity Federation, has received funds for performing clinical trials from the NHMRC, SFI, the Australian Egg Corporation, NovoNordisk, BMS and Pfizer, and has given talks on obesity for Servier Laboratories and Ache Pharmaceuticals. P.H. receives/has received sessional fees and lecture fees from the Australian Medical Council, Therapeutic Guidelines publication, and New South Wales Institute of Psychiatry and royalties/honoraria from Hogrefe and Huber, McGraw Hill Education, and Blackwell Scientific Publications, Biomed Central and PlosMedicine, and has received research grants from the NHMRC and ARC. She is Deputy Chair of the National Eating Disorders Collaboration Steering Committee in Australia (2012-) and Member of the ICD-11 Working Group for Eating Disorders (2012-) and was Chair of the Clinical Practice Guidelines Project Working Group (Eating Disorders) of RANZCP (2012–2015). She is a consultant to Shire Pharmaceuticals. A.S. is the author of *The Don't Go Hungry Diet* (Bantam, Australia and New Zealand, 2007) and *Don't Go Hungry For Life* (Bantam, Australia and New Zealand, 2011). She has also received payment from Eli Lilly, the Pharmacy Guild of Australia, Novo Nordisk, the Dietitians Association of Australia, Shoalhaven Family Medical Centers and the Pharmaceutical Society of Australia for presentation at conferences, and has served on the Nestlé Health Science Optifast® VLCD™ Advisory Board since 2016. For the TEMPO Diet Trial, Prima Health Solutions, Brookvale, NSW, Australia, provided in-kind support in the form of below-cost KicStart™ meal replacement products (shakes) and a gift of associated adherence tools (shakers). Prima Health Solutions had no involvement in the design or analysis of the research. This relationship with Prima Health Solutions was established after the dietary protocol for the TEMPO Diet Trial had been established.

## References

1. Afshin, A.; Forouzanfar, M.H.; Reitsma, M.B.; Sur, P.; Estep, K.; Lee, A.; Marczak, L.; Mokdad, A.H.; Moradi-Lakeh, M.; Naghavi, M.; et al. Health effects of overweight and obesity in 195 countries over 25 years. *N. Engl. J. Med.* **2017**, *377*, 13–27. [PubMed]

2. Lauby-Secretan, B.; Scoccianti, C.; Loomis, D.; Grosse, Y.; Bianchini, F.; Straif, K. Body fatness and cancer–viewpoint of the iarc working group. *N. Engl. J. Med.* **2016**, *375*, 794–798. [CrossRef] [PubMed]

3. Ng, M.; Fleming, T.; Robinson, M.; Thomson, B.; Graetz, N.; Margono, C.; Mullany, E.C.; Biryukov, S.; Abbafati, C.; et al. Global, regional, and national prevalence of overweight and obesity in children and adults during 1980–2013: A systematic analysis for the global burden of disease study 2013. *Lancet* **2014**, *384*, 766–781. [CrossRef]

4. Colagiuri, S.; Lee, C.M.; Colagiuri, R.; Magliano, D.; Shaw, J.E.; Zimmet, P.Z.; Caterson, I.D. The cost of overweight and obesity in australia. *Med. J. Aust.* **2010**, *192*, 260–264. [PubMed]

5. Cawley, J.; Meyerhoefer, C. The medical care costs of obesity: An instrumental variables approach. *J. Health Econ.* **2012**, *31*, 219–230. [CrossRef] [PubMed]

6. Wang, Y.C.; McPherson, K.; Marsh, T.; Gortmaker, S.L.; Brown, M. Health and economic burden of the projected obesity trends in the USA and the UK. *Lancet* **2011**, *378*, 815–825. [CrossRef]

7.  Yanovski, S.Z.; Yanovski, J.A. Long-term drug treatment for obesity: A systematic and clinical review. *JAMA* **2014**, *311*, 74–86. [CrossRef] [PubMed]

8.  Adams, T.D.; Gress, R.E.; Smith, S.C.; Halverson, R.C.; Simper, S.C.; Rosamond, W.D.; Lamonte, M.J.; Stroup, A.M.; Hunt, S.C. Long-term mortality after gastric bypass surgery. *N. Engl. J. Med.* **2007**, *357*, 753–761. [CrossRef] [PubMed]

9.  Mingrone, G.; Panunzi, S.; De Gaetano, A.; Guidone, C.; Iaconelli, A.; Nanni, G.; Castagneto, M.; Bornstein, S.; Rubino, F. Bariatric-metabolic surgery versus conventional medical treatment in obese patients with type 2 diabetes: 5 year follow-up of an open-label, single-centre, randomised controlled trial. *Lancet* **2015**, *386*, 964–973. [CrossRef]

10. Jensen, M.D.; Ryan, D.H.; Apovian, C.M.; Ard, J.D.; Comuzzie, A.G.; Donato, K.A.; Hu, F.B.; Hubbard, V.S.; Jakicic, J.M.; Kushner, R.F.; et al. 2013 AHA/ACC/TOS guideline for the management of overweight and obesity in adults: A report of the american college of cardiology/american heart association task force on practice guidelines and the obesity society. *J. Am. Coll. Cardiol.* **2014**, *63*, 2985–3023. [CrossRef] [PubMed]

11. Cefalu, W.T.; Bray, G.A.; Home, P.D.; Garvey, W.T.; Klein, S.; Pi-Sunyer, F.X.; Hu, F.B.; Raz, I.; Van Gaal, L.; Wolfe, B.M.; et al. Advances in the science, treatment, and prevention of the disease of obesity: Reflections from a diabetes care editors' expert forum. *Diabetes Care* **2015**, *38*, 1567–1582. [CrossRef] [PubMed]

12. Atukorala, I.; Makovey, J.; Lawler, L.; Messier, S.P.; Bennell, K.; Hunter, D.J. Is there a dose-response relationship between weight loss and symptom improvement in persons with knee osteoarthritis? *Arthritis Care Res.* **2016**, *68*, 1106–1114. [CrossRef] [PubMed]

13. De Luis, D.A.; Izaola, O.; Garcia Alonso, M.; Aller, R.; Cabezas, G.; de la Fuente, B. Effect of a hypocaloric diet with a commercial formula in weight loss and quality of life in obese patients with chronic osteoarthritis. *Nutricion Hospitalaria* **2012**, *27*, 1648–1654. [PubMed]

14. Hall, K.D.; Kahan, S. Maintenance of lost weight and long-term management of obesity. *Med. Clin. N. Am.* **2018**, *102*, 183–197. [CrossRef] [PubMed]

15. Sainsbury, A.; Zhang, L. Role of the hypothalamus in the neuroendocrine regulation of body weight and composition during energy deficit. *Obes. Rev.* **2012**, *13*, 234–257. [CrossRef] [PubMed]

16. Anton, S.D.; Hida, A.; Heekin, K.; Sowalsky, K.; Karabetian, C.; Mutchie, H.; Leeuwenburgh, C.; Manini, T.M.; Barnett, T.E. Effects of popular diets without specific calorie targets on weight loss outcomes: Systematic review of findings from clinical trials. *Nutrients* **2017**, *9*, 822. [CrossRef] [PubMed]

17. Harris, L.; Hamilton, S.; Azevedo, L.B.; Olajide, J.; De Brun, C.; Waller, G.; Whittaker, V.; Sharp, T.; Lean, M.; Hankey, C.; et al. Intermittent fasting interventions for treatment of overweight and obesity in adults: A systematic review and meta-analysis. *JBI Database Syst. Rev. Implement. Rep.* **2018**, *16*, 507–547. [CrossRef] [PubMed]

18. Anderson, J.W.; Konz, E.C.; Frederich, R.C.; Wood, C.L. Long-term weight-loss maintenance: A meta-analysis of US studies. *Am. J. Clin. Nutr.* **2001**, *74*, 579–584. [CrossRef] [PubMed]

19. Delbridge, E.; Proietto, J. State of the science: Vled (very low energy diet) for obesity. *Asia Pac. J. Clin. Nutr.* **2006**, *15*, 49–54. [PubMed]

20. Mustajoki, P.; Pekkarinen, T. Very low energy diets in the treatment of obesity. *Obes. Rev.* **2001**, *2*, 61–72. [CrossRef] [PubMed]

21. Gibson, A.A.; Seimon, R.V.; Lee, C.M.; Ayre, J.; Franklin, J.; Markovic, T.P.; Caterson, I.D.; Sainsbury, A. Do ketogenic diets really suppress appetite? A systematic review and meta-analysis. *Obes. Rev.* **2015**, *16*, 64–76. [CrossRef] [PubMed]

22. Purcell, K.; Sumithran, P.; Prendergast, L.A.; Bouniu, C.J.; Delbridge, E.; Proietto, J. The effect of rate of weight loss on long-term weight management: A randomised controlled trial. *Lancet Diabetes Endocrinol.* **2014**, *2*, 954–962. [CrossRef]

23. Astrup, A.; Rossner, S. Lessons from obesity management programmes: Greater initial weight loss improves long-term maintenance. *Obes. Rev.* **2000**, *1*, 17–19. [CrossRef] [PubMed]

24. Nackers, L.M.; Ross, K.M.; Perri, M.G. The association between rate of initial weight loss and long-term success in obesity treatment: Does slow and steady win the race? *Int. J. Behav. Med.* **2010**, *17*, 161–167. [CrossRef] [PubMed]

25. Casazza, K.; Brown, A.; Astrup, A.; Bertz, F.; Baum, C.; Brown, M.B.; Dawson, J.; Durant, N.; Dutton, G.; Fields, D.A.; et al. Weighing the evidence of common beliefs in obesity research. *Crit. Rev. Food Sci. Nutr.* **2015**, *55*, 2014–2053. [CrossRef] [PubMed]

26. Casazza, K.; Fontaine, K.R.; Astrup, A.; Birch, L.L.; Brown, A.W.; Bohan Brown, M.M.; Durant, N.; Dutton, G.; Foster, E.M.; Heymsfield, S.B.; et al. Myths, presumptions, and facts about obesity. *N. Engl. J. Med.* **2013**, *368*, 446–454. [CrossRef] [PubMed]

27. Wadden, T.A.; Foster, G.D.; Letizia, K.A.; Stunkard, A.J. A multicenter evaluation of a proprietary weight reduction program for the treatment of marked obesity. *Arch. Intern. Med.* **1992**, *152*, 961–966. [CrossRef] [PubMed]

28. Purcell, K. The Rate of Weight Loss Does Not Influence Long Term Weight Maintenance. Ph.D. Thesis, The University of Melbourne, Melbourne, Australia, 2014.

29. Gibson, A.A.; Franklin, J.; Pattinson, A.L.; Cheng, Z.G.; Samman, S.; Markovic, T.P.; Sainsbury, A. Comparison of very low energy diet products available in australia and how to tailor them to optimise protein content for younger and older adult men and women. *Healthcare* **2016**, *4*, 71. [CrossRef] [PubMed]

30. Collins, C. Survey of dietetic management of overweight and obesity and comparison with best practice criteria. *Nutr. Diet.* **2003**, *60*, 177–184.

31. Da Luz, F.Q.; Hay, P.; Gibson, A.A.; Touyz, S.W.; Swinbourne, J.M.; Roekenes, J.A.; Sainsbury, A. Does severe dietary energy restriction increase binge eating in overweight or obese individuals? A systematic review. *Obes. Rev.* **2015**, *16*, 652–665. [CrossRef] [PubMed]

32. Saris, W.H. Very-low-calorie diets and sustained weight loss. *Obes. Res.* **2001**, *9* (Suppl. 4), 295S–301S. [CrossRef] [PubMed]

33. Toubro, S.; Astrup, A. Randomised comparison of diets for maintaining obese subjects' weight after major weight loss: Ad lib, low fat, high carbohydrate diet v fixed energy intake. *BMJ* **1997**, *314*, 29–34. [CrossRef] [PubMed]

34. Chaston, T.B.; Dixon, J.B.; O'Brien, P.E. Changes in fat-free mass during significant weight loss: A systematic review. *Int. J. Obes.* **2007**, *31*, 743–750. [CrossRef] [PubMed]

35. Senechal, M.; Arguin, H.; Bouchard, D.R.; Carpentier, A.C.; Ardilouze, J.L.; Dionne, I.J.; Brochu, M. Effects of rapid or slow weight loss on body composition and metabolic risk factors in obese postmenopausal women. A pilot study. *Appetite* **2012**, *58*, 831–834. [CrossRef] [PubMed]

36. Ashtary-Larky, D.; Ghanavati, M.; Lamuchi-Deli, N.; Payami, S.A.; Alavi-Rad, S.; Boustaninejad, M.; Afrisham, R.; Abbasnezhad, A.; Alipour, M. Rapid weight loss vs. Slow weight loss: Which is more effective on body composition and metabolic risk factors? *Int. J. Endocrinol. Metab.* **2017**, *15*, e13249. [CrossRef] [PubMed]

37. Garthe, I.; Raastad, T.; Refsnes, P.E.; Koivisto, A.; Sundgot-Borgen, J. Effect of two different weight-loss rates on body composition and strength and power-related performance in elite athletes. *Int. J. Sport Nutr. Exerc. Metab.* **2011**, *21*, 97–104. [CrossRef] [PubMed]

38. Bryson, J.M.; King, S.E.; Burns, C.M.; Baur, L.A.; Swaraj, S.; Caterson, I.D. Changes in glucose and lipid metabolism following weight loss produced by a very low calorie diet in obese subjects. *Int. J. Obes. Relat. Metab. Disord.* **1996**, *20*, 338–345. [PubMed]

39. Byrne, N.M.; Meerkin, J.D.; Laukkanen, R.; Ross, R.; Fogelholm, M.; Hills, A.P. Weight loss strategies for obese adults: Personalized weight management program vs. Standard care. *Obesity* **2006**, *14*, 1777–1788. [CrossRef] [PubMed]

40. McMillan-Price, J.; Petocz, P.; Atkinson, F.; O'Neill, K.; Samman, S.; Steinbeck, K.; Caterson, I.; Brand-Miller, J. Comparison of 4 diets of varying glycemic load on weight loss and cardiovascular risk reduction in overweight and obese young adults: A randomized controlled trial. *Arch. Intern. Med.* **2006**, *166*, 1466–1475. [CrossRef] [PubMed]

41. Hsu, M.S.H.; Harper, C.; Gibson, A.A.; Sweeting, A.N.; McBride, J.; Markovic, T.P.; Caterson, I.D.; Byrne, N.M.; Sainsbury, A.; Seimon, R.V. Recruitment strategies for a randomised controlled trial comparing fast versus slow weight loss in postmenopausal women with obesity—The tempo diet trial. *Healthcare (Basel)* **2018**, *6*. [CrossRef] [PubMed]

42. Cooper, C.; Melton, L.J., 3rd. Epidemiology of osteoporosis. *Trends Endocrinol. Metab.* **1992**, *3*, 224–229. [CrossRef]

43. City of Sydney. Metropolitan Sydney. Available online: www.cityofsydney.nsw.gov.au/learn/research-and-statistics/the-city-at-a-glance/metropolitan-sydney (accessed on 12 February 2017).

44. Australian Bureau of Statistics. Frequently Asked Questions: How Does the ABS Define Metropolitan and Non-Metropolitan? Available online: www.abs.gov.au/websitedbs/d3310114.nsf/home/frequently+asked+questions#Anchor8 (accessed on 12 February 2017).

45. American Diabetes Association. Diagnosis and classification of diabetes mellitus. *Diabetes Care* **2014**, *37* (Suppl. 1), S81–S90.

46. Australian Government National Health and Medical Research Council. Healthy Eating for Adults. 2013. Available online: http://www.eatforhealth.gov.au/sites/default/files/files/ (accessed on 20 June 2018).

47. Gibson, A.A.; Seimon, R.V.; Franklin, J.; Markovic, T.P.; Byrne, N.M.; Manson, E.; Caterson, I.D.; Sainsbury, A. Fast versus slow weight loss: Development process and rationale behind the dietary interventions for the tempo diet trial. *Obes. Sci. Pract.* **2016**, *2*, 162–173. [CrossRef] [PubMed]

48. Chan, A.W.; Tetzlaff, J.M.; Gotzsche, P.C.; Altman, D.G.; Mann, H.; Berlin, J.A.; Dickersin, K.; Hrobjartsson, A.; Schulz, K.F.; Parulekar, W.R.; et al. Spirit 2013 explanation and elaboration: Guidance for protocols of clinical trials. *BMJ* **2013**, *346*, e7586. [CrossRef] [PubMed]

49. Toombs, R.J.; Ducher, G.; Shepherd, J.A.; De Souza, M.J. The impact of recent technological advances on the trueness and precision of dxa to assess body composition. *Obesity* **2012**, *20*, 30–39. [CrossRef] [PubMed]

50. Ritz, P.; Salle, A.; Audran, M.; Rohmer, V. Comparison of different methods to assess body composition of weight loss in obese and diabetic patients. *Diabetes Res. Clin. Pract.* **2007**, *77*, 405–411. [CrossRef] [PubMed]

51. Pourhassan, M.; Schautz, B.; Braun, W.; Gluer, C.C.; Bosy-Westphal, A.; Muller, M.J. Impact of body-composition methodology on the composition of weight loss and weight gain. *Eur. J. Clin. Nutr.* **2013**, *67*, 446–454. [CrossRef] [PubMed]

52. Wang, Z.; Pi-Sunyer, F.X.; Kotler, D.P.; Wielopolski, L.; Withers, R.T.; Pierson, R.N., Jr.; Heymsfield, S.B. Multicomponent methods: Evaluation of new and traditional soft tissue mineral models by in vivo neutron activation analysis. *Am. J. Clin. Nutr.* **2002**, *76*, 968–974. [CrossRef] [PubMed]

53. Schoeller, D.A.; van Santen, E.; Peterson, D.W.; Dietz, W.; Jaspan, J.; Klein, P.D. Total body water measurement in humans with 18O and 2H labeled water. *Am. J. Clin. Nutr.* **1980**, *33*, 2686–2693. [CrossRef] [PubMed]

54. Roberts, H.C.; Denison, H.J.; Martin, H.J.; Patel, H.P.; Syddall, H.; Cooper, C.; Sayer, A.A. A review of the measurement of grip strength in clinical and epidemiological studies: Towards a standardised approach. *Age Ageing* **2011**, *40*, 423–429. [CrossRef] [PubMed]

55. Ross, R.; Berentzen, T.; Bradshaw, A.J.; Janssen, I.; Kahn, H.S.; Katzmarzyk, P.T.; Kuk, J.L.; Seidell, J.C.; Snijder, M.B.; Sorensen, T.I.; et al. Does the relationship between waist circumference, morbidity and mortality depend on measurement protocol for waist circumference? *Obes. Rev.* **2008**, *9*, 312–325. [CrossRef] [PubMed]

56. Johnson, N.A.; Walton, D.W.; Sachinwalla, T.; Thompson, C.H.; Smith, K.; Ruell, P.A.; Stannard, S.R.; George, J. Noninvasive assessment of hepatic lipid composition: Advancing understanding and management of fatty liver disorders. *Hepatology* **2008**, *47*, 1513–1523. [CrossRef] [PubMed]

57. Vanhamme, L.; van den Boogaart, A.; Van Huffel, S. Improved method for accurate and efficient quantification of mrs data with use of prior knowledge. *J. Magn. Reson.* **1997**, *129*, 35–43. [CrossRef] [PubMed]

58. Touboul, P.J.; Hennerici, M.G.; Meairs, S.; Adams, H.; Amarenco, P.; Bornstein, N.; Csiba, L.; Desvarieux, M.; Ebrahim, S.; Hernandez Hernandez, R.; et al. Mannheim carotid intima-media thickness and plaque consensus (2004-2006-2011). An update on behalf of the advisory board of the 3rd, 4th and 5th watching the risk symposia, at the 13th, 15th and 20th European stroke conferences, Mannheim, Germany, 2004, Brussels, Belgium, 2006, And Hamburg, Germany, 2011. *Cerebrovasc. Dis.* **2012**, *34*, 290–296. [PubMed]

59. Fairburn, C. *Cognitive Behavior Therapy and Eating Disorders*; Guilford: New York, NY, USA, 2008.

60. Beglin, S.J.; Fairburn, C.G. Evaluation of a new instrument for the detection of eating disorders in community samples. *Psychiatry Res.* **1992**, *44*, 191–201. [CrossRef]

61. Mond, J.M.; Hay, P.J.; Rodgers, B.; Owen, C.; Beumont, P.J. Validity of the eating disorder examination questionnaire (EDE-Q) in screening for eating disorders in community samples. *Behav. Res. Ther.* **2004**, *42*, 551–567. [CrossRef]

62. Goldfein, J.A.; Devlin, M.J.; Kamenetz, C. Eating disorder examination-questionnaire with and without instruction to assess binge eating in patients with binge eating disorder. *Int. J. Eat. Disord.* **2005**, *37*, 107–111. [CrossRef] [PubMed]

63. Palavras, M.A.; Hay, P.J.; Lujic, S.; Claudino, A.M. Comparing symptomatic and functional outcomes over 5 years in two nonclinical cohorts characterized by binge eating with and without objectively large episodes. *Int. J. Eat. Dis.* **2015**, *48*, 1158–1165. [CrossRef] [PubMed]

64. American Psychiatric Association. *Diagnostic and Statistical Manual of Mental Disorders: Fifth Edition*, 5th ed.; American Psychiatric Association: Washington, DC, USA, 2013.

65. Latner, J.D.; Mond, J.M.; Kelly, M.C.; Haynes, S.N.; Hay, P.J. The loss of control over eating scale: Development and psychometric evaluation. *Int. J. Eat. Disord.* **2014**, *47*, 647–659. [CrossRef] [PubMed]

66. Cappelleri, J.C.; Bushmakin, A.G.; Gerber, R.A.; Leidy, N.K.; Sexton, C.C.; Lowe, M.R.; Karlsson, J. Psychometric analysis of the three-factor eating questionnaire-r21: Results from a large diverse sample of obese and non-obese participants. *Int. J. Obes.* **2009**, *33*, 611–620. [CrossRef] [PubMed]

67. Stunkard, A.J.; Messick, S. The three-factor eating questionnaire to measure dietary restraint, disinhibition and hunger. *J. Psychosom. Res.* **1985**, *29*, 71–83. [CrossRef]

68. Burton, A.L.; Abbott, M.J.; Modini, M.; Touyz, S. Psychometric evaluation of self-report measures of binge-eating symptoms and related psychopathology: A systematic review of the literature. *Int. J. Eat. Disord.* **2016**, *49*, 123–140. [CrossRef] [PubMed]

69. Van Strien, T.; Frijters, J.E.R.; Bergers, G.P.A.; Defares, P.B. The dutch eating behavior questionnaire (DEBQ) for assessment of restrained, emotional, and external eating behavior. *Int. J. Eat. Disord.* **1986**, *5*, 295–315. [CrossRef]

70. Van Strien, T. *DEBQ Dutch Eating Behaviour Questionnaire Manual*; Boom Test Publishers: Amsterdam, The Netherlands, 2010.

71. Sheehan, D.; Janavs, J.; Baker, R.; Sheehan, K.H.; Knapp, E.; Sheehan, M. Mini International Neuropsychiatric Interview—Version 7.0.0 DSM-5. 2015. Available online: www.medical-outcomes.com (accessed on 10 July 2018).

72. Rosenberg, M. *Society and the Adolescent Self-Image*; Princeton University Press: Princeton, NJ, USA, 1965.

73. Ware, J.E., Jr.; Sherbourne, C.D. The mos 36-item short-form health survey (SF-36). I. Conceptual framework and item selection. *Med. Care* **1992**, *30*, 473–483. [CrossRef] [PubMed]

74. Lovibond, S.H.; Lovibond, P.F. *Manual for the Depression Anxiety Stress Scales*, 2nd ed.; Psychology Foundation: Sydney, NSW, Australia, 1995.

75. Henry, J.D.; Crawford, J.R. The short-form version of the depression anxiety stress scales (DASS-21): Construct validity and normative data in a large non-clinical sample. *Br. J. Clin. Psychol.* **2005**, *44*, 227–239. [CrossRef] [PubMed]

76. Antony, M.M.; Bieling, P.J.; Cox, B.J.; Enns, M.W.; Swinson, R.P. Psychometric properties of the 42-item and 21-item versions of the depression anxiety stress scales in clinical groups and a community sample. *Psychol. Assess.* **1998**, *10*, 176–181. [CrossRef]

77. Haigh, E.; Moore, M.; Kashdan, T.; Fresco, D. Examination of the factor structure and concurrent validity of the langer mindfulness/mindlessness scale. *Assessment* **2011**, *18*, 11–26. [CrossRef] [PubMed]

78. Bodner, T.E. On the Assessment of Individual Differences in Mindful Information Processing. Ph.D. Thesis, Harvard University, Cambridge, MA, USA, 2000.

79. Baer, R.A.; Smith, G.T.; Hopkins, J.; Krietemeyer, J.; Toney, L. Using self-report assessment methods to explore facets of mindfulness. *Assessment* **2006**, *13*, 27–45. [CrossRef] [PubMed]

80. John, O.P.; Naumann, L.P.; Soto, C.J. *Paradigm Shift to the Integrative Big-Five Trait Taxonomy: History, Measurement, and Conceptual Issues*; Guilford Press: New York, NY, USA, 2008.

81. John, O.P.; Donahue, E.M.; Kentle, R.L. *The Big Five Inventory—Versions 4a and 54*; University of California: Berkeley, CA, USA, 1991.

82. Benet-Martinez, V.; John, O.P. Los cinco grandes across cultures and ethnic groups: Multitrait multimethod analyses of the big five in Spanish and English. *J. Personal. Soc. Psychol.* **1998**, *75*, 729–750. [CrossRef]

83. Basiotis, P.P.; Welsh, S.O.; Cronin, F.J.; Kelsay, J.L.; Mertz, W. Number of days of food intake records required to estimate individual and group nutrient intakes with defined confidence. *J. Nutr.* **1987**, *117*, 1638–1641. [CrossRef] [PubMed]

84. Nijs, I.M.; Franken, I.H.; Muris, P. The modified trait and state food-cravings questionnaires: Development and validation of a general index of food craving. *Appetite* **2007**, *49*, 38–46. [CrossRef] [PubMed]

85. Bandura, A. *Guide for Constructing Self-Efficacy Scales*; Pajares, F., Urdan, T., Eds.; Information Age Publishing: Greenwich, CT, USA, 2006.

86.   Glynn, S.M.; Ruderman, A.J. The development and validation of an eating self-efficacy scale. *Cognit. Ther. Res.* **1986**, *10*, 403–420. [CrossRef]

87.   Gibbons, C.; Caudwell, P.; Finlayson, G.; King, N.; Blundell, J. Validation of a new hand-held electronic data capture method for continuous monitoring of subjective appetite sensations. *Int. J. Behav. Nutr. Phys. Act.* **2011**, *8*, 57. [CrossRef] [PubMed]

88.   Donnelly, J.E.; Blair, S.N.; Jakicic, J.M.; Manore, M.M.; Rankin, J.W.; Smith, B.K. American college of sports medicine position stand. Appropriate physical activity intervention strategies for weight loss and prevention of weight regain for adults. *Med. Sci. Sports Exerc.* **2009**, *41*, 459–471. [CrossRef] [PubMed]

89.   BaHammam, A.; Alrajeh, M.; Albabtain, M.; Bahammam, S.; Sharif, M. Circadian pattern of sleep, energy expenditure, and body temperature of young healthy men during the intermittent fasting of ramadan. *Appetite* **2010**, *54*, 426–429. [CrossRef] [PubMed]

90.   Johns, M.W. A new method for measuring daytime sleepiness: The epworth sleepiness scale. *Sleep* **1991**, *14*, 540–545. [CrossRef] [PubMed]

91.   Johns, M.W. Reliability and factor analysis of the epworth sleepiness scale. *Sleep* **1992**, *15*, 376–381. [CrossRef] [PubMed]

92.   Buysse, D.J.; Reynolds, C.F., 3rd; Monk, T.H.; Berman, S.R.; Kupfer, D.J. The pittsburgh sleep quality index: A new instrument for psychiatric practice and research. *Psychiatry Res.* **1989**, *28*, 193–213. [CrossRef]

93.   Byrne, N.M.; Wood, R.E.; Schutz, Y.; Hills, A.P. Does metabolic compensation explain the majority of less-than-expected weight loss in obese adults during a short-term severe diet and exercise intervention? *Int. J. Obes.* **2012**, *36*, 1472–1478. [CrossRef] [PubMed]

94.   Landsberg, L. Core temperature: A forgotten variable in energy expenditure and obesity? *Obes. Rev.* **2012**, *13* (Suppl. 2), 97–104. [CrossRef] [PubMed]

# 6

# Associations between Parents' Health Literacy and Sleeping Hours in Children

**Hiroto Ogi** [1,2], **Daisuke Nakamura** [2,3], **Masato Ogawa** [2,3,4], **Teruhiko Nakamura** [5] and
**Kazuhiro P. Izawa** [2,3,*]

[1] Department of Physical Therapy, Faculty of Health Sciences, Kobe University School of Medicine,
7-10-2 Tomogaoka, Suma-ku, Kobe 654-0142, Japan; ogihiroto6062@gmail.com

[2] Cardiovascular stroke Renal Project (CRP), 7-10-2 Tomogaoka, Suma-ku, Kobe 654-0142, Japan;
nakadai525@gmail.com (D.N.); mogawa@med.kobe-u.ac.jp (M.O.)

[3] Department of International Health, Graduate School of Health Sciences, Kobe University,
7-10-2 Tomogaoka, Suma-ku, Kobe 654-0142, Japan

[4] Division of Rehabilitation Medicine, Kobe University Hospital, 7-5-2 Kusunoki-cho, Chuo-ku,
Kobe 650-0017, Japan

[5] Educational Corporation Tsukushi Gakuen, 2-3-11 Takadai, Chitose 066-0035, Japan;
nakamura_00_00@yahoo.co.jp

* Correspondence: izawapk@harbor.kobe-u.ac.jp

**Abstract:** Background: Sleep in preschool children is an important factor for their health and active lives. The lack of adequate sleep in preschool children is a serious public problem in Japan. The relationship between health literacy (HL) and health status is well recognized. The purpose of this study was to investigate the association between the sleep duration of preschool children and the HL of their parents. Methods: In the present study, participants were preschool children (3–6 years) and their parents. We assessed the HL of the parents with the 14-item Health Literacy Scale (HLS-14) questionnaire. Sleep duration of the children was reported by their parents. We divided parents into two groups according to HLS-14 score and analyzed children's sleeping time separately. Results: Data from 279 parents and their children were ultimately analyzed. The high HL group comprised 210 families (75.3%) and the low HL group comprised 69 families (24.7%). Average children's sleep duration was significantly longer in the high HL group (9.5 ± 0.9 h) than in the low HL group (9.1 ± 1.1 h) ($p = 0.013$). A positive correlation was found in the low HL group between parents' HL and their children's sleeping times ($p < 0.01$, r = 0.32) but the difference was not significant in the high HL group ($p = 0.98$, r = −0.0009). Conclusion: The HL of parents appears to affect their children's sleep duration, suggesting that parental HL may be an appropriate target for interventions aiming to lengthen children's sleeping time.

**Keywords:** parents' health literacy; sleeping hours; children

## 1. Introduction

Short sleep duration has been linked to a wide array of poor mental and physical health outcomes [1]. In children, sleep has a significant influence on developmental outcomes and is commonly overlooked as an ecological influence on their development [2]. Previous studies suggested that the shortening of nocturnal sleep is associated with cardiac autonomic hypofunction and low systolic blood pressure in preschool children [3,4]. In addition, the poor sleep schedules of preschool-aged children were found to predict behavioral problems during the primary school years [5]. Sleep problems of 5–6-year-olds have been associated with poor behavior, obesity and negative secondary effects on maternal and family well-being [6]. Collectively, sleep in preschool children is an important factor for their health and active lives.

Adequate sleeping time for children has not been fully elucidated but the National Sleep Foundation (NSF) in the US proposed sleep duration recommendations for preschool-aged children (3–5 years) of 10–13 h [7]. In contrast, the lack of sleep in preschool children is a serious public health problem in Japan. A previous study in Japan showed that the percentage of children aged 3.5 years old who slept for less than 10 h was 39.5% [8]. Another study in Japan suggested that the percentage of preschool children who went to sleep before 9 p.m. was only around 15% (3 years old: 14.6%, 4 years old: 16.9%, 5–6 years old: 12.9%) [9], suggesting insufficient sleep duration in the majority of Japanese preschoolers. It is interesting to note that children's bedtime correlated with their parent's bedtime in Japan [10]. This study suggested that parents' inadequate sleeping and life habits were associated with their children's insufficient sleep duration. Thus, parents can have a great influence on their children's sleep duration.

The relation between health literacy (HL) and health status is now well recognized and better understood [11]. HL is defined as a person's ability to access, understand, evaluate, communicate and use health information to make decisions for one's health [12]. According to previous studies, an adult's low HL has been associated with their own insufficient health status and insufficient health outcomes [13,14] and parents' low HL has also been associated with insufficient health outcomes for their children [15–19]. Previous studies in Japan suggested that the people with higher HL were positively associated with adult healthy lifestyle characteristics [20] and that people with insomnia were less likely to seek help for their problem [21].

Improvement of parents' HL encourages improvement of their own lives and sleep habits and it may help to improve the sleep duration of their children. Thus, it is important to investigate the association between parents' HL and their children's sleep duration in Japan. Although one study in the US investigated the association between parents' HL and children's sleep issues [22], due to the lack of knowledge on this subject in Japan, no consensus has been reached on parents' HL and their children's sleep issues. Therefore, the hypothesis of the present study was that the low HL of parents would be associated with the insufficient sleep duration of their children. The purpose of this study was to investigate the association between the sleep duration of preschool children and the HL of their parents in Japan.

## 2. Methods

### 2.1. Participants

This was a multicenter cross-sectional cohort study using a convenience sample. The participants included preschool children (3–6 years old) and their parents who lived in Chitose city, Hokkaido, Japan. They attended kindergarten, nursery school, or a center for early childhood education and care: two kindergartens, one nursery school and one center for early childhood education and care. To invite them to participate, we asked the school staff to distribute materials that included the intention of the study, the consent for participation in the study, the withdrawal of consent to participate and the questionnaire to parents in September 2016. If the parents had more than one child in the same school, we asked them to answer the questionnaire for their oldest child. We excluded parents for whom a questionnaire had missing values. Participants voluntarily provided written informed consent. This study received prior approval from the Research Ethics Committee of Kobe University (approval number 498).

### 2.2. Demographic and Socioeconomic Characteristics

The following demographic and socioeconomic characteristics were investigated: parent sex; parent age; parent height and weight; parent alcohol and smoking behavior; marital status, married or not; education level (up to high school, 2-year college or vocational college, college graduate or above);

household income level (<5 million yen, ≥5 million yen); child age; child birthweight; and number of siblings.

### 2.3. Health Literacy of Parents

We assessed the HL of parents with the 14-item Health Literacy Scale (HLS-14) questionnaire, which was created in Japan (Table 1) [23]. A previous study on the HLS-14 indicated that it is an adequate questionnaire with which to evaluate comprehensive HL [24]. Every question is estimated at 5 stages. The total score is calculated by totaling the scores of all answers. The scores range from 14 to 70 and were analyzed as continuous variables. The higher the score, the better the comprehensive HL is. The validity and reliability of this method was already shown [23]. We divided the participants into two groups according to an HLS-14 score >50 (high HL group) and an HLS-14 score <50 (low HL group) [23,25].

**Table 1.** The 14-item Health Literacy Scale.

| | When you read instructions or leaflets from hospitals or pharmacies, how do you agree or disagree about the following? | | | | |
|---|---|---|---|---|---|
| | | Strongly Disagree | Disagree | Not Sure | Agree | Strongly Agree |
| 1 | I find characters that I cannot read | 5 | 4 | 3 | 2 | 1 |
| 2 | The print is too small for me (even though I wear glasses) | 5 | 4 | 3 | 2 | 1 |
| 3 | The content is too difficult for me | 5 | 4 | 3 | 2 | 1 |
| 4 | It takes a long time to read them | 5 | 4 | 3 | 2 | 1 |
| 5 | I need someone to help me read them | 5 | 4 | 3 | 2 | 1 |
| | If you are diagnosed as having a disease and you have little information about the disease and its treatment, how to you agree or disagree about the following? | | | | |
| | | Strongly Disagree | Disagree | Not sure | Agree | Strongly Agree |
| 6 | I collect information from various sources | 1 | 2 | 3 | 4 | 5 |
| 7 | I extract the information I want | 1 | 2 | 3 | 4 | 5 |
| 8 | I understand the obtained information | 1 | 2 | 3 | 4 | 5 |
| 9 | I tell my opinion about my illness to my doctor, family or friends | 1 | 2 | 3 | 4 | 5 |
| 10 | I apply the obtained information to my daily life | 1 | 2 | 3 | 4 | 5 |
| | If you are diagnosed as having a disease and you can obtain information about the disease and its treatment how do you agree or disagree about the following? | | | | |
| | | Strongly Disagree | Disagree | Not sure | Agree | Strongly Agree |
| 11 | I consider whether the information if applicable to me | 1 | 2 | 3 | 4 | 5 |
| 12 | I consider whether the information is credible | 1 | 2 | 3 | 4 | 5 |
| 13 | I check whether the information is valid and reliable | 1 | 2 | 3 | 4 | 5 |
| 14 | I collect information to make my healthcare decisions | 1 | 2 | 3 | 4 | 5 |

Table taken from Ref. [23].

### 2.4. Children's Sleeping Duration

Although sleep duration is a continuous variable, it can be difficult for participants to provide the time in minutes and seconds. Therefore, we asked the parents to provide their average children's sleeping hours and minutes per day during the previous one month.

### 2.5. Statistical Analysis

The differences in the clinical characteristics between the low and the high HL groups were determined by the Student $t$-test or Mann-Whitney U test. Pearson correlation analysis was performed to compare the parents' HL and the children's sleeping times. The median HL score of the HLS-14 in Japanese adults was 50 points [23]. Furthermore, the trend of the children's sleeping time was greatly different at 50 points or less. As such, to investigate the parent's HL and their child's sleeping time in detail, we divided the parents' HL into two groups according to a score above or below 50 points on the HLS-14 and analyzed children's sleeping time separately. All statistical analyses were performed using EZR (Saitama Medical Center, Jichi Medical University, Saitama, Japan), which is a graphical user interface for R (The R Foundation for Statistical Computing, Vienna, Austria). Differences and correlations were considered significant when $p < 0.05$.

## 3. Results

Figure 1 shows participant flow during this study. The original response rate of the target population was 68.9% (351/509) but after the 72 parents were excluded, the final response rate was 54.8% of the target population).

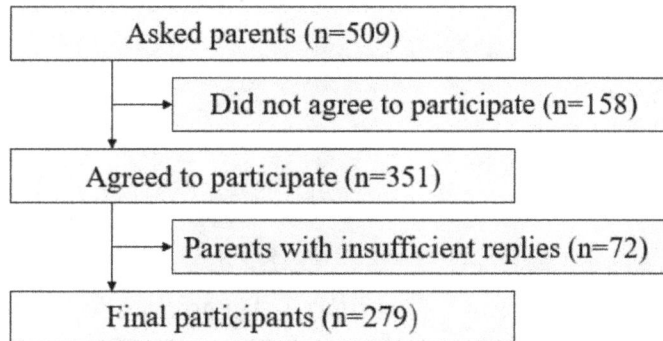

**Figure 1.** Chart of participant flow during the study.

Table 2 shows the demographic differences between the low HL group and high HL group. The number of participants in the high HL group was 210 (75.3%) and that in the low HL group was 69 (24.7%). The average sleep duration of the children was 9.4 ± 0.9 h and it was significantly longer in the high HL group (9.5 ± 0.9 h) than in the low HL group (9.1 ± 1.1 h) ($p = 0.01$). In addition, the number of siblings ($p = 0.03$), parent's age ($p = 0.05$) and the percentage of females ($p = 0.01$) were greater in the high HL group than in the low HL group.

The correlation between parents' HL and children's sleeping times is shown in Figures 2 and 3. In the low HL group, a positive correlation was shown between the parents' HL and children's sleeping times ($p = 0.01$, r = 0.32). However, in high HL group, there were no statistically significant differences between parents' HL and children's sleeping times ($p = 0.98$, r = $-0.0009$).

**Table 2.** Characteristics Differences between the High Health Literacy and Low Health Literacy Groups.

| Characteristic | Total (n = 279) | High Health Literacy Group (n = 210) | Low Health Literacy Group (n = 69) | t-Value or $\chi^2$ Value * | p Value |
|---|---|---|---|---|---|
| **Child** | | | | | |
| Age (months) | 56.4 ± 10.0 | 56.3 ± 9.9 | 56.6 ± 10.6 | −0.15 | 0.88 |
| Sex (girls) | 119 (42.7%) | 89 (42.3%) | 30 (43.4%) | 0.15 * | 0.87 |
| BMI (kg/m$^2$) | 15.6 ± 1.3 | 15.5 ± 1.2 | 15.7 ± 1.6 | −0.65 | 0.52 |
| Birth weight (g) | 3012.0 ± 451.1 | 2995.3 ± 431.8 | 3063.7 ± 506.2 | −1.09 | 0.28 |
| Number of siblings (n) | 1.2 ± 0.8 | 1.3 ± 0.8 | 1.1 ± 0.8 | 2.20 * | 0.03 |
| Sleep duration (Continuous h) | 9.4 ± 0.9 | 9.5 ± 0.9 | 9.1 ± 1.1 | 2.50 | 0.01 |
| Breakfast (everyday eater) | 261 (93.6%) | 199 (94.8%) | 62 (89.6%) | 1.47 * | 0.14 |
| **Parent** | | | | | |
| Age (years) | 36.2 ± 5.1 | 35.9 ± 5.2 | 37.2 ± 4.9 | −2.02 | 0.05 |
| Sex (female) | 258 (92.4%) | 199 (94.7%) | 59 (85.5%) | 2.58 * | 0.01 |
| BMI (kg/m$^2$) | 21.1 ± 2.9 | 21.1 ± 2.8 | 21.1 ± 3.1 | −0.19 | 0.85 |
| Marital status (married) | 258 (92.4%) | 195 (92.8%) | 63 (91.3%) | 0.70 * | 0.50 |
| Education (years) | 13.3 ± 1.6 | 13.3 ± 1.6 | 13.2 ± 1.7 | −0.59 | 0.56 |
| Household income <5 million Yen (n) | 143 (51.3%) | 111 (52.9%) | 32 (46.4%) | 0.93 * | 0.35 |
| Alcohol consumption (non-everyday drinker) | 255 (91.4%) | 193 (91.9%) | 62 (89.9%) | 1.02 * | 0.31 |
| Smoking behavior (non-smoking) | 225 (80.6%) | 170 (81.0%) | 55 (79.7%) | 0.22 * | 0.82 |
| Sleep duration (h) | 6.4 ± 1.1 | 6.4 ± 1.2 | 6.4 ± 1.1 | −0.53 | 0.60 |

The study subjects were divided into two groups according to a total health literacy score of above or below the cutoff value of 50. Data are expressed as mean ± standard deviation or number (percentage). BMI, body mass index.

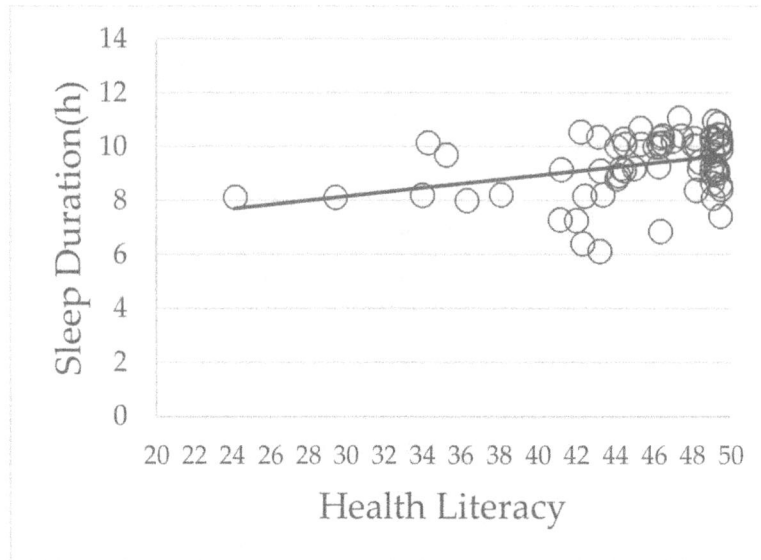

**Figure 2.** The correlation between parents' health literacy and their children's sleep duration in the low health literacy group. The *p* value was 0.01 and the correlation coefficient (r) was 0.32.

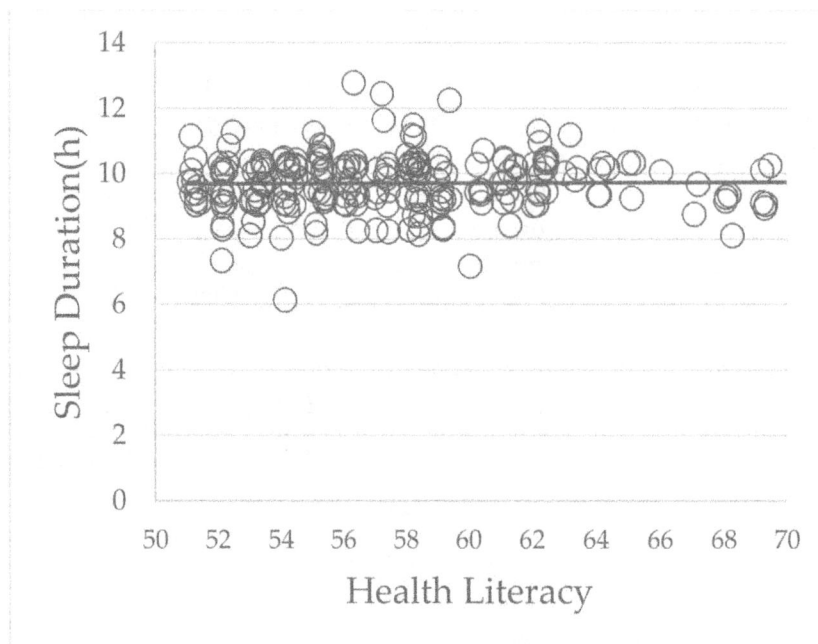

**Figure 3.** The correlation between parents' health literacy and their children's sleep duration in the high health literacy group. The *p* value was 0.98 and the correlation coefficient (r) was 0.0009.

## 4. Discussion

This is the first study, to our knowledge, to show that parents' comprehensive HL correlated positively with the sleep duration of their children in Japan. Moreover, this correlation was observed only in the low HL group. A similar study in the US suggested that if the parents' functional HL was low, the sleep duration of their children was likely to be short [22]. In the Japanese population, even though the level of functional HL is high [24], comprehensive HL is relatively lower than that of other populations [26]. In the present study, comprehensive HL was assessed with the HLS-14, so this study should have great significance in Japan.

There are three possible explanations for the observed associations between parents' HL and their child's sleep duration in this study. First, Japanese parents with low HL may not be able to access health and medical professionals to obtain the appropriate health information of their children. One study suggested that those with low (vs. adequate) HL were significantly less likely to access health information about their children [27]. Second, Japanese parents with low HL may not be able to understand the importance of sleep for their children. Parents, particularly pregnant and new mothers, rely on obstetric and pediatric providers, along with parenting books and online sources, for information on common parenting questions, especially with respect to their children's sleep [28]. Another study suggested that parents with low HL also have greater difficulty understanding and acting on health recommendations [14,18]. Thus, if the parents' HL is low in Japan, they may less likely to understand the health information pertaining to their children. Third, parenting behavior may be associated with the sleep duration of children in Japan. It was already proven that parental intervention positively influenced developmentally appropriate bedtime routines, sleep-related behaviors and sleep duration of infants [29]. Another study indicated that low parent HL has been linked to poor parenting practices and to inadequate parenting behavior such as putting a TV in the room where their child sleeps [22]. Lo suggested that it was easy for preschool-aged children without a bedtime TV-viewing habit to have an adequate quantity of sleep [30]. Thus, we believe that low HL in some Japanese parents may result in poor parenting, which may then be associated with the sleep duration of their preschool children. However, we did not investigate variables relevant to childhood development, sleep quality and individual family patterns of sleep behaviors, which are significant factors for sleep in children and the issue of poor parenting. Therefore, additional study is needed to investigate this association in the future.

The results of the present study are not consistent with other previous studies that showed significant relationships between the low HL of parents and their own insufficient sleep duration [21], high body mass index (BMI) and drinking and smoking behaviors [31,32]. A possible explanation is that most (92.4%) of the participating parents in the present study were mothers. An earlier study suggested that the HL of Japanese women was not associated with their healthy lifestyle characteristics, such as alcohol consumption, smoking behavior, exercise frequency, obesity (BMI), sleep duration, breakfast and snacking between meals [20]. Also, the results of the present study are not consistent with other previous studies that showed significant relationships between the low HL of parents and their own low educational level. A possible explanation for this is that the proportion of parents whose education was at high school or 2-year college level was extremely high (81.7%). Moreover, we regarded education level as a continuous variable in our analysis. Consequently, we found no significant relationships between the low HL of the parents and their own health behaviors such as those listed above and their own low educational level.

However, parents' sex and age and the number of siblings were associated with the parents' HL. There are two possible explanations for these observed associations with parents' sex. First, we think the difference is related to the material used by men or women to obtain health information. A previous study suggested that more women get nutritional information from books/magazines or from health professionals, whereas more men get this information from their friends [33]. Second, it is easier for mothers than fathers to have good relations with their neighbors, with whom they can talk about health. In Japan, almost all domestic work and child care is performed by mothers and there are almost no cases of a father doing such tasks. Therefore, we think that it is easier for a mother than a father to form relationships in which information on the health of their children can be shared with their friends or neighbors. The reason that the HL of young parents was significantly higher than that of older parents relates to the greater percentage of men in the low HL group than in the high HL group. In 2010, the average age of first marriage was 30.5 years in Japanese men and 28.8 years in Japanese women. So, the age of the men in the low HL group, which had a proportionately greater number of men, was high. Finally, we consider the reason for the association with the number of siblings. In Chitose, every child undergoes five yearly checkups, from years 1 to 5, so parents with more than one child have more chances to obtain information about their children's health. As well, when they raise more than one child, they can put the knowledge and methods learned to resolve various health problems.

According to Figures 2 and 3, parents' higher HL scores were associated with longer sleep duration of their children only in the low HL group. A previous study showed that Japanese adults with lower HLS-14 scores were significantly less likely to recognize problems such as the risk of illness, the need for preventive action and the reluctance to take preventive action in compliance with their doctor's advice [25]. In other words, parents with low HL were less likely to understand and use health information to make decisions for their own or their children's health. In contrast, parents with high HL were more likely to have these abilities. Consequently, parents' HL correlated positively with children's sleep duration only in the low HL group. This result suggested that to improve the sleep duration of preschool children, parents with low HL need to be open to all interventions. However, the positive correlation between parents' low HL and the reduced sleep duration in their children was weak ($r = 0.32$; $r < 0.4$, weak; $r \geq 0.4$ but $r < 0.6$, moderate; $r \geq 0.6$ but $r < 0.8$, strong [34]). Therefore, there is a need for further studies to confirm our findings in a larger population and to determine a causal relationship between parents' HL and their children's sleep duration.

There are some limitations in this study. First, this is a cross-sectional study and thus, we cannot determine the causality of various factors. Second, we collected data in only one small area of Japan, so the results obtained may not apply to other parts of Japan or the world. Third, the sample size was small, so we did not perform multivariate analysis to adjust for potential confounding factors. Moreover, we did not detect cut off points of HL. Fourth, The HLS-14 has been used for an adult population in previous studies, not for an adult parent population. Fifth, it could be possible that the parents who did not agree to participate had relatively had low HL compared with those who did participate. Sixth, previous studies suggested that long naps affect nighttime sleep patterns [35,36] and the quality of sleep [37]. Not only the total sleeping time but also the quality of the sleep is important [38–42]. However, we did not collect information relevant to childhood development, sleep quality and individual family patterns of sleep behavior, which are significant factors for the sleep of children and the issue of poor parenting. Also, we did not investigate factors that are important variables relating to childhood development, sleep quality, sleep behaviors, sleep duration such as parents' working patterns, dwelling and residential conditions, location of sleep of the children, parent and child health, physical activity and screen time. Seventh, one study suggested that parents tended to overestimate the sleep duration of their children [43] and this study used a parent-reported questionnaire. Eighth, an important variable that relates to sleep duration would also include sleep location of the child but we did not specifically investigate this.

Finally, it is important to go to sleep at a regular time [10,44–46] but we also did not collect this information. Therefore, even though the duration of sleep may be long, the quality of the sleep is unknown.

## 5. Conclusions

There was a statistically significant difference between parents' HL and the sleep duration of their preschool children. A weak positive correlation between parents' HL and their children's sleep duration was observed only in the low HL group. These results suggested that parental HL may be an appropriate target for interventions aiming to lengthen children's sleeping time. In the future, prospective and longitudinal studies to investigate the clinical effects of parents' HL will be warranted.

**Acknowledgments:** We are indebted to the large number of parents and children and the school staff of Tsukushi Gakuen in Hokkaido, Japan for their agreement to take part and cooperate in this study. This study was benefitted by the support and encouragement of Taku Shinoda (Kobe University Graduate School of Health Sciences, Kobe University), Masashi Kanai (Kobe University Graduate School of Health Sciences) and Masahiro Kitamura (Kobe University Graduate School of Health Sciences).

**Author Contributions:** Hiroto Ogi and Daisuke Nakamura conceptualized and designed the study, collected data, drafted the initial manuscript and approved the final manuscript as submitted; Masato Ogawa carried out the initial analyses, reviewed and revised the manuscript and approved the final manuscript as submitted; Teruhiko Nakamura collected data and approved the final manuscript as submitted; Kazuhiro P. Izawa reviewed and revised the manuscript and approved the final manuscript as submitted; All authors approved the final manuscript as submitted and agree to be accountable for all aspects of the work.

## Abbreviations

| | |
|---|---|
| CI | confidence interval |
| HL | health literacy |
| HLS-14 | 14-item Health Literacy Scale |
| NSF | National Sleep Foundation |

## References

1. Dietch, J.R.; Taylor, D.J.; Smyth, J.M.; Ahn, C.; Smith, T.W.; Uchino, B.N.; Allison, M.; Ruiz, J.M. Gender and racial/ethnic differences in sleep duration in the North Texas heart study. *Sleep Health* **2017**, *3*, 324–327. [CrossRef] [PubMed]

2. Schlieber, M.; Han, J. The sleeping patterns of Head Start children and the influence on developmental outcomes. *Child Care Health Dev.* **2017**. [CrossRef] [PubMed]

3. Sampei, M.; Dakeishi, M.; Wood, D.C.; Murata, K. Impact of total sleep duration on blood pressure in preschool children. *Biomed. Res.* **2006**, *27*, 111–115. [CrossRef] [PubMed]

4. Sampei, M.; Murata, K.; Dakeishi, M.; Wood, D.C. Cardiac autonomic hypofunction in preschool children with short nocturnal sleep. *Tohoku J. Exp. Med.* **2006**, *208*, 235–242. [CrossRef] [PubMed]

5. Kobayashi, K.; Yorifuji, T.; Yamakawa, M.; Oka, M.; Inoue, S.; Yoshinaga, H.; Doi, H. Poor toddler-age sleep schedules predict school-age behavioral disorders in a longitudinal survey. *Brain Dev.* **2015**, *37*, 572–578. [CrossRef] [PubMed]

6. Bathory, E.; Tomopoulos, S. Sleep Regulation, Physiology and Development, Sleep Duration and Patterns, and Sleep Hygiene in Infants, Toddlers, and Preschool-Age Children. *Curr. Probl. Pediatr. Adolesc. Health Care* **2017**, *47*, 29–42. [CrossRef] [PubMed]

7. Hirshkowitz, M.; Whiton, K.; Albert, S.M.; Alessi, C.; Bruni, O.; DonCarlos, L.; Hazen, N.; Herman, J.; Katz, E.S.; Kheirandish-Gozal, L.; et al. National Sleep Foundation's sleep time duration recommendations: Methodology and results summary. *Sleep Health* **2015**, *1*, 40–43. [CrossRef] [PubMed]

8. The 4th The General Condition Which Is Birth Child Running through Survey Result in the 21st Century. Available online: www.wam.go.jp/wamappl/bb16GS70.nsf/0/3baf55ad7af95af5492570cf001e6a58/$FILE/siryou_all.pdf (accessed on 10 March 2018).

9. A Continual Comparative Study about the Degree of Infant Health. Available online: http://jschild.or.jp/book/pdf/2010_kenkochousa.pdf (accessed on 10 March 2018).

10. Shinkoda, H.; Suetsugu, Y.; Asami, E.; Kato, N.; Kohyama, J.; Uchimura, N.; Chishaki, A.; Nishioka, K.; Okubo, I.; Matsumoto, K.; et al. Analysis of parent-child sleeping and living habits related to later bedtimes in children. *Fukuoka Igaku Zasshi* **2012**, *103*, 12–23. [PubMed]

11. Nutbeam, D. The evolving concept of health literacy. *Soc. Sci. Med.* **2008**, *67*, 2072–2078. [CrossRef] [PubMed]

12. Shum, J.; Poureslami, I.; Doyle-Waters, M.M.; FitzGerald, J.M. The application of health literacy measurement tools (collective or individual domains) in assessing chronic disease management: A systematic review protocol. *Syst. Rev.* **2016**, *5*, 97. [CrossRef] [PubMed]

13. Kutner, M.; Greenberg, E.; Jin, Y.; Paulsen, C. *The Health Literacy of America's Adults: Results from the 2003 National Assessment of Adult Literacy*; National Center for Education Statistics: Washington, DC, USA, 2006.

14. Berkman, N.D.; Sheridan, S.L.; Donahue, K.E.; Halpern, D.J.; Viera, A.; Crotty, K.; Holland, A.; Brasure, M.; Lohr, K.N.; Harden, E.; et al. Health literacy interventions and outcomes: An updated systematic review. *Evid. Rep. Technol. Assess. (Full Rep.)* **2011**, *199*, 1–941.

15. Yin, H.S.; Forbis, S.G.; Dreyer, B.P. Health literacy and pediatric health. *Curr. Probl. Pediatr. Adolesc. Health Care* **2007**, *37*, 258–286. [CrossRef] [PubMed]

16. Heerman, W.J.; Perrin, E.M.; Yin, H.S.; Sanders, L.M.; Eden, S.K.; Shintani, A.; Coyne-Beasley, T.; Bronaugh, A.B.; Barkin, S.L.; Rothman, R.L. Health literacy and injury prevention behaviors among caregivers of infants. *Am. J. Prev. Med.* **2014**, *46*, 449–456. [CrossRef] [PubMed]

17. Harrington, K.F.; Zhang, B.; Magruder, T.; Bailey, W.C.; Gerald, L.B. The Impact of Parent's Health Literacy on Pediatric Asthma Outcomes. *Pediatr. Allergy Immunol. Pulmonol.* **2015**, *28*, 20–26. [CrossRef] [PubMed]

18. DeWalt, D.A.; Hink, A. Health literacy and child health outcomes: A systematic review of the literature. *Pediatrics* **2009**, *124* (Suppl. 3), S265–S274. [CrossRef] [PubMed]

19. Chari, R.; Warsh, J.; Ketterer, T.; Hossain, J.; Sharif, I. Association between health literacy and child and adolescent obesity. *Patient Educ. Couns.* **2014**, *94*, 61–66. [CrossRef] [PubMed]

20. Yokokawa, H.; Fukuda, H.; Yuasa, M.; Sanada, H.; Hisaoka, T.; Naito, T. Association between health literacy and metabolic syndrome or healthy lifestyle characteristics among community-dwelling Japanese people. *Diabetol. Metab. Syndr.* **2016**, *8*, 30. [CrossRef] [PubMed]

21. Suka, M.; Yamauchi, T.; Sugimori, H. Help-seeking intentions for early signs of mental illness and their associated factors: Comparison across four kinds of health problems. *BMC Public Health* **2016**, *16*, 301. [CrossRef] [PubMed]

22. Bathory, E.; Tomopoulos, S.; Rothman, R.; Sanders, L.; Perrin, E.M.; Mendelsohn, A.; Dreyer, B.; Cerra, M.; Yin, H.S. Infant Sleep and Parent Health Literacy. *Acad. Pediatr.* **2016**, *16*, 550–557. [CrossRef] [PubMed]

23. Suka, M.; Odajima, T.; Kasai, M.; Igarashi, A.; Ishikawa, H.; Kusama, M.; Nakayama, T.; Sumitani, M.; Sugimori, H. The 14-item health literacy scale for Japanese adults (HLS-14). *Environ. Health Prev. Med.* **2013**, *18*, 407–415. [CrossRef] [PubMed]

24. Suka, M.; Odajima, T.; Okamoto, M.; Sumitani, M.; Igarashi, A.; Ishikawa, H.; Kusama, M.; Yamamoto, M.; Nakayama, T.; Sugimori, H. Relationship between health literacy, health information access, health behavior, and health status in Japanese people. *Patient Educ. Couns.* **2015**, *98*, 660–668. [CrossRef] [PubMed]

25. Suka, M.; Odajima, T.; Okamoto, M.; Sumitani, M.; Nakayama, T.; Sugimori, H. Reading comprehension of health checkup reports and health literacy in Japanese people. *Environ. Health Prev. Med.* **2014**, *19*, 295–306. [CrossRef] [PubMed]

26. Nakayama, K.; Osaka, W.; Togari, T.; Ishikawa, H.; Yonekura, Y.; Sekido, A.; Matsumoto, M. Comprehensive health literacy in Japan is lower than in Europe: A validated Japanese-language assessment of health literacy. *BMC Public Health* **2015**, *15*, 505. [CrossRef] [PubMed]

27. Liechty, J.M.; Saltzman, J.A.; Musaad, S.M. Health literacy and parent attitudes about weight control for children. *Appetite* **2015**, *91*, 200–208. [CrossRef] [PubMed]

28. Bernhardt, J.M.; Felter, E.M. Online pediatric information seeking among mothers of young children: Results from a qualitative study using focus groups. *J. Med. Internet Res.* **2004**, *6*, e7. [CrossRef] [PubMed]

29. Paul, I.M.; Savage, J.S.; Anzman-Frasca, S.; Marini, M.E.; Mindell, J.A.; Birch, L.L. INSIGHT Responsive Parenting Intervention and Infant Sleep. *Pediatrics* **2016**, *138*, e20160762. [CrossRef] [PubMed]

30. Lo, M.J. Relationship between Sleep Habits and Nighttime Sleep among Healthy Preschool Children in Taiwan. *Ann. Acad. Med. Singap.* **2016**, *45*, 549–556. [PubMed]

31. Mitsutake, S.; Shibata, A.; Ishii, K.; Oka, K. Associations of eHealth Literacy With Health Behavior Among Adult Internet Users. *J. Med. Internet Res.* **2016**, *18*, e192. [CrossRef] [PubMed]

32. Curtis, L.M.; Revelle, W.; Waite, K.; Wilson, E.A.; Condon, D.M.; Bojarski, E.; Park, D.C.; Baker, D.W.; Wolf, M.S. Development and validation of the comprehensive health activities scale: A new approach to health literacy measurement. *J. Health Commun.* **2015**, *20*, 157–164. [CrossRef] [PubMed]

33. Aihara, Y.; Minai, J. Barriers and catalysts of nutrition literacy among elderly Japanese people. *Health Promot. Int.* **2011**, *26*, 421–431. [CrossRef] [PubMed]

34. Campbell, M.J. *Statistics at Square Two*, 2nd ed.; BMJ Books; Blackwell: London, UK, 2006.

35. Wamsley, E.J.; Tucker, M.; Payne, J.D.; Benavides, J.A.; Stickgold, R. Dreaming of a learning task is associated with enhanced sleep-dependent memory consolidation. *Curr. Biol.* **2010**, *20*, 850–855. [CrossRef] [PubMed]

36. Fukuda, K.; Ishihara, K. Routine evening naps and night-time sleep patterns in junior high and high school students. *Psychiatry Clin. Neurosci.* **2002**, *56*, 229–230. [CrossRef] [PubMed]

37. Sasaki, T.; Matsumoto, S. Actual conditions of work, fatigue and sleep in non-employed, home-based female information technology workers with preschool children. *Ind. Health* **2005**, *43*, 142–150. [CrossRef] [PubMed]

38. Xiao, G.; Ye, Q.; Han, T.; Yan, J.; Sun, L.; Wang, F. Study of the sleep quality and psychological state of patients with hepatitis B liver cirrhosis. *Hepatol. Res.* **2017**, *48*, E275–E282. [CrossRef] [PubMed]

39. Sedov, I.D.; Cameron, E.E.; Madigan, S.; Tomfohr-Madsen, L.M. Sleep quality during pregnancy: A meta-analysis. *Sleep Med. Rev.* **2017**, *38*, 168–176. [CrossRef] [PubMed]

40. Menear, A.; Elliott, R.; Aitken, L.A.; Lal, S.; McKinley, S. Repeated sleep-quality assessment and use of sleep-promoting interventions in ICU. *Nurs. Crit. Care* **2017**, *22*, 348–354. [CrossRef] [PubMed]

41. Iwadare, Y.; Kamei, Y.; Usami, M.; Ushijima, H.; Tanaka, T.; Watanabe, K.; Kodaira, M.; Saito, K. Behavioral symptoms and sleep problems in children with anxiety disorder. *Pediatr. Int.* **2015**, *57*, 690–693. [CrossRef] [PubMed]

42. Angelhoff, C.; Edell-Gustafsson, U.; Morelius, E. Sleep quality and mood in mothers and fathers accommodated in the family-centred paediatric ward. *J. Clin. Nurs.* **2017**, *27*, e544–e550. [CrossRef] [PubMed]

43. Sekine, M.; Chen, X.; Hamanishi, S.; Wang, H.; Yamagami, T.; Kagamimori, S. The validity of sleeping hours of healthy young children as reported by their parents. *J. Epidemiol.* **2002**, *12*, 237–242. [CrossRef] [PubMed]

44. Takemura, T.; Funaki, K.; Kanbayashi, T.; Kawamoto, K.; Tsutsui, K.; Saito, Y.; Aizawa, R.; Inomata, S.; Shimizu, T. Sleep habits of students attending elementary schools, and junior and senior high schools in Akita prefecture. *Psychiatry Clin. Neurosci.* **2002**, *56*, 241–242. [CrossRef] [PubMed]

45. Kohyama, J.; Shiiki, T.; Hasegawa, T. Sleep duration of young children is affected by nocturnal sleep onset time. *Pediatr. Int.* **2000**, *42*, 589–591. [CrossRef] [PubMed]

46. Kitamura, S.; Enomoto, M.; Kamei, Y.; Inada, N.; Moriwaki, A.; Kamio, Y.; Mishima, K. Association between delayed bedtime and sleep-related problems among community-dwelling 2-year-old children in Japan. *J. Physiol. Anthropol.* **2015**, *34*, 12. [CrossRef] [PubMed]

# 7

# Allostatic Load Biomarker Associations with Depressive Symptoms Vary among US Black and White Women and Men

**Ganga S. Bey \*, Bill M. Jesdale, Christine M. Ulbricht, Eric O. Mick and Sharina D. Person**

Department of Quantitative Health Sciences, University of Massachusetts Medical School, Worcester, MA 01655, USA; bill.jesdale@umassmed.edu (B.M.J.); christine.ulbricht@umassmed.edu (C.M.U.); Eric.mick@umassmed.edu (E.O.M.); sharina.person@umassmed.edu (S.D.P.)
\* Correspondence: ganga.bey@umassmed.edu

**Abstract:** The prevalence and severity of depression differ in women and men and across racial groups. Psychosocial factors such as chronic stress have been proposed as contributors, but causes of this variation are not fully understood. Allostatic load, a measure of the physiological burden of chronic stress, is known to be associated with depression. Using data from the National Health and Nutrition Examination Survey 2005–2010, we examined the associations of nine allostatic load biomarkers with depression among US black and white adults aged 18–64 years ($n = 6431$). Depressive symptoms were assessed using the Patient Health Questionaire-9; logistic models estimated adjusted odds of depression based on allostatic load biomarkers. High-risk levels of c-reactive protein were significantly associated with increased odds of depression among white women (adjusted odds ratio (aOR) = 1.7, 95% CI: 1.1–2.5) and men (aOR = 1.8, 95% CI: 1.1–2.8) but not black women (aOR = 0.8, 95% CI: 0.6–1.1) or men (aOR = 0.9, 95% CI: 0.5–1.5). Among black men, hypertension (aOR = 1.7, 95% CI: 1.1–2.7) and adverse serum albumin levels (aOR = 1.7, 95% CI: 1.0–2.9) predicted depression, while high total cholesterol was associated with depression among black women (aOR = 1.6, 95% CI: 1.0–2.7). The associations between allostatic load biomarkers and depression varies with gendered race, suggesting that, despite consistent symptomatology, underlying disease mechanisms may differ between these groups.

**Keywords:** chronic stress; allostatic load; depression; gender; race; intersectionality

---

## 1. Introduction

A large proportion of the United States chronic disease burden is attributed to depressive disorders [1]. Major depressive disorder (MDD), the most common form of depression, is the leading cause of disability among those aged 15 years and older [2]. Of central public health concern are racial and gender disparities in who develops depression; differences in the prevalence and incidence of MDD diagnosis and depressive symptomatology between black and white women and men have been well documented [3–6]. Specifically, rates of MDD diagnosis are higher among white persons. Yet, black women and men report a higher prevalence of depressive symptoms. Further, there is evidence that somatic symptoms are more common among black persons, while affective symptoms of depression are more frequently reported among whites [7].

Consensus has yet to be reached on what proportion of this disparity can be attributed to true differences in disease prevalence and manifestation between these groups as opposed to cultural and social factors yielding underreporting, underdiagnosis, and undertreatment of depression in black persons and men [8]. A host of genetic and social factors are thought to be associated with the likelihood of developing depression [4,9–14], further underscoring a need for additional investigation. In concert with potential surveillance inconsistencies, persistent uncertainty about the mechanisms for these risk factors [9] render efforts to characterize and alleviate true racial and gender disparities in depression particularly challenging.

One approach to identifying mechanisms for an effect of social status on the development of depression is the use of allostatic load, a measure of the physiological wear and tear accumulating from sustained stress exposure. The concept of allostatic load within the epidemiological discipline has improved efforts to evaluate the role of race and gender inequity in yielding depression disparities [10]. Social environment theories for gender differences in depression attribute much of the increased risk for depression among women to chronic strain associated with the subordinate social position women occupy [4,11,15]. A growing body of evidence supports a number of key physiological measures as markers of chronic stress burden associated with psychosocial exposures stemming from membership in a disadvantaged social group. Adverse levels of neuroendocrine, cardiovascular, metabolic, and immunological biomarkers comprising AL have been linked to perception of social rejection, marginalization, and exclusion [11,16–19]. Specifically, this research emphasizes the role of inflammatory processes in mediating the effect of threatening social stimuli, such as identity threat stemming from perceived racial or gender discrimination, on health [11,16]. As evidence for depression as an inflammatory disease emerges [11,20,21], studies linking psychosocial risk factors with inflammatory indicators of chronic stress offer biologically plausible mechanisms for depression as a manifestation of the chronic stress associated with exposure to structural inequity.

"Paradoxical" findings of lower rates of MDD among black persons [22,23], who, like women, occupy marginalized social positions [24], complicate social environment theories. The impact of socioeconomic factors on depression varies between black and white communities [3], with socioeconomic position largely accounting for gender disparities among black persons but not white. More work is needed to understand these divergent findings in regard to the pathogenesis of depression across these groups.

In efforts to account for gender–race differences in the relationship of chronic psychosocial stress with depression, etiologic inquiry has increasingly turned to epigenetic explanations, centering the interdependency of biological and social risk factors for disease [9]. Within such sociobiological frameworks, further consideration of the psychosocial exposures individuals encounter at the junction of gender and race ("gendered racial" exposures) becomes integral to clarifying the causes of persistent differences in depression morbidity. Examined through the lens of intersectionality theory [25], intersecting axes of structured inequity on the basis of gender and race impose a set of chronic social stressors whose effects on health cannot be reasonably separated into individual racial and gendered components. Acting concomitantly with biological vulnerability, these unique gendered racial exposures may serve as catalysts for psychopathology among certain populations but not others, as proposed by the differential effect hypothesis [26], in addition to shaping the way psychological distress manifests within these groups. Research investigating the nature of social group variation in the effects of chronic strain on mental health may therefore provide valuable insight into the causes and magnitude of gendered racial differences in risk for depression and elucidate opportunities for improvement in treatment efficacy.

Although previous literature has identified an association of inflammation with depression among white but not black persons [27,28], to our knowledge no US study has examined the extent to which gender and race simultaneously moderate the association of individual allostatic load components with depression. To address this lacuna, this analysis uses a nationally representative sample to explore variation in the relationships between nine allostatic load biomarkers of chronic stress and depressive symptoms among black and white women and men.

## 2. Materials and Methods

### 2.1. Data

We used data from the National Health and Nutrition Examination Survey (NHANES), 2005–2010. These years were combined to maximize sample size; the analysis was limited to this time period because a different depression measure was used prior to 2005 and all biomarkers of interest were not included after 2010. Conducted by the National Center for Health Statistics (NCHS), NHANES uses weighted samples to provide national estimates of health and nutritional status for the noninstitutionalized population of the United States. Study staff use specially designed and equipped mobile health centers that travel to locations throughout the country to take health measurements on about 5000 participants in 15 counties annually. NHANES data collection methodology has been further documented elsewhere [29].

### 2.2. Participants

Our analytic sample included men and women aged 18–64 years who self-identified as non-Hispanic black or non-Hispanic white (referred to hereafter as "black" and "white") from options provided by investigators that included Mexican-American, Other Hispanic, Non-Hispanic White, Non-Hispanic Black, and Other Race—including Multi-Racial. Pregnant women ($n = 490$) were excluded, as pregnancy can alter a number of physiological measures comprising allostatic load [30,31]. Of the 14,050 participants aged 18–64 years in NHANES 2005–2010, we further excluded participants whose reported race was not black or white ($n = 5025$), those missing information on any of the questions included in the depression measure ($n = 1824$), AL biomarkers of interest ($n = 2530$), and/or family poverty–income ratio (PIR, $n = 1120$).

### 2.3. Depressive Symptoms

Participants completed the 9-item Patient Health Questionnaire (PHQ), a validated screen for depression [32]. Each question on this self-reported assessment of Diagnostic and Statistical Manual of Mental Disorders 4th edition signs and symptoms of depression is scored from 0 (not at all) to 3 (nearly every day), with a total possible score of 27 calculated by summing the scores of the nine individual questions. A total score of ten or higher is considered indicative of major depression [32].

### 2.4. Allostatic Load Biomarkers

The biomarkers included in this analysis as comprising the allostatic load (AL) are consistent with previous research [10,33,34]. These include three cardiovascular biomarkers (systolic and diastolic blood pressure (BP), and pulse rate); four metabolic markers (glycosolated hemoglobin, body mass index (BMI), high-density lipoprotein (HDL) cholesterol, and total cholesterol); and two immunological markers (serum albumin and c-reactive protein (CRP)). Systolic and diastolic BP values were calculated as the average of three readings. Biomarkers with values above the 75th percentile of nationally weighted empirical cutoffs were categorized as "high-risk", with the exception of serum albumin and HDL cholesterol, which were categorized as "high-risk" for values below the 25th percentile empirical cutoff, as lower values of these biomarkers are considered indicative of poor physiological function. High-risk thresholds were as follows: systolic BP > 127.3 mmHG; diastolic BP > 76 mmHG; pulse rate > 82 bpm; glycosylated hemoglobin > 5.7%; BMI > 30.6; HDL cholesterol < 42 mg/dL; total cholesterol > 216 mg/dL; serum albumin < 4.1 g/dL; CRP > 0.37 mg/dL. Previous research indicates these cutoffs as the preferred method of calculating the components of AL [28,34,35]. To calculate total AL score, one point was assigned for each high-risk biomarker value, with a total possible score of 9. In accordance with the literature [10], we consider AL scores of 4 or higher as "high-risk".

*2.5. Covariates*

In consideration of potential over-controlling for mediating variables, we strictly limited the covariates for which we adjusted [36]. We included age, family poverty-to-income ratio (PIR), and each biomarker as covariates in our primary analysis based on prior literature showing associations of age and socioeconomic status (SES) with both depression [22] and allostatic load [33]. Age was stratified into five groups (18–24, 25–34, 35–44, 45–54, and 55–64 years) across which AL is known to vary [22]. PIR is an index for the ratio of household income to the federal poverty level based on family size and state of residence. NHANES provides PIR for each participant [26]. We stratified our analysis into five categories of PIR—"At or below", ">1 and $\leq 2\times$", ">2 and $\leq 3\times$", ">3 and $\leq 4\times$", and ">4$\times$" the federal poverty threshold—to better capture the distribution of the biomarkers and depression across socioeconomic status.

*2.6. Statistical Analysis*

Statistical analysis was conducted between 1 August 2016 and 15 October 2016. All analyses were weighted to represent black and white women and men nationally following National Center for Health Statistics guidelines. For univariate analyses, means or frequencies (%) were reported; Pearson's chi-square was used to test for statistically significant differences of categorical variables. Four multivariable logistic models with a significance level of $\alpha = 0.05$ estimated the odds of depression as a function of each biomarker stratified by gendered race, adjusting for age, PIR, and all other biomarkers. All analyses were conducted using STATA version 14 (StataCorp LLC, College Station, TX, USA); code is available in Supplementary Materials (Supplementary S1) [37].

## 3. Results

Exclusions resulted in an analytic sample of 6431 US adults, which represents approximately 113 million black and white women and men nationally. Sociodemographics, depression, and high-risk levels of each of the nine included biomarkers are reported in Table 1 by gendered race. Black persons were more likely to be hypertensive and women had higher pulse rates. Half of black women were obese, while the prevalence of obesity ranged from 30% to 34% in the other three groups. A greater percentage of black women also had low serum album (52%) and elevated CRP (45%) levels. At 35%, the prevalence of high levels of glyco-hemoglobin was highest among black men. White men had the highest prevalence of high total cholesterol (44%) and low HDL cholesterol (39%). With the exception of low HDL cholesterol, white women had the lowest prevalence of high-risk biomarker levels of all groups. Black persons and women were more likely to report elevated depressive symptoms.

The adjusted odds of depression associated with high-risk levels of each biomarker is reported in Table 2 stratified by gendered race. Adjusting for age, socioeconomic status, and all other biomarkers, high-risk CRP, serum album, and total cholesterol levels, as well as high-risk pulse rate were differentially associated with increased risk for depression across the four groups. High-risk CRP levels increased odds of depression among white women (aOR = 1.7, 95% CI: 1.1–2.6) and white men (aOR = 1.8, 95% CI: 1.1–2.8), while no statistically significant associations were found among black women (aOR = 0.8, 95% CI: 0.6–1.1) or black men (aOR = 0.9, 95% CI: 0.5–1.5). Similarly, adjusted odds ratios for high-risk pulse rates were 1.5 (95% CI: 1.1–2.2) and 1.8 (95% CI: 1.1–2.9) for white women and white men, respectively, but not statistically significant among black women (1.1, 95% CI: 0.7–1.6) or men (1.2, 95% CI: 0.6–2.4). Among black men only, high-risk levels of systolic BP (aOR = 1.7, 95% CI: 1.1–2.7) and serum albumin (aOR = 1.7, 95% CI: 1.0–2.9) predicted depression. High levels of total cholesterol were associated with depression among black women (aOR = 1.6, 95% CI: 1.0–2.7).

**Table 1.** Sample characteristics by gendered race in NHANES 2005–2010, weighted %.

| Measures | Black Women | White Women | Black Men | White Men | $P$ [d] |
|---|---|---|---|---|---|
| Sample $N$ | 980 | 2147 | 1028 | 2276 | |
| Weighted $N$ | 7,895,277 | 48,156,035 | 7,129,498 | 49,990,472 | |
| Age, mean (SD) | 40.7 (14.4) | 41.7 (13.2) | 40.2 (14.8) | 41.4 (13.5) | |
| Family PIR [a] | | | | | <0.001 |
| $\leq 1$ | 25.3 | 10.7 | 19.6 | 8.3 | |
| >1 and $\leq 2\times$ | 25.5 | 14.0 | 25.8 | 13.6 | |
| >2 and $\leq 3\times$ | 15.6 | 13.4 | 18.4 | 13.9 | |
| >3 and $\leq 4\times$ | 13.4 | 15.4 | 14.0 | 14.8 | |
| >4 | 20.2 | 46.4 | 22.1 | 49.4 | |
| High-risk AL Biomarkers [b] | | | | | |
| Systolic BP | 46.5 | 33.7 | 48.3 | 42.3 | <0.001 |
| Diastolic BP | 50.3 | 40.4 | 50.7 | 50.2 | <0.001 |
| Pulse | 25.9 | 24.0 | 13.5 | 16.0 | <0.001 |
| BMI | 50.1 | 31.4 | 34.8 | 30.2 | <0.001 |
| Total cholesterol | 36.4 | 43.7 | 36.3 | 44.4 | <0.001 |
| HDL cholesterol | 12.5 | 14.3 | 27.3 | 39.3 | <0.001 |
| Glyco-hemoglobin | 29.3 | 14.6 | 35.4 | 14.8 | <0.001 |
| Serum Albumin | 52.4 | 29.8 | 23.1 | 10.5 | <0.001 |
| CRP | 44.7 | 32.0 | 26.2 | 18.6 | <0.001 |
| High-risk AL | 17.1 | 15.3 | 10.1 | 7.4 | <0.001 |
| Depression [c] | 14.6 | 8.6 | 7.1 | 4.9 | <0.001 |

Abbreviations: AL = allostatic load; BP = blood pressure; BMI = body mass index; HDL = high-density lipoprotein; CRP = c-reactive protein; PIR = poverty-to-income ratio; [a] PIR is a ratio of household income to the US poverty threshold based on family size and state of residence; [b] "High-risk" thresholds for each biomarker were: systolic BP > 127.3 mmHG; diastolic BP > 76 mmHG; pulse rate > 82 bpm; glycosylated hemoglobin > 5.7%; BMI > 30.6; HDL cholesterol < 42 mg/dL; total cholesterol > 216 mg/dL; serum albumin < 4.1 g/dL; and CRP > 0.37 mg/dL; [c] PHQ-9 scores of $\geq 10$; [d] $p$-value from Pearson's chi-square test.

**Table 2.** Adjusted [a] odds of depression [b] with high-risk allostatic load and biomarker levels by gendered race in NHANES 2005–2010, OR (95% CI) [c].

| Biomarker | Black Women | White Women | Black Men | White Men |
|---|---|---|---|---|
| Systolic BP | 1.2 (0.6, 2.5) | 1.1 (0.6, 2.0) | 1.7 (1.1, 2.7) * | 1.4 (0.8, 2.5) |
| Diastolic BP | 1.1 (0.6, 2.1) | 1.3 (0.8, 2.2) | 1.2 (0.8, 1.9) | 1.3 (0.8, 2.1) |
| Pulse | 1.1 (0.7, 1.6) | 1.5 (1.1, 2.2) * | 1.2 (0.6, 2.4) | 1.8 (1.1, 2.9) * |
| BMI | 0.8 (0.5, 1.2) | 1.1 (0.7, 1.7) | 1.1 (0.6, 2.0) | 0.9 (0.6, 1.3) |
| Total cholesterol | 1.6 (1.0, 2.7) * | 1.1 (0.8, 1.5) | 1.0 (0.5, 2.0) | 0.8 (0.4, 1.3) |
| HDL cholesterol | 1.2 (0.6, 2.3) | 1.1 (0.7, 1.7) | 1.7 (0.9, 3.4) | 1.3 (0.8, 1.9) |
| Glyco-hemoglobin | 1.1 (0.8, 1.7) | 1.0 (0.6, 1.7) | 0.9 (0.5, 1.6) | 0.8 (0.5, 1.4) |
| Serum Albumin | 0.9 (0.6, 1.3) | 1.0 (0.7, 1.6) | 1.7 (1.0, 2.9) * | 1.3 (0.7, 2.5) |
| CRP | 0.8 (0.6, 1.1) | 1.7 (1.1, 2.6) * | 0.9 (0.5, 1.5) | 1.8 (1.1, 2.8) * |
| High-risk AL [d] | 1.1 (0.6, 2.0) | 2.1 (1.5, 3.0) * | 1.7 (1.0, 2.9) * | 1.4 (0.8, 2.5) |

Abbreviations: BP = blood pressure; BMI = body mass index; HDL = high-density lipoprotein; CRP = c-reactive protein; [a] models adjusted for PIR (ratio of household income to the US poverty threshold), age, and all biomarkers; [b] PHQ-9 scores of $\geq 10$; [c] results are from four separate regression models. The reference category for the biomarkers in each model is "low-risk"; [d] AL scores of $\geq 4$ were considered "high-risk".

## 4. Discussion

Our results support the differential effect hypothesis. The relationship between a number of physiological markers of chronic stress and depressive symptoms varied with respect to gendered race. While the prevalence of depression and high-risk inflammation indicators were notably higher among black women than white women, black men, or white men, black women were the only of the four groups among whom inflammation was not associated with depression. The biomarkers associated with depression were also consistent among white women and men, but not among black persons. Adverse levels of serum album and systolic BP predicted depression in black men, while among black women, high-risk levels of total cholesterol were associated with depression.

### 4.1. Gendered Racial Variation in Manifestations of Chronic Stress

An extensive body of literature supports gender and racial differences in the prevalence of inflammation [37–41], as well as in the cardiovascular and metabolic biomarkers comprising the allostatic load [13,18–20]. Our findings are consistent with prior literature showing that the prevalence of elevated pulse rate and inflammation tends to be higher among women regardless of race [13,42]. Even accounting for socioeconomic position, black women are particularly susceptible to premature aging, chronic inflammation, and associated conditions such as obesity [10,20,33], results that are supported in this analysis. In line with extant research, we also found high levels of total cholesterol and low levels of HDL cholesterol to be more prevalent among men and white persons [43].

Data linking adverse social exposures to increased risk of inflammation and subsequently depression [13,43] provide some support for the differential effect hypothesis but fall short of accounting for the concomitant effects of gender and race on the experience of social stimuli and for how this interaction influences variability in risk for psychiatric disorder. In contrast, research grounded in intersectionality theory has identified gendered racial differences in the effects of stress on mental health, finding a stronger association between stressful life events and major depressive episodes among white men than black men while identifying no such interaction among women [44]. Another study examined how allostatic load differentially predicts depressive symptoms in black and white women and men, finding an association only among black men and white women [45]. In accordance with these findings, our results indicate different underlying disease relationships among black and white women and men, divergence in the predictors of depressive symptoms potentially steered by unmeasured psychosocial exposures that are unique to each gendered race. Such variability in the experience of stress and its psychiatric presentation may indicate the necessity for more nuanced approaches to patient evaluation and prescribing practices.

### 4.2. Divergence in the Pathways from Chronic Stress to Depression

As noted earlier, treatment efficacy among black and white women and men contributes to disparities in morbidity [6] and is likely complicated by differences in the neurobiological processes associated with depression between these groups. In this study, inflammatory markers predicted depression in all groups except black women. Specifically, CRP, elevated levels of which have been increasingly identified as a risk factor for depression [13,18], was associated with increased odds only among whites. Previous findings [27,28] have identified an association of CRP with depressive symptoms only among whites and not blacks. Our study further builds on this evidence by identifying within-race gender differences in the association of inflammation with depression, as well as in other gendered race group-specific markers of chronic stress predictive of depression which have been earlier noted in the literature [46]. These findings are of particular interest in light of other literature demonstrating symptom-specific associations of CRP with depression. In one study, investigators found that higher levels of inflammation are more likely to underlie depressive symptoms indicative of sickness behavior including fatigue, reduced appetite, withdrawal, and inhibited motivation [29]. As black persons are more likely to report these somatic symptoms, our findings stand in contrast to this evidence, providing further indication of distinct physiological pathways from stress associated with social inequity to the development of depression among black and white women and men.

These disparate relationships suggest that, while a genetic predisposition may contribute to the likelihood of developing risk factors for depression such as inflammation [42], the particular experience of the social environment that is predicated upon one's gendered race plays an integral part in depression pathogenesis [47]. This assertion is consistent with evidence for an interactive effect of genotype and social context on depression that varies with gender [15]. Such social environmental exposures moderating the experience of stress and subsequent effects on mental health may include cultural influences on racially informed gender roles and expectations, as well as the frequency and severity of perceived prejudice [47–50].

Research suggests that white women are more likely to ruminate and self-blame following identity threat (e.g., following discrimination exposure) than black women or white men [4,47–51], a socialized stress response [49] that may contribute to a greater proclivity for affective symptoms of depression under certain kinds of chronic stress [48]. In contrast, coping with the co-occurrence of racial and gender identity-based stressors may have allowed for the development of a psychological fortitude that is protective against depression, or affective symptoms of depression, under these conditions among black women [52,53], despite greater exposure to genetic and psychosocial risk factors for inflammation. The chronic strain-inflammation pathway of depression may therefore be more applicable to those operating within sociocultural paradigms that yield psychological and behavioral responses to social status-based stress—responses that may in turn exacerbate biological vulnerability to depression. Given potentially diverging mechanisms, approaches to evaluating and developing treatment plans for patients presenting with depressive symptoms should consider the sociocultural factors associated with gendered race as drivers of differences in underlying disease causes.

### 4.3. Limitations

This study has important limitations requiring acknowledgement. While the PHQ-9 has been validated and shown to have strong reliability and validity within a range of racial and ethnic populations [53], and among women and men [54], the instrument assesses depression based on current symptoms. Depressed individuals being successfully treated with medication or therapy may not be captured by the PHQ-9. Accordingly, our estimates of the association between allostatic load biomarkers and depression may be underestimated, particularly among white women, who are most likely of the groups under study to seek and undergo treatment for depression [55–58]. Our analysis was limited to NHANES 2005–2010 because the 2005–2006 surveys were the first to include the PHQ-9, and 2009–2010 was the latest wave to include all nine biomarkers used to calculate AL. This limited sample size prevented further analysis of interactive effects within stratified models. Research examining these associations among larger and more contemporary cohorts of US adults is therefore needed.

The number of participants excluded for missing data could raise concern about the representativeness of our sample. However, among those excluded due to missing data on biomarkers, missingness was distributed independently such that excluding one biomarker would not recover a significant number of respondents. Similarly, family PIR missingness was approximately equally distributed across AL biomarkers, race, and gender. Among participants missing depression scores, approximately 24% were black and 36% white. This missingness by race was distributed approximately equally across men and women, although not across income categories; participants excluded for missing information on depression had lower family PIRs (data are not shown).

## 5. Conclusions

Our findings provide some evidence of fundamental differences in the underlying neurological processes leading to depression pathogenesis among US black and white women and men. Interventions designed to eradicate social inequities remain important to reduce racial and gender disparities in a number of chronic diseases. However, implementing such interventions are challenging due in part to sociopolitical barriers and a lack of consensus among policy makers for best practices. Additional approaches at the individual level may complement system-level efforts by targeting the specific pathways over which chronic, identity-based, psychosocial stressors act to cause depression in different sociodemographic groups. On the importance of causal frameworks in the treatment of psychiatric disorders, Aaron Lazare opined: "The complexity of the decision-making process resulting from the use of several models may unnecessarily limit the treatment options of the psychiatrist [ ... ] If the conceptual models and their use in clinical psychiatry are made explicit, a broader range of treatment modalities should be made available" [59].

This study raises important concerns about the efficacy of psychiatric treatments which neglect sociocultural influences on the presentation of both chronic stress and depressive symptoms. Refining drug and psychotherapies as appropriate for distinct depression etiologies may yield improved treatment outcomes and reduce disparities between black and white women and men. We also suggest that prevention efforts should further focus on building resilience that targets the specific vulnerabilities associated with an individual's gendered race. Additional research exploring the psychosocial and cultural exposures that contribute to the varied manifestations of chronic stress and depression would significantly strengthen subsequent research investigating the nature of gendered racial differences in depression etiology.

**Author Contributions:** Conceptualization, G.S.B. and C.M.U.; Methodology, G.S.B., B.M.J. and S.D.P.; Software, G.S.B.; Validation, C.M.U., E.O.M., B.M.J. and S.D.P.; Formal Analysis, G.S.B.; Investigation, G.S.B. and C.M.U.; Resources, S.D.P.; Data Curation, G.S.B.; Writing—Original Draft Preparation, G.S.B.; Writing—Review & Editing, G.S.B., E.O.M. and B.M.J.; Visualization, G.S.B.; Supervision, S.D.P.

**Funding:** This research received no external funding.

## References

1. Pratt, L.A.; Brody, D.J. Depression in the, U.S. household population, 2009–2012. In *NCHS Data Brief*; National Center for Health Statistics: Hyattsville, MD, USA, 2014.

2. Murray, C.J.; Abraham, J.; Ali, M.K.; Alvarado, M.; Atkinson, C.; Baddour, L.M.; Bartels, D.H.; Benjamin, E.J.; Bhalla, K.; Birbeck, G.; et al. The state of US health, 1999–2010: Burden of diseases, injuries, and risk factors. *JAMA* **2013**, *310*, 591–608. [CrossRef] [PubMed]

3. Dunlop, D.D.; Song, J.; Lyons, J.S.; Manheim, L.M.; Chang, R.W. Racial/ethnic differences in rates of depression among preretirement adults. *Am. J. Public Health* **2003**, *93*, 1945–1952. [CrossRef] [PubMed]

4. Nolen-Hoeksema, S.; Larson, J.; Grayson, C. Explaining the gender difference in depressive symptoms. *J. Pers. Soc. Psychol.* **1999**, *77*, 1061–1072. [CrossRef] [PubMed]

5. Riolo, S.A.; Nguyen, T.A.; Greden, J.F.; King, C.A. Prevalence of depression by race/ethnicity: Findings from the National Health and Nutrition Examination Survey III. *Am. J. Public Health* **2005**, *95*, 998–1000. [CrossRef] [PubMed]

6. Blazer, D.G.; Kessler, R.C. The prevalence and distribution of major depression in a national community sample: The National Comorbidity Survey. *Am. J. Psychiatry* **1994**, *151*, 979–986. [PubMed]

7. Ayalon, L.; Young, M.A. Comparison of depressive symptoms in African Americans and Caucasian Americans. *J. Cross Cult. Psychol.* **2003**, *34*, 111–124. [CrossRef]

8. Shao, Z.; Richie, W.D.; Bailey, R.K. Racial and ethnic disparity in major depressive disorder. *J. Racial Ethnic Health Dispar.* **2016**, *3*, 692–705. [CrossRef] [PubMed]

9. Menke, A.; Binder, E. Epigenetic alterations in depression and antidepressant treatment. *Dialogues Clin. Neurosci.* **2014**, *16*, 395–404. [PubMed]

10. Geronimus, A.T.; Hicken, M.; Keene, D.; Bound, J. 'Weathering' and age patterns of allostatic load scores among blacks and whites in the United States. *Am. J. Public Health* **2006**, *96*, 826–833. [CrossRef] [PubMed]

11. Slavich, G.M.; Irwin, M.R. From stress to inflammation and major depressive disorder: A social signal transduction theory of depression. *Psychol. Bull.* **2014**, *140*, 774–815. [CrossRef] [PubMed]

12. Uddin, M.; Koenen, K.C.; de los Santos, R.; Bakshis, E.; Aiello, A.E.; Galea, S. Gender differences in the genetic and environmental determinants of adolescent depression. *Depress. Anxiety* **2010**, *27*, 658–666. [CrossRef] [PubMed]

13. Piccinelli, M.; Wilkinson, G. Gender differences in depression. *Br. J. Psychiatry* **2000**, *177*, 486–492. [CrossRef] [PubMed]

14. Lohoff, F.W. Overview of the genetics of major depressive disorder. *Curr. Psychiatr. Rep.* **2010**, *12*, 539–546. [CrossRef] [PubMed]

15. Bey, G.S.; Ulbricht, C.M.; Person, S.D. Theories for race and gender differences in management of social-identity related stressors: A systematic review. *J. Racial Ethn. Health Disparities* **2018**. [CrossRef] [PubMed]

16. Glaser, R.; Kiecolt-Glaser, J.K. Stress-induced immune dysfunction: Implications for health. *Nat. Rev. Immunol.* **2005**, *5*, 243–251. [CrossRef] [PubMed]

17. Krieger, N.; Sidney, S. Racial discrimination and blood pressure: The CARDIA study of young black and white adults. *Am. J. Public Health* **1996**, *86*, 1370–1378. [CrossRef] [PubMed]

18. Powell, L.R.; Jesdale, W.M.; Lemon, S.C. On the edge: The impact of race-related vigilance on obesity status in African-Americans. *Obes. Sci. Pract.* **2016**. [CrossRef] [PubMed]

19. Troxel, W.M.; Matthews, K.A.; Bromberger, J.T.; Sutton-Tyrrell, K. Chronic stress burden, discrimination, and subclinical carotid artery disease in African American and Caucasian women. *Health Psychol.* **2003**, *22*, 300–309. [CrossRef] [PubMed]

20. Kobrosly, R.W.; Van Wijngaarden, E.; Seplaki, C.L.; Cory-Sletcha, D.A.; Moynihan, J. Depressive symptoms are associated with allostatic load among community-dwelling older adults. *Physiol. Behav.* **2014**, *123*, 223–230. [CrossRef] [PubMed]

21. Raison, C.L.; Miller, A.H. Is depression an inflammatory disorder? *Curr. Psychiatry Rep.* **2011**, *13*, 467–475. [CrossRef] [PubMed]

22. Assari, S.; Burgard, S.; Zivin, K. Long-term reciprocal associations between depressive symptoms and number of chronic medical conditions: Longitudinal support for Black–White health paradox. *J. Racial Ethnic Health Dispar.* **2015**, *2*, 589–597. [CrossRef] [PubMed]

23. Barnes, D.M.; Keyes, K.K.; Bates, L.M. Racial differences in depression in the United States: How do subgroup analyses inform a paradox? *Soc. Psychiatry Psychiatr. Epidemiol.* **2013**, *48*, 1941–1949. [CrossRef] [PubMed]

24. Keyes, C.L. The Black-White paradox in health: Flourishing in the face of social inequality and discrimination. *J. Pers. Soc. Psychol.* **2009**, *77*, 1677–1706. [CrossRef] [PubMed]

25. Crenshaw, K. Demarginalizing the intersection of race and sex: A black feminist critique of antidiscrimination doctrine, feminist theory and antiracist politics. *Univ. Chic. Legal Forum* **1989**, *140*, 139–167.

26. Assari, S.; Lankarani, M.M. Stressful life events and risk of depression 25 years later: Race and gender differences. *Front. Public Health* **2016**. [CrossRef] [PubMed]

27. Stewart, J.C. One size does not fit all—Is the depression-inflammation link missing in racial/ethnic minority individuals? *JAMA Psychiatry* **2016**, *73*, 301–302. [CrossRef] [PubMed]

28. Stewart, J.C.; Rand, K.L.; Muldoon, M.F.; Kamarck, T.W. A prospective evaluation of the directionality of the depression-inflammation relationship. *Brain Behav. Immunity* **2009**, *23*, 936–944. [CrossRef] [PubMed]

29. Jokela, M.; Virtanen, M.; Batty, G.D.; Kivimäki, M. Inflammation and specific symptoms of depression. *JAMA Psychiatry* **2016**, *73*, 1199–1201. [CrossRef] [PubMed]

30. Zipf, G.; Chiappa, M.; Porter, K.S.; Ostchega, Y.; Lewis, B.G.; Dostal, J. National Health and Nutrition Examination Survey: Plan and operations, 1999–2010. *Vital Health Stat.* **2013**, *1*, 1–37.

31. Gunderson, E.P. Childbearing and obesity in women: Weight before, during, and after pregnancy. *Obstet. Gynecol. Clin. N. Am.* **2009**, *36*, 317–332. [CrossRef] [PubMed]

32. Zamorski, M.A.; Green, L.A. NHBPEP report on high blood pressure in pregnancy: A summary for family physicians. *Am. Fam. Phys.* **2001**, *64*, 263–271.

33. Kroenke, K.; Spitzer, R.L. The PHQ-9: A new depression and diagnostic severity measure. *Psychiatr. Ann.* **2002**, *32*, 509–521. [CrossRef]

34. Chyu, L.; Upchurch, D.M. Racial and ethnic patterns of allostatic load among adult women in the United States: Findings from the National Health and Nutrition Examination Survey 1999–2004. *J. Women Health* **2011**, *20*, 575–583. [CrossRef] [PubMed]

35. Wexler Rainisch, B.K.; Upchurch, D.M. Sociodemographic correlates of allostatic load among a national sample of adolescents: Findings from the National Health and Nutrition Examination Survey, 1999–2008. *J. Adolesc. Health* **2013**, *53*, 506–511. [CrossRef] [PubMed]

36. Kaufman, J.; Cooper, R. Seeking causal explanations in social epidemiology. *Am. J. Epidemiol.* **1999**, *150*, 113–120. [CrossRef] [PubMed]

37. StataCorp LP. *Stata/IC 13.1 for Windows*; StataCorp LP: College Station, TX, USA, 2014.

38. Albert, M.A.; Glynn, R.J.; Buring, J.; Ridker, P.M. Impact of traditional and novel risk factors on the relationship between socioeconomic status and incident cardiovascular events. *Circulation* **2006**, *114*, 2619–2626. [CrossRef] [PubMed]

39. Khera, A.; McGuire, D.K.; Murphy, S.A.; Stanek, H.G.; Das, S.R.; Vongpatanasin, W.; Wians, F.H.; Grundy, S.M.; de Lemos, J.A. Race and gender differences in C-reactive protein levels. *J. Am. Coll. Cardiol.* **2005**, *46*, 464–469. [CrossRef] [PubMed]

40. Ranjit, N.; Diez-Roux, A.V.; Shea, S.; Cushman, M.; Ni, H.; Seeman, T. Socioeconomic position, race/ethnicity, and inflammation in the multi-ethnic study of atherosclerosis. *Circulation* **2007**, *116*, 2383–2390. [CrossRef] [PubMed]

41. Lakoski, S.G.; Cushman, M.; Siscovick, D.S.; Blumenthal, R.S.; Palmas, W.; Burke, G.; Harrington, D.M. The relationship between inflammation, obesity, and risk for hypertension in the multi-ethnic study of atherosclerosis (MESA). *J. Hum. Hypertens.* **2006**, *25*, 73–79. [CrossRef] [PubMed]

42. Rainer, A.P.; Beleza, S.; Franceschini, N.; Auer, P.L.; Robinson, J.G.; Kooperberg, U.P.; Tang, H. Genome-wide association and population genetic analysis of C-reactive protein in African American and Hispanic American women. *Am. J. Hum. Genet.* **2012**, *91*, 502–512. [CrossRef] [PubMed]

43. Sharpley, C.F. Differences in pulse rate and heart rate and effects on the calculation of heart rate reactivity during periods of mental stress. *J. Behav. Med.* **1994**, *17*, 99–109. [CrossRef] [PubMed]

44. Morris, A.; Ferdinand, K.C. Hyperlipidemia in racial/ethnic minorities: Differences in lipid profiles and the impact of statin therapy. *Clin. Lipidol.* **2009**, *4*, 741–754. [CrossRef]

45. Assari, S.; Lankarani, M.M. Association between stressful life events and depression; Intersection of race and gender. *J. Racial Ethnic Health Dispar.* **2015**, 1–8. [CrossRef] [PubMed]

46. Hicken, M.T.; Lee, H.; Mezuk, B.; Kershaw, K.N.; Rafferty, J.; Jackson, J.S. Racial and ethnic differences in the association between obesity and depression in women. *J. Women Health* **2013**, *22*, 445–452. [CrossRef] [PubMed]

47. Bey, G.S.; Waring, M.E.; Jesdale, B.M.; Person, S.D. Gendered race modification of the association between chronic stress and depression among black and white US adults. *Am. J. Orthopsychiatr.* **2018**, *88*, 151–160. [CrossRef] [PubMed]

48. Mezo, P.G.; Baker, R.M. The moderating effect of stress and rumination on depressive symptoms in women and men. *Stress Health* **2012**, *28*, 333–339. [CrossRef] [PubMed]

49. Buchanan, T.; Selmon, N. Race and gender differences in self-efficacy: Assessing the role of gender role attitudes and family background. *Sex Roles* **2008**, *58*, 822–836. [CrossRef]

50. Woods-Giscombe, C.L. Superwoman schema: African American women's views on stress, strength, and health. *Qual. Health Res.* **2010**, *20*, 668–683. [CrossRef] [PubMed]

51. Felsten, G. Gender and coping: Use of distinct strategies and associations with stress and depression. *Anxiety Stress Coping* **1998**, *11*, 289–309. [CrossRef]

52. Watson, N.N.; Hunter, C.D. Anxiety and depression among African American women: The costs of strength and negative attitudes toward psychological help-seeking. *Cult. Divers. Ethnic Minor. Psychol.* **2015**, *21*, 604–612. [CrossRef] [PubMed]

53. Huang, F.Y.; Chung, H.; Kroenke, K.; Delucchi, K.L.; Spirtzer, R.L. Using the patient health questionnaire-9 to measure depression among racially and ethnically diverse primary care patients. *J. Gener. Intern. Med.* **2006**, *21*, 547–552. [CrossRef] [PubMed]

54. Kroenke, K.; Spitzer, R.L.; Williams, J.B.W. The PHQ-9: Validity of a brief depression severity measure. *J. Gener. Intern. Med.* **2001**, *16*, 606–613. [CrossRef]

55. Cooper, L.A.; Gonzales, J.J.; Gallo, J.J.; Rost, K.M.; Meredith, L.S.; Rubenstein, L.V.; Wang, N.; Ford, D.E. The acceptability of treatment for depression among African American, Hispanic, and white primary care patients. *Med. Care* **2003**, *41*, 479–489. [CrossRef] [PubMed]

56. Möller-Leimkühler, A.M. Barriers to help-seeking by men: A review of sociocultural and clinical literature with particular reference to depression. *J. Affect. Disord.* **2002**, *71*, 1–9. [CrossRef]

57. Sussman, L.K.; Robins, L.N.; Earls, F. Treatment-seeking for depression by black and white Americans. *Soc. Sci. Med.* **1987**, *42*, 187–196. [CrossRef]

58. Select Statistical Services. Available online: https://select-statistics.co.uk/calculators/sample-size-calculator-odds-ratio/ (accessed on 21 January 2018).

59.   Lazare, A. Hidden conceptual models in clinical psychiatry. *N. Engl. J. Med.* **1973**, *288*, 345–351. [CrossRef] [PubMed]

# 8

# Recruitment Strategies for a Randomised Controlled Trial Comparing Fast Versus Slow Weight Loss in Postmenopausal Women with Obesity—The TEMPO Diet Trial

Michelle S.H. Hsu [1], Claudia Harper [1] (iD), Alice A. Gibson [1] (iD), Arianne N. Sweeting [1,2], John McBride [1], Tania P. Markovic [1,2], Ian D. Caterson [1,2] (iD), Nuala M. Byrne [3], Amanda Sainsbury [1,*,†] (iD) and Radhika V. Seimon [1,*,†] (iD)

[1] The Boden Institute of Obesity, Nutrition, Exercise & Eating Disorders, Sydney Medical School, Charles Perkins Centre, The University of Sydney, Camperdown, NSW 2006, Australia; michelle.hsu@sydney.edu.au (M.S.H.H.); claudia.harper@sydney.edu.au (C.H.); alice.gibson@sydney.edu.au (A.A.G.); arianne.sweeting@sydney.edu.au (A.N.S.); johnpresmb@hotmail.com (J.M.); tania.markovic@sydney.edu.au (T.P.M.); ian.caterson@sydney.edu.au (I.D.C.)

[2] Metabolism & Obesity Services, Royal Prince Alfred Hospital, Camperdown, NSW 2050, Australia

[3] School of Health Sciences, College of Health and Medicine, University of Tasmania, Launceston, TAS 7250, Australia; nuala.byrne@utas.edu.au

* Correspondence: amanda.salis@sydney.edu.au (A.S.); radhika.seimon@sydney.edu.au (R.V.S.)

† These authors contributed equally to this work.

**Abstract:** Current research around effective recruitment strategies for clinical trials of dietary obesity treatments have largely focused on younger adults, and thus may not be applicable to older populations. The TEMPO Diet Trial (**T**ype of **E**nergy **M**anipulation for **P**romoting optimal metabolic health and body composition in **O**besity) is a randomised controlled trial comparing the long-term effects of fast versus slow weight loss on body composition and cardio-metabolic health in postmenopausal women with obesity. This paper addresses the recruitment strategies used to enrol participants into this trial and evaluates their relative effectiveness. 101 post-menopausal women aged 45–65 years, with a body mass index of 30–40 kg/m$^2$ were recruited and randomised to either fast or slow weight loss. Multiple strategies were used to recruit participants. The total time cost (labour) and monetary cost per randomised participant from each recruitment strategy was estimated, with lower values indicating greater cost-effectiveness and higher values indicating poorer cost-effectiveness. The most cost-effective recruitment strategy was word of mouth, followed (at equal second place) by free publicity on TV and radio, and printed advertorials, albeit these avenues only yielded 26/101 participants. Intermediate cost-effective recruitment strategies were flyer distribution at community events, hospitals and a local tertiary education campus, internet-based strategies, and clinical trial databases and intranets, which recruited a further 40/101 participants. The least cost-effective recruitment strategy was flyer distribution to local health service centres and residential mailboxes, and referrals from healthcare professionals were not effective. Recruiting for clinical trials involving postmenopausal women could benefit from a combination of recruitment strategies, with an emphasis on word of mouth and free publicity via radio, TV, and print media, as well as strategic placement of flyers, supplemented with internet-based strategies, databases and intranets if a greater yield of participants is needed.

**Keywords:** weight loss; clinical trial; diet—reducing; recruitment; obesity

## 1. Introduction

Obesity is a major healthcare burden for both individuals and society, associated with adverse consequences in multiple aspects of wellbeing and quality of life [1,2]. Having a higher body mass index (BMI) is a key risk factor for various non-communicable chronic diseases including cardiovascular disease, type 2 diabetes mellitus and certain cancers [3]. Lifestyle interventions which incorporate dietary and/or physical activity modifications have been demonstrated to be effective in eliciting reductions in body weight and associated risk factors in individuals with overweight and obesity [4]. However, physiological and hormonal changes during the life course, in conjunction with behavioural and lifestyle factors, can promote weight gain and pose challenges to achieving weight reduction goals. A key example are women who have undergone the menopausal transition, which can result in shifts in body composition and fat deposition which are associated with health risk factors in this population group [1]. Hence, there is scope to undertake clinical trials of dietary obesity treatments in postmenopausal population groups.

With any clinical trial, including those of lifestyle-based interventions, recruitment is a crucial determinant of the trial's success. It has been reported that up to 50% of randomised controlled trials in health and healthcare research fail to recruit their target number of participants, and only half of the trials that successfully reach their target do so within their original timeframe [5]. Current research around effective recruitment strategies in weight loss and nutrition intervention trials have largely been focussed with younger adult groups and thus may not be applicable to older populations [5–8]. The effectiveness of specific recruitment methods varies depending on characteristics of the population group, such as age, sex and ethnicity, as well as other sociodemographic factors [6–8]. Research into recruitment of older people to date has largely focused on clinical trials conducted in primary care, which have traditionally drawn on cancer registries and aged centre facilities to recruit participants. Thus, knowledge about effective ways to recruit free-living non-clinical populations into community-based clinical trials has been limited due to a lack of systematic collection and reporting of recruitment data [9]. Compared to clinical populations, community-based trial participants may be more challenging to recruit due to their diverse behaviours and characteristics. Insights into successful methods for recruitment of such populations would likely benefit research regarding lifestyle-based treatment of obesity and other chronic conditions, as these trials often require non-clinical populations [9,10].

The current paper describes and assesses the relative effectiveness of the recruitment strategies that were used to enrol participants into the TEMPO Diet Trial (**T**ype of **E**nergy **M**anipulation for **P**romoting optimal metabolic health and body composition in **O**besity). In light of the above-mentioned challenges of recruitment for clinical trials, our evaluation of the multi-strategy recruitment process used for the present trial will not only provide insights into the effectiveness of various recruitment strategies, it will also provide information to obesity and health researchers in planning more cost-effective recruitment strategies (both in terms of time and monetary costs), thereby helping to improve the time, resource and financial efficiencies of health research.

## 2. Methods

### 2.1. Ethics

The TEMPO Diet Trial is a randomised controlled trial designed to assess the long-term effects of fast versus slow weight loss on body composition and cardio-metabolic health in postmenopausal women aged 45–65 years with a BMI of 30–40 $kg/m^2$. Ethical approval was obtained from the Sydney Local Health District, Royal Prince Alfred Hospital Human Research Ethics Committee. The trial was prospectively registered with the Australian New Zealand Clinical Trials Registry (ANZCTR Reference Number 12612000651886). The inclusion and exclusion criteria for the TEMPO Diet Trial, and the screening methods used to investigate them, are listed in Table 1.

**Table 1.** Screening methods used to investigate inclusion and exclusion criteria for the TEMPO Diet Trial.

| Inclusion Criteria | E-mail Screening | Telephone Screening | Face-To-Face Medical Screening |
|---|---|---|---|
| Female | X | X | X |
| 45–65 years of age | X | X | X |
| Postmenopausal for ≥5 years (calculated from date of last menses) | X | X | X |
| Body Mass Index (BMI) 30–40 kg/m² | X | X | X |
| Weight stable (±2 kg) for ≥past 6 months | | X | X |
| English-speaking | | X | |
| Living in the Sydney metropolitan area (defined by the City of Sydney Statistical Division [11,12]) and able to attend all in-person appointments at the University of Sydney Camperdown campus | X | X | |
| Sedentary (defined as <3 h of structured physical activity per week) | | X | X |
| Asked if they were capable of completing activities required for the trial (e.g., keeping a food, activity and sleep diary, wearing accelerometers for 7 days at a time, etc.) | | | X* |
| **Exclusion Criteria** | | | |
| Not ambulatory, or having restrictions to physical movement that would impede completion of trial activities | | X | X |
| Osteoporosis | | | X |
| Extreme anaemia that could be exacerbated by the fast weight loss intervention (very low energy diet) to be used in the trial | | | X |
| Hyperthyroidism or hypothyroidism | | | X |
| Diabetes mellitus (defined by self-report during e-mail screening and by fasting blood glucose level ≥7.0 mmol/L and glycated haemoglobin (HbA₁c) ≥6.5% at the face-to-face medical screening) [13] | X | X | X |
| Cardiovascular disease | | X | |
| Gastrointestinal disease | | X | |
| Previous gastric or other surgery that may affect appetite | | X | |
| Any loose metal in the body (e.g., pacemaker or bullet) that is contraindicated for magnetic resonance imaging for safety reasons, or which may result in artefacts in medical imaging | | X | X |
| Planning to undertake any major surgery in the next three years | | X | |
| Tobacco use | | X | |
| Alcohol or drug dependency | | X | |
| Taking medication that affects heart rate, body composition or bone mass (e.g., beta-blockers, glucocorticoids) | | X | X |

**Table 1.** *Cont.*

| | | |
|---|---|---|
| Having taken anti-resorptive therapy within the last 3 years | X | X |
| Having taken medication that affects appetite, metabolism, or weight within the past 6 months | X | X |
| Any of the following contraindications for following a total meal replacement diet: lactose intolerance; following a strict vegan diet; or unwillingness to be randomised to one of the two diets | X | X |
| Donated whole blood within 3 months prior to trial commencement | X | |
| Liver or kidney impairments (which may render fast weight loss unsuitable) | | X |

* This was also verified prior to randomization and enrolment into the trial, which occurred 1 week prior to commencement of the dietary interventions (−1 weeks). X = applicable.

## 2.2. Recruitment of Potential Participants

Multiple strategies were used to recruit participants into the trial over a 3-year period (Table 2). The recruitment strategy mentioned in the prospective participant's initial email or telephone expression of interest was determined to be the source of trial information which ultimately led to their decision to contact the research team. If prospective participants did not indicate their source of information about the trial in their first communication with our team, this was asked by the research team in subsequent correspondence.

## 2.3. E-mail Screening

Expressions of interest in participation, and subsequent correspondence, were managed through a trial e-mail account. A generic response, which doubled as an 'e-mail screening', was e-mailed to all enquirers. It included the following questions, which addressed 6 key eligibility criteria:

1.    Do you live in the Sydney metropolitan area?
2.    Are you female?
3.    Are you 45–65 years of age?
4.    Are you at least 5 years postmenopausal?
5.    Are you free from diabetes?
6.    Do you have a body mass index (BMI) of 30–40 kg/m$^2$?

Attached to the e-mail screening message was a participant information sheet with details of the trial purpose and procedures, and the e-mail also contained an invitation to undertake a telephone screening if the recipient was still interested in participating in the trial and could answer 'Yes' to all of the above 6 questions.

## 2.4. Telephone Screening

Eligible respondents to the e-mail screening were invited to participate in a 20-min telephone screening, during which they were given details of the trial and were asked a series of standardised questions based on the full eligibility criteria. The standardised questions were asked in the order of the inclusion and exclusion criteria as listed in Table 1. If the potential participant did not meet a particular criterion, the telephone screening was terminated, and that criterion was recorded as the reason for ineligibility. If the individual was classified as eligible after completing the telephone screening, a 1-h face-to-face medical screening was arranged.

## 2.5. Face-to-Face Medical Screening

Written informed consent was obtained, prospective participants were asked to complete and sign a magnetic resonance imaging (MRI) safety questionnaire, and a face-to-face screening interview and medical tests were conducted (or results from any recent medical tests were examined), in order to fully assess the eligibility of prospective participants. They were asked to provide (either in person at the face-to-face medical screening, or via e-mail), a copy of their results from any bone density scans of the hip that they had undergone in the past 2 years, and any fasting blood tests that they had undergone in the past 6 months. If no bone density results were available, a bone density scan of the left hip was conducted in our facility. The bone density scan results were reviewed by one of our endocrinologist co-authors (A.N.S. or T.P.M.) to check for osteoporosis. Any available fasting pathology results were also reviewed by T.P.M. or A.N.S. to determine whether tests for the following conditions had been undertaken, and—if yes—whether the results showed the prospective participant was eligible for inclusion. Specifically, this included full blood count (to exclude extreme anaemia that could be exacerbated by the fast weight loss diet to be used in the trial), plus circulating concentrations of thyroid stimulating hormone (to exclude hyperthyroidism or hypothyroidism), glucose and glycosylated haemoglobin (HbA$_{1c}$, to exclude diabetes mellitus), as well as markers of hepatic and renal function (to exclude hepatic or renal impairment, which may render fast weight loss unsuitable). If any or all of the required fasting pathology results were not available, a pathology request form from a pathology service accredited with the National Association of Testing Authorities (NATA; Douglas Hanly Moir, Sydney, Australia) was given to prospective participants, including request for any fasting pathology tests that were missing from tests undertaken in the past 6 months. Prospective participants were reimbursed for the cost of any pathology tests requested at the face-to-face medical screening, if they were found to be ineligible for the trial, or—if eligible for the trial—at 36 months, once they had completed all trial outcome measurements.

### 2.6. Interventions

Eligible participants were randomised to either a total meal replacement diet (KicStart$^{TM}$ meal replacement shakes and soups from Prima Health Solutions Pty Ltd., Brookvale, NSW, Australia) involving severe energy restriction (target range for energy restriction was 65–75% relative to estimated energy expenditure) for 16 weeks, or until a BMI of no lower than 20 kg/m$^2$ was reached, whichever came first, followed by slow weight loss (as for the SLOW intervention) for the remaining time up until 52 weeks ("FAST" intervention), or they were randomised to a prescribed food-based diet involving moderate energy restriction (target range for energy restriction was 25–35% relative to estimated energy expenditure) for a total of 52 weeks ("SLOW" intervention). A protein intake of 1 g per kg of actual body weight per day was prescribed for both interventions. Full details of the dietary interventions have been published previously [14].

The number of participants to be recruited for the trial ($n = 100$) was determined based on power calculations, allowing for up to 20% attrition as seen in previously-published weight loss interventions [15–17].

## 3. Results

### 3.1. Participant Recruitment

Participants were recruited from March 2013 to July 2016. The recruitment period resulted in a total of 2514 e-mail enquiries, out of which 401 (16.0%) proceeded to undertake a telephone screening (Figure 1). Of the 2113 enquirers who did not proceed to telephone screening, over half (56%) did not provide any further reasoning or correspondence. For the remaining 44%, reasons for not proceeding with their enquiry included self-reported ineligibility based on the 6 key trial criteria (see Methods, 'Recruitment of potential participants'), no longer being interested in the trial due to the requirements of the trial, as well as medical conditions, medication or a history of gastric surgery, which were revealed after further email correspondence prior to arranging a telephone screening appointment with prospective participants. For the 401 individuals who proceeded to a telephone screening, 151 (6.0%) attended a face-to-face medical screening, and 101 (4.0%) were randomised (and enrolled) into the trial (Figure 1), fulfilling our original recruitment target of 100 women.

Of the 401 women who underwent telephone screening, almost two thirds did not proceed to face-to-face medical screening ($n = [193 + 57 = 250]/401$, 62.3%) (Figure 1), primarily due to exclusion for not meeting the eligibility criteria ($n = 193/250$, 77.2%). Of the women who did not meet the eligibility criteria, BMI was the most common reason for ineligibility ($n = [32 + 16 = 48]/193$, 24.9%) (Figure 1). At the face-to-face medical screening step, the main reason for not proceeding to enrolment into the trial was prospective participants' refusal to participate ($n = 32/[18 + 32 = 50]$, 64.0%) rather than exclusion for not meeting the eligibility criteria ($n = 18/50$, 36.0%). The main reason for refusal to participate, cited at the face-to-face medical screening ($n = 11/32$, 34.4%) as well as at the telephone screening ($n = 28/57$, 49.1%), was the inability to commit to the trial. Any other reasons are not known, as prospective participants ceased further correspondence after the telephone ($n = 18$) or face-to-face medical ($n = 17$) screening.

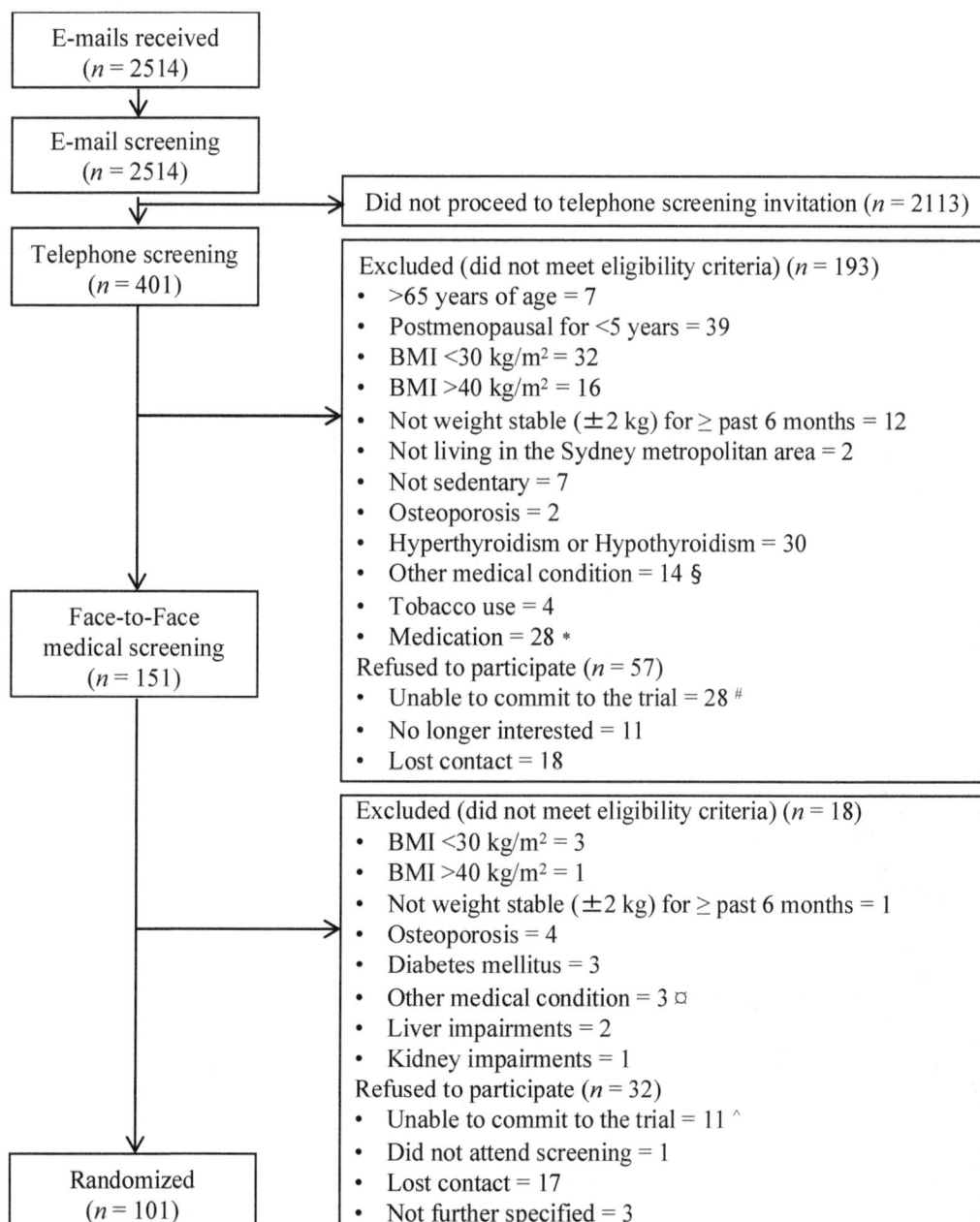

**Figure 1.** Recruitment flowchart. BMI = body mass index. § History of abnormal liver function = 2, metal in body that was incompatible with magnetic resonance imaging = 5, chronic heart failure = 1, gastric banding = 6. * Anti-depressants = 21, anti-anxiety = 2, anti-epileptic = 1, anti-diabetic = 3, other medication = 1. # Time commitment = 18, not willing to undertake dietary intervention = 6, not willing to undertake trial procedures (blood tests, magnetic resonance imaging, body composition measurements) = 3, not willing to abstain from alcohol = 1. Taking anti-depressants = 2, hip replacement = 1. ^Time commitment = 8, not willing to undertake dietary intervention = 1, not willing to undertake trial procedure (magnetic resonance imaging) = 1, commenced a diet by themselves = 1.

### 3.2. Recruitment Strategies

Different recruitment strategies were used concurrently throughout the recruitment period as summarised in Table 2. All but one strategy (print media, namely flyers) were utilised intermittently throughout the 2.5-year recruitment period and print media (flyers) were used throughout the 2.5 years.

**Table 2.** Relative effectiveness of recruitment strategies used in the TEMPO Diet Trial.

| Strategies | Description | Number of Instances Used | Total Response n (% of Total Response from all Strategies) | Screened n (% of Total Responses from Strategy) | Eligible n (% of Total Responses from Strategy) | Randomised n (% of Total Responses from Strategy) | Total Time Invested (Active Recruitment/Correspondence Time) (hours) | Time cost per Randomised Participant * (hours) |
|---|---|---|---|---|---|---|---|---|
| All strategies | | - | 2514 (100.0) | 401 (16.0) | 151 (6.0) | 101 (4.0) | 1828 (828/1000) | 18 |
| **Other** | | | | | | | | |
| • Word of mouth | Informally used throughout the trial through individuals directly involved with the trial (researchers, students, volunteers, ineligible participants and enrolled participants) and indirect associates (health practitioners, family, friends, acquaintances who may have learnt about the trial through the other recruitment strategies). | Continuous | 29 (1.2) | 17 (58.6) | 11 (37.9) | 5 (17.2) | 10 (NA/10) | 2 |
| • Not further specified | Individuals did not specify or could not recall their source of information in their initial enquiry. | - | 1009 (40.1) | 156 (15.5) | 44 (4.4) | 26 (2.6) | 401 (NA/401) | 15 |
| **Free publicity on radio and TV (total)** | TV and radio programs that invited trial researchers to provide commentary on health topics featured a free advertorial about the trial in exchange for accepting the interview. The suggested content of advertorials included brief description of the trial and trial e-mail address, which was announced verbally on air or as a web link on the channel website. Trial recruitment information was mentioned on radio stations 2GB and | 9 | 58 (2.3) | 21 (36.2) | 16 (27.6) | 15 (25.9) | 65 (42/23) | 4 |
| • Radio (local and national) | ABC, during/at the end of segments involving guest researcher and was included on the radio station website. | 6 | 17 (0.7) | 8 (47.1) | 8 (47.1) | 8 (47.1) | 25 (18/7) | 3 |
| • TV (local and national) | Brief advertisement was included for stories about weight loss and health featuring trial researchers. | 3 | 41 (1.6) | 13 (31.7) | 8 (19.5) | 7 (17.1) | 40 (24/16) | 6 |
| **Print media (total)** | Printed advertorials in magazines and a local newspaper, and flyers. Commercial advertisements included as part of magazine and newspaper articles featuring expert commentary from trial researchers. Advertisements were free | - | 78 (3.1) | 61 (78.2) | 40 (51.3) | 22 (28.2) | 588 (556/32) | 27 |
| • Printed advertorials (total) | of charge in exchange for providing expert commentary. Advertisement mentioned brief description of trial, key eligibility criteria and trial e-mail address, but was ultimately determined by the journalist or media liaison. | 6 | 9 (0.4) | 7 (77.8) | 6 (66.7) | 6 (66.7) | 22 (18/4) | 4 |

**Table 2.** *Cont.*

| Strategy | Description | | | | | | | |
|---|---|---|---|---|---|---|---|---|
| ○ University magazine, newsletter | University of Sydney alumni magazine and newsletter. | 2 | 4 (0.2) | 4 (100.0) | 4 (100.0) | 3 (75.0) | 8 (6/2) | 3 |
| ○ Newspaper and magazine advertisements | Local and national newspaper and magazines, including one paid advertisement (AU$500) for a free local newspaper, entitled Mx, that was available to train commuters in Sydney metropolitan area. | 4 | 5 (0.2) | 3 (60.0) | 3 (60.0) | 3 (60.0) | 14 (12/2) | 5 |
| ● Flyers (total) | A4 and brochure-sized flyers were printed using university facilities free of charge and distributed to locations in the Sydney metropolitan area by researchers, volunteers and students. The flyer included a brief description of the trial, key eligibility criteria and trial e-mail address. Over 17,000 flyers delivered in total, at AU$0.05 per flyer (total of AU$850). | - | 69 (2.7) | 27 (39.1) | 17 (24.6) | 16 (23.2) | 566 (538/28) | 35 |
| ○ Community events | Annual Sydney Craft & Quilt Fair held over 4 consecutive days (300 flyers delivered per day). | 1 | 14 (0.6) | 5 (35.7) | 3 (21.4) | 3 (21.4) | 20 (14/6) | 7 |
| ○ Hospitals | Hospitals in the Sydney metropolitan area, in waiting rooms, staff rooms and common areas. | Continuous | 6 (0.2) | 3 (50.0) | 2 (33.3) | 2 (33.3) | 22 (20/2) | 11 |
| ○ Local tertiary education campus | Libraries, common rooms and study spaces within the University of Sydney campus. | Continuous | 5 (0.2) | 3 (60.0) | 2 (40.0) | 2 (40.0) | 22 (20/2) | 11 |
| ○ Local health service centres | 50–70 pharmacy and/or chemist sites (10 flyers delivered per site) and 100 medical practices (10 flyers delivered per site). | Continuous | 8 (0.3) | 4 (50.0) | 4 (50.0) | 4 (50.0) | 243 (240/3) | 61 |
| ○ Residential mailboxes^ | Houses and unit complexes (15,000 flyers delivered in total). | Continuous | 10 (0.4) | 4 (40.0) | 2 (20.0) | 2 (20.0) | 244(240/4) | 122 |
| ○ Not further specified | Individual did not specify or could not recall where they found flyer. | - | 19 (0.8) | 7 (36.8) | 4 (21.1) | 3 (15.8) | 8 (NA/8) | 3 |
| ○ Local community areas | 6 libraries, 10–20 grocery stores/shopping centres, gyms and women's centre (10 flyers delivered per site). | Continuous | 7 (0.3) | 1 (14.3) | 0 (0.0) | 0 (0.0) | 7 (4/3) | NE |
| **Internet-based (total)** | **Free advertisements were featured in online health articles and social networking sites. Researchers requested a brief advertisement of the trial to be included in the footer of articles or as social media posts, including at least a brief description of the trial and e-mail address.** | - | **1082 (43.0)** | **128 (11.8)** | **40 (3.7)** | **24 (2.2)** | **541 (110/431)** | **23** |

**Table 2.** *Cont.*

| Strategy | Description | | | | | | | |
|---|---|---|---|---|---|---|---|---|
| • Health columns of news websites # | Free advertisements were featured at the bottom of online health and nutrition-related articles of news and magazine sites which requested expert commentary from trial researchers. | 37 | 1,033 (41.1) | 127 (12.3) | 40 (3.9) | 24 (2.3) | 521 (110/411) | 22 |
| • Social media pages | Image of the trial flyer was posted on Facebook health pages related to women's health and fitness. | 1 | 32 (1.3) | 0 (0.0) | 0 (0.0) | 0 (0.0) | 13 (NA/13) | NE |
| • Other | Individual read about trial through other online source which referred to an article or media release that advertised the trial. | Continuous | 17 (0.7) | 1 (5.9) | 0 (0.0) | 0 (0.0) | 7 (NA/7) | NE |
| Clinical trial databases and intranets | Advertisements and trial flyer were featured on staff intranets and portals of the University of Sydney, local tertiary hospitals (St Vincent's Hospital and Royal Prince Alfred Hospital) and a local health network (Human Services Network). An ongoing advertisement was also listed on the University of Sydney clinical trials webpage which includes a database for research volunteers. Registrants in the database who met the trial criteria were invited by e-mail to arrange a telephone screening. | Continuous | 248 (9.9) | 40 (16.1) | 17 (6.9) | 9 (3.6) | 199 (100/99) | 22 |
| Referrals from healthcare professionals | Personal letter invitations and trial information packs (10 flyers and a participant information sheet per pack) sent to healthcare professionals in medical clinics across Sydney metropolitan suburbs requesting referrals of suitable patients. Follow-up packs were sent to healthcare professionals or clinics that responded to initial invitations or referred individual(s). Participants enrolled into the trial provided details of referring healthcare professionals. ~50 professionals or clinics were sent packs, at AU$1.10 per pack (total of AU$55). | Continuous | 10 (0.4) | 5 (50.0) | 0 (0.0) | 0 (0.0) | 24 (20/4) | NE |

All strategies were unpaid except one local newspaper advertisement which cost AU$500 and printing material which cost AU$905. NA = not applicable; NE = not effective, did not yield any randomised participants. * Time invested in active recruitment and correspondence (e-mails, telephone calls and telephone screenings) per randomised participant for each recruitment strategy, whereby smaller value indicates a more time effective strategy. # Health news column of websites including the Australian Broadcasting Commission, Huffington Post Australia, Body and Soul, News.com, Ninemsn, the Conversation, Yahoo7 and the Sydney Morning Herald. ^ Delivered to residential properties in the Northern Beaches, Inner West, Eastern and Inner Sydney metropolitan areas.

*3.3. Time or Monetary Cost per Randomised Participant, and Yield of Recruitment Strategies*

To compare the overall success of different recruitment strategies, the time cost (labour) and monetary cost per randomised participant from each recruitment strategy was estimated, whereby lower values indicate greater cost-effectiveness and higher values indicate poorer cost-effectiveness (Table 2) [18,19]. The total number of prospective participants who made initial enquiries, were telephone screened, eligible, or recruited into the trial was also calculated for each recruitment strategy and is shown in Table 2, because yield is just as important as cost effectiveness. In the current trial, time cost per randomised participant is almost synonymous with the total time or monetary cost per randomised participant, because all recruitment strategies, except for one printed local newspaper advertisement in a circular entitled *MX* (AU$500) were free of monetary cost. Although printing of flyers and referral packs for healthcare professionals was provided by the University of Sydney, we estimated a cost of AU$905 for this print material (approximately 17,000 flyers × AU$0.05/flyer + 50 referral packs × AU$1.10/pack). In addition, the trial was supported by students and volunteers which significantly reduced the cost of hiring additional personnel. An estimated total of 828 h was spent on active recruitment, while approximately 1000 h (6–8 h/week) were spent managing e-mail and telephone enquiries and correspondences, including telephone screenings, each of which ranged from 5–60 min in duration. Assuming a casual pay rate of AU$40/h, the total cost of recruitment would have been AU$74,525 ([1828 h × AU$40/h] + AU$500 [for the local newspaper advertisement] + AU$905 [for printed materials]). Thus, over 98% of the costs for recruitment for this trial was the cost of time. While this equated to an average of 18 h (+AU$14 in advertisement and printing), or AU$738, invested for every participant randomised into the trial, the time cost per randomised participant varied between 0–122 h for different strategies (Table 2).

The recruitment strategy with the lowest time cost per randomised participant, and which was therefore the most cost-effective strategy, was word of mouth, which occurred passively and informally throughout the trial and consequently did not require any time or monetary investment for active recruitment and yielded 5 randomised participants.

The recruitment strategies with the equal-second-lowest time cost per randomised participant were free publicity on radio and TV, as well as printed advertorials (a sub-strategy of print media). Free publicity on radio and TV cost an average of 4 h per randomised participant and yielded a total of 15 randomised participants (radio *n* = 8; TV *n* = 7) (Table 2). It is noteworthy that radio publicity cost half as much as TV publicity (3 h per randomised participant versus 6 h for TV) and was used on twice as many instances as TV publicity (*n* = 6 versus *n* = 3, respectively) and received less than half as many responses as TV publicity (*n* = 17 versus *n* = 41, respectively). This difference is likely related to a greater proportion of respondents to radio than to TV publicity being eligible for the trial (47.1% versus 19.5%, respectively), as shown in Table 2. Like the average of radio and TV publicity, printed advertorials also cost an average of 4 h per randomised participant. This recruitment strategy yielded a total of 6 randomised participants.

Two recruitment strategies with intermediate time cost per randomised participant were internet-based strategies, and clinical trial databases and intranets (Table 2). Internet-based recruitment strategies yielded 24 randomised participants, which was the greatest of all recruitment strategies, although they cost an average of 23 h per randomised participant, which is almost six times greater than for free publicity on radio and TV or printed advertorials. Similarly, clinical trial databases and intranets cost an average of 22 h per randomised participant. This recruitment strategy only yielded 9 randomised participants.

The recruitment strategy with the overall greatest total time cost per randomised participant was flyers (a sub-strategy of print media), with an average cost of 35 h per randomised participant, albeit yielding 16 randomised participants, which is the second greatest yield of all strategies used. Approximately 17,000 flyers were distributed, equating to 1063 flyers per recruited participant. It is noteworthy that flyer distribution at community events, hospitals and the local tertiary education campus had intermediate time cost effectiveness, costing between 7–11 h per randomised participant.

Also noteworthy is our observation that distributing flyers to local health service centres cost 61 h per randomised participant, while flyer distribution to residential mailboxes cost 122 h per randomised participant and only yielded 2 randomised participants.

Recruitment via referrals from healthcare professionals was not effective, incurring 24 h of investment but yielding 0 randomised participants (Table 2).

*3.4. Level of Detail Provided in Recruitment Strategies and Impact on Time Cost per Randomised Participant*

We hypothesised that recruitment strategies that provided greater detail about the trial (e.g., eligibility criteria and requirements) would have a lower time cost per randomised participant by enabling prospective participants to 'self-screen' prior to enquiring about the trial. Due to the nature of word of mouth information, the level of detail which was shared informally by individuals involved in the trial (researchers, students, participants, previous enquirers) and associates (family, friends, people who had learned about the trial through other recruitment strategies) could not be determined. For other recruitment strategies, the level of detail provided varied, mainly because media bodies decided on the final content. Free publicity on radio and TV only included detailed information about the trial in 2 of the 9 instances (22%), while printed advertorials included detailed information in 50% of instances, although both recruitment strategies were equal second in terms of the time cost per randomised participant. Internet-based strategies (which were intermediate in terms of the time cost per randomised participant) included detailed information about the trial in 6 of 37 instances (16%), and clinical trial databases and intranets (which had an intermediate time cost per randomised participant), flyers (which had the greatest time cost per randomised participant) and referrals from healthcare professional (which were not effective) provided detailed information about the trial in 100% of instances, as the trial researchers had complete control over the content in all copies. Taken together, these findings suggest that the level of detail provided in recruitment strategies did not influence the cost-effectiveness of a recruitment strategy.

## 4. Discussion

The current paper details the protocol for the TEMPO Diet Trial and describes and evaluates the effectiveness of recruitment strategies used to enrol participants into the trial. This trial found word of mouth to be the recruitment strategy with the lowest time cost per randomised participant, while free publicity on radio and TV, as well as printed advertorials, had the equal-second-lowest time cost per randomised participant. Despite being cost-effective, these recruitment strategies yielded only 26/101 participants. Internet-based and clinical trial databases and intranets had intermediate time cost per randomised participant, and yielded a further 33/101 participants. Another recruitment strategy that was intermediately cost-effective was flyer distribution at community events, hospitals and the local tertiary education campus, with a yield of 7/101 participants, while flyer distribution to local health service centres and residential mailboxes had the greatest time cost per randomised participant and yielded 6/101 participants. Recruitment via referrals from healthcare professionals was not effective. Taking into account both the cost-effectiveness of the different recruitment strategies and their yield, we conclude that clinical trials involving postmenopausal women with obesity could benefit from a combination of recruitment strategies, with an emphasis on word of mouth, free publicity via radio, TV and print media, and strategic placement of flyers, supplemented (if a greater yield of participants is needed) with internet-based strategies, databases and intranets.

Our finding that word of mouth was the most cost-effective recruitment strategy for women aged 45–65 years for the current randomised controlled trial of dietary obesity treatment extends previous findings in younger women with overweight or obesity, which showed that word of mouth was a more cost-effective recruitment strategy than radio, TV, printed advertorials and flyers, e-mails or mass snail mail [20]. The instances of reported word of mouth recruitments were sporadic in the current trial and did not increase over time, perhaps because strategic effort was not invested into this recruitment strategy. It is also possible that some participants who may have initially been referred to the trial by word of mouth were classified as having been recruited by other strategies, as they may have also learned about the trial via other recruitment avenues and reported these as their source of trial information. Future trials in this field could benefit from concerted efforts to enhance word of mouth recruitment alongside other strategies, as a highly cost-effective source of participant recruitment. While researchers in the current trial occasionally encouraged randomised participants and associates to share information about the trial, word of mouth could be further enhanced in future trials by actively providing trial details on distributable items. Such details could be included on items such as regular e-mailed newsletters to participants (including notification of up-coming public seminars by the research team on topics of relevance to weight loss), business cards, pens, and reusable folders and bags that participants and researchers could use as reference when discussing with others. However, it would be important to avoid overcapitalizing on trial-specific merchandise, as excessive spending in this domain would reduce the cost effectiveness of word of mouth recruitment.

Free publicity on radio and TV, as well as printed advertorials, were the equal-second most cost-effective strategies for recruiting older women with obesity into the current randomised controlled trial, possibly due to the nature of the announcements. Trial researchers leveraged long-term relationships with media contacts, including journalists and personnel in the university media office, to find opportunities for free publicity via avenues such as national radio, TV, magazines and newspapers that would otherwise be costly. Providing expert opinion on trial-related health news topics was a valuable form of reciprocity that further helped to develop collaborative relationships with media contacts. After announcements were made, contact was maintained with responsible media contacts (e.g., to give feedback on their media stories, to give thanks if an announcement generated a particularly strong number of enquiries about the trial, and to let them know that we were available for expert comment on any future media stories about weight management that they may be preparing), and this undoubtedly led to our ongoing opportunities for collaboration. Therefore, recruitment for future trials could benefit by establishing or maintaining long-term, strong, positive, mutually beneficial, collaborative relationships with media contacts, and soliciting opportunities for free publicity during recruitment drives.

Flyer distribution—overall—was the least cost-effective recruitment strategy in the current trial. While this is not true of flyers distributed to community events, hospitals and the local tertiary education campus, which had intermediate cost-effectiveness, it was true of distributing flyers to local health service centres and residential mailboxes. A previous study involving postmenopausal women in primary care interventions reported considerable success from residential mailbox flyers [9]. However, unlike our anonymous residential mailbox deliveries, that study used clinical cancer registries and senior community service organisation lists to address recruitment announcements to individuals who may have already held an interest in the topic of the trial [9]. Such registries may not be accessible to research groups due to privacy laws [9], and purchasing commercial lists of mailing contacts would be costly and would not guarantee an interested population. Although flyers were high in cost investment, not only in time for production and delivery, but also for printing materials, for future trials for this demographic, flyer distribution at community events, hospitals and local tertiary education campus could be specifically targeted, along with the other recruitment strategies listed above.

In the present trial, internet-based strategies and clinical trial databases and intranets also demonstrated intermediate cost-effectiveness. Internet-based strategies had a high influx of non-specific enquiries, which lead to a time cost per randomised participant that was almost 6 times greater than that of free publicity on radio and TV, or printed advertorials. Nonetheless, internet-based recruitment was a valuable strategy, as it contributed the largest number of randomised participants to the trial. For future trials, internet-based strategies could be used to supplement word of mouth recruitment and free publicity on radio and TV and printed advertorials, but could be better harnessed (and the cost-effectiveness improved) by implementing an automated response to direct initial enquirers to a web page from which they could learn more about the trial, including key eligibility criteria, and then—if still interested and if they consider that they meet these criteria—to register through an ethically-approved and secure online screening. Such automated systems would assist researchers to refine the sample of interested individuals they choose to contact based on pre-filled demographic and other details, thereby rendering this recruitment strategy more cost-effective. As mentioned above for trial-specific merchandise, it would be important not to overcapitalize on any such automated systems. Commercial options for automating and managing clinical trial recruitment are available to researchers, but these are often expensive. In contrast, many research organizations (e.g., universities, hospitals, and research institutes) have cost-effective bulk subscriptions to software that enables researchers to conduct surveys securely via the Internet, and these could be explored and cheaply deployed for clinical trial recruitment.

Contacting prospective participants through clinical trials databases and intranets was less cost-effective than expected. This may be explained by the lapse in time between prospective participants' initial registration with the database, which may have been in response to announcement about the present or another clinical trial several months before contact by the research team or trial commencement. Evidence for this comes from one instance of free publicity on national TV, which had approximately 6 million viewers. While prospective participants were contacted within several days after their initial expression of interest, the trial commencement was not until five months or more afterwards, by which time ~58% of initial enquirers were either no longer interested or contactable.

Working through healthcare professionals to recruit participants via referrals yielded no contribution to the overall recruitment effort. Healthcare professionals may not have the time and resources to actively and conscientiously refer suitable patients to trials, and this method of recruitment may therefore be deprioritised for future trials unless they require clinical populations [5,9]. It should also be noted that the current trial invested less time and other resources into engaging and informing healthcare professionals about the trial, compared to free publicity on radio and TV, or print media and internet-based strategies or clinical trial databases and intranets. Thus, future trials, at least in those targeting participants with the demographic of the current trial, may benefit from minimising or completely avoiding recruitment via referrals from healthcare professionals.

The cost-effectiveness of the recruitment strategies implemented in the current trial could potentially be improved in future trials by including a trial telephone number, in addition to the e-mail address provided, to increase the number of initial enquiries. This is because people reading a printed article in a magazine or newspaper may find it easier to call a telephone number rather than to send an e-mail, by avoiding any delay that may be required to gain access to a device connected to the Internet. However, providing a trial telephone number would need to be supported by automated systems that do not lead to a greater time cost of recruitment, such as providing an automated message inviting prospective participants to leave a voice message with their mobile telephone number or e-mail address so that researchers can send participant information via short mobile messaging (SMS) or e-mail, including a link to conduct cost-effective surveys securely via the Internet as mentioned above.

This recruitment analysis has several strengths and limitations. To our knowledge, the current study is the first to evaluate the relative effectiveness of multiple recruitment strategies to engage and recruit postmenopausal women for a randomised controlled trial of dietary obesity treatments, as previous research has focused on younger adults [21,22]. However, the generalisability of the current results is limited to our target demographic, and results may differ for trials aiming to recruit people of other age or sex, or for different areas of clinical research. Time and monetary cost and cost-effectiveness were synonymous in the current study, because all strategies, except one paid newspaper advertisement, as well as printing costs which was provided by the University of Sydney, were free of monetary charge. This is because the current trial was well supported with students and volunteers, which significantly reduced the need to allocate limited government grant funding towards hiring additional personnel. In this sense, the current results are only applicable to other trials that also have access to the valuable contributions of students and volunteers, such as those conducted in universities, hospitals and research institutes. Hence, labour costs of recruitment for trials with limited access to students and volunteers were simulated using a casual pay rate for an average research assistant. A combination of cost effectiveness and yield of participants from different recruitment strategies need to be considered when researchers determine the overall suitability of recruitment methods for their specific research question, trial design and available resources. A further limitation of our recruitment time cost (or cost-effectiveness) calculations is that they do not predict conscientious and successful participants in terms of commitment and trial outcomes, as has previously been reported [22]. In addition, 40.1% of initial enquirers did not specify any details regarding their source of trial information, and others discontinued contact with the research team after the initial telephone screening invitation, rendering some self-reported recruitment data unobtainable—although it is likely that many of these enquiries were derived from Internet advertorials. Greater detail and rigour in documentation of recruitment data in future trials would reduce missing data and provide more refined insights into the recruitment process. Since the current recruitment analysis was conducted post-hoc, a randomised comparison of recruitment strategies was not conducted, and some avenues of recruitment were not fully assessed. While the trial incorporated some newer forms of popular media to recruit participants (Facebook, health blogs, Internet-based health articles), social media platforms and paid online advertisements were not explored in-depth, and may be subject to future investigation into the relative effectiveness of different Internet-based strategies. Moreover, commercial recruitment avenues were not explored at all in the current trial due to funding limitations. These may have resulted in faster recruitment. The current work is thus mostly relevant to research teams with limited access to research funds, but with strong access to students and volunteers, as is the case in many universities, hospitals and research institutes around the world.

## 5. Conclusions

The present findings highlight the inherent challenges of recruiting free-living older women with obesity into a randomised controlled trial of dietary obesity treatments, and illustrate a path forward for more cost-effective recruitment. In summary and conclusion, recruitment for future trials in this area will likely benefit by investing time into creative word of mouth recruitment strategies, building relationships with media contacts (including journalists and personnel in the university media office) to facilitate free publicity at the time when it is required for trial recruitment, only using flyers if they can be strategically placed in locations that the target demographic are known to utilise such as at community events, hospitals and local tertiary education campuses and—if recruitment yields with these three cost-effective strategies are not sufficient—internet-based strategies, all supported by automated online systems to reduce the time cost of screening to improve the cost-effectiveness of all recruitment strategies. These current results may provide important strategies and factors that could be considered in planning recruitment for future clinical weight loss trials.

**Author Contributions:** Conceptualization, A.S. and R.V.; Methodology, M.S.H.H., C.H., A.A.G., A.N.S., J.M., T.P.M., A.S. and R.V.S.; Formal Analysis, M.S.H.H., A.S. and R.V.S.; Writing—Original Draft Preparation, M.S.H.H., A.S. and R.V.S.; Writing-Review & Editing, M.S.H.H., C.H., A.A.G., A.N.S., T.P.M., I.D.C., N.M.B., A.S. and R.V.S.

**Funding:** This work was supported by the National Health and Medical Research Council (NHMRC) of Australia via an Early Career Research Fellowship to R.V.S. (1072771) and A.N.S. (1148952), as well as a Project Grant (1026005) to A.S., N.M.B. and I.D.C., and Senior Research Fellowships (1042555 and 1135897) to A.S. The Endocrine Society of Australia additionally supported this work via a Postdoctoral Award to R.V.S. The Australian Government's Department of Education & Training also supported this research through an Australian Postgraduate Award to A.A.G.

**Conflicts of Interest:** A.A.G. has received payment for oral presentations from the Pharmacy Guild of Australia and Nestlé Health Science. A.N.S has received funds for performing clinical trials from NovoNordisk. T.P.M. is on the NovoNordisk Obesity Advisory Board and Health Science Optifast® VLCD™ Advisory Board, has received funds for performing clinical trials from Pfizer, NovoNordisk, SFI, Australia Egg Corporation and has given talks on obesity for NovoNordisk. I.D.C. is past-president of the World Obesity Federation, has received funds for performing clinical trials from the NHMRC, SFI, the Australia Egg Corporation, NovoNordisk, BMS and Pfizer, and has given talks on obesity for Servier Laboratories, Ache Pharmaceuticals. A.S. is the author of *The Don't Go Hungry Diet* (Bantam, Australia and New Zealand, 2007) and *Don't Go Hungry For Life* (Bantam, Australia and New Zealand, 2011). She has also received payment from Eli Lilly, the Pharmacy Guild of Australia, Novo Nordisk, the Dietitians Association of Australia, Shoalhaven Family Medical Centres and the Pharmaceutical Society of Australia for presentation at conferences, and has served on the Nestlé Health Science Optifast® VLCD™ Advisory Board since 2016. For the TEMPO Diet Trial, Prima Health Solutions, Brookvale, NSW, Australia, provided in-kind support in the form of below-cost KicStart™ meal replacement products (shakes) and a gift of associated adherence tools (shakers). Prima Health Solutions had no involvement in the design or analysis of the research. This relationship with Prima Health Solutions was established after the protocol for the TEMPO Diet Trial had been established.

## References

1.  Davis, S.R.; Castelo-Branco, C.; Chedraui, P.; Lumsden, M.A.; Nappi, R.E.; Shah, D.; Villaseca, P. Understanding weight gain at menopause. *Climacteric* **2012**, *15*, 419–429. [CrossRef] [PubMed]
2.  Baker, A.; Sirois-Leclerc, H.; Tulloch, H. The impact of long-term physical activity interventions for overweight/obese postmenopausal women on adiposity indicators, physical capacity, and mental health outcomes: A systematic review. *J. Obes.* **2016**, *2016*, 6169890. [CrossRef] [PubMed]
3.  Afshin, A.; Forouzanfar, M.H.; Reitsma, M.B.; Sur, P.; Estep, K.; Lee, A.; Marczak, L.; Mokdad, A.H.; Moradi-Lakeh, M.; Naghavi, M.; et al. Health effects of overweight and obesity in 195 countries over 25 years. *N. Engl. J. Med.* **2017**, *377*, 13–27. [PubMed]
4.  Hassan, Y.; Head, V.; Jacob, D.; Bachmann, M.O.; Diu, S.; Ford, J. Lifestyle interventions for weight loss in adults with severe obesity: A systematic review. *Clin. Obes.* **2016**, *6*, 395–403. [CrossRef] [PubMed]
5.  Fletcher, B.; Gheorghe, A.; Moore, D.; Wilson, S.; Damery, S. Improving the recruitment activity of clinicians in randomised controlled trials: A systematic review. *BMJ Open* **2012**, *2*, e000496. [CrossRef] [PubMed]
6.  Nguyen, T.T.; Jayadeva, V.; Cizza, G.; Brown, R.J.; Nandagopal, R.; Rodriguez, L.M.; Rother, K.I. Challenging recruitment of youth with type 2 diabetes into clinical trials. *J. Adolesc. Health* **2014**, *54*, 247–254. [CrossRef] [PubMed]
7.  Robinson, L.; Adair, P.; Coffey, M.; Harris, R.; Burnside, G. Identifying the participant characteristics that predict recruitment and retention of participants to randomised controlled trials involving children: A systematic review. *Trials* **2016**, *17*, 294. [CrossRef] [PubMed]
8.  Lindenstruth, K.A.; Curtis, C.B.; Allen, J.K. Recruitment of African American and white postmenopausal women into clinical trials: The beneficial effects of soy trial experience. *Ethn. Dis.* **2006**, *16*, 938–942. [PubMed]
9.  Butt, D.A.; Lock, M.; Harvey, B.J. Effective and cost-effective clinical trial recruitment strategies for postmenopausal women in a community-based, primary care setting. *Contemp. Clin. Trials* **2010**, *31*, 447–456. [CrossRef] [PubMed]
10. Warner, E.T.; Glasgow, R.E.; Emmons, K.M.; Bennett, G.G.; Askew, S.; Rosner, B.; Colditz, G.A. Recruitment and retention of participants in a pragmatic randomized intervention trial at three community health clinics: Results and lessons learned. *BMC Public Health* **2013**, *13*, 192. [CrossRef] [PubMed]
11. City of Sydney. Metropolitan Sydney. Available online: www.cityofsydney.nsw.gov.au/learn/research-and-statistics/the-city-at-a-glance/metropolitan-sydney (accessed on 12 February 2017).
12. Australian Bureau of Statistics. Frequently Asked Questions: How Does the Abs Define Metropolitan and Non-Metropolitan? Available online: www.abs.gov.au/websitedbs/d3310114.nsf/home/frequently+asked+questions#Anchor8 (accessed on 12 February 2017).
13. American Diabetes Association. Diagnosis and classification of diabetes mellitus. *Diabetes Care* **2014**, *37* (Suppl. 1), S81–S90.
14. Gibson, A.A.; Seimon, R.V.; Franklin, J.; Markovic, T.P.; Byrne, N.M.; Manson, E.; Caterson, I.D.; Sainsbury, A. Fast versus slow weight loss: Development process and rationale behind the dietary interventions for the tempo diet trial. *Obes. Sci. Pract.* **2016**, *2*, 162–173. [CrossRef] [PubMed]
15. Bryson, J.M.; King, S.E.; Burns, C.M.; Baur, L.A.; Swaraj, S.; Caterson, I.D. Changes in glucose and lipid metabolism following weight loss produced by a very low calorie diet in obese subjects. *Int. J. Obes. Relat. Metab. Disord.* **1996**, *20*, 338–345. [PubMed]
16. Byrne, N.M.; Meerkin, J.D.; Laukkanen, R.; Ross, R.; Fogelholm, M.; Hills, A.P. Weight loss strategies for obese adults: Personalized weight management program vs. Standard care. *Obesity* **2006**, *14*, 1777–1788. [CrossRef] [PubMed]

17. McMillan-Price, J.; Petocz, P.; Atkinson, F.; O'Neill, K.; Samman, S.; Steinbeck, K.; Caterson, I.; Brand-Miller, J. Comparison of 4 diets of varying glycemic load on weight loss and cardiovascular risk reduction in overweight and obese young adults: A randomized controlled trial. *Arch. Intern. Med.* **2006**, *166*, 1466–1475. [CrossRef] [PubMed]

18. Krusche, A.; Rudolf von Rohr, I.; Muse, K.; Duggan, D.; Crane, C.; Williams, J.M. An evaluation of the effectiveness of recruitment methods: The staying well after depression randomized controlled trial. *Clin. Trials* **2014**, *11*, 141–149. [CrossRef] [PubMed]

19. Chin Feman, S.P.; Nguyen, L.T.; Quilty, M.T.; Kerr, C.E.; Nam, B.H.; Conboy, L.A.; Singer, J.P.; Park, M.; Lembo, A.J.; Kaptchuk, T.J.; et al. Effectiveness of recruitment in clinical trials: An analysis of methods used in a trial for irritable bowel syndrome patients. *Contemp. Clin. Trials* **2008**, *29*, 241–251. [CrossRef] [PubMed]

20. Tate, D.F.; LaRose, J.G.; Griffin, L.P.; Erickson, K.E.; Robichaud, E.F.; Perdue, L.; Espeland, M.A.; Wing, R.R. Recruitment of young adults into a randomized controlled trial of weight gain prevention: Message development, methods, and cost. *Trials* **2014**, *15*, 326. [CrossRef] [PubMed]

21. Lam, E.; Partridge, S.R.; Allman-Farinelli, M. Strategies for successful recruitment of young adults to healthy lifestyle programmes for the prevention of weight gain: A systematic review. *Obes. Rev.* **2016**, *17*, 178–200. [CrossRef] [PubMed]

22. Frandsen, M.; Thow, M.; Ferguson, S.G. The effectiveness of social media (facebook) compared with more traditional advertising methods for recruiting eligible participants to health research studies: A randomized, controlled clinical trial. *JMIR Res. Protoc.* **2016**, *5*, e161. [CrossRef] [PubMed]

# 9

# Stakeholder Views on Active Cascade Screening for Familial Hypercholesterolemia

Carla G. van El [1,*], Valentina Baccolini [2] , Peter Piko [3,4] and Martina C. Cornel [1]

[1] Department of Clinical Genetics and APH Research Institute, Amsterdam UMC,
   Vrije Universiteit Amsterdam, 1081 GT Amsterdam, The Netherlands; mc.cornel@vumc.nl

[2] Department of Public Health and Infectious Diseases, Sapienza University of Rome, 00185 Rome, Italy;
   valentina.baccolini@uniroma1.it

[3] MTA-DE Public Health Research Group of the Hungarian Academy of Sciences, Faculty of Public Health,
   University of Debrecen, 4028 Debrecen, Hungary; piko.peter@sph.unideb.hu

[4] Department of Preventive Medicine, Faculty of Public Health, University of Debrecen,
   4028 Debrecen, Hungary

* Correspondence: cg.vanel@vumc.nl

**Abstract:** In familial hypercholesterolemia (FH), carriers profit from presymptomatic diagnosis and early treatment. Due to the autosomal dominant pattern of inheritance, first degree relatives of patients are at 50% risk. A program to identify healthy relatives at risk of premature cardiovascular problems, funded by the Netherlands government until 2014, raised questions on privacy and autonomy in view of the chosen active approach of family members. Several countries are building cascade screening programs inspired by Dutch experience, but meanwhile, the Netherlands' screening program itself is in transition. Insight in stakeholders' views on approaching family members is lacking. Literature and policy documents were studied, and stakeholders were interviewed on pros and cons of actively approaching healthy relatives. Sociotechnical analysis explored new roles and responsibilities, with uptake, privacy, autonomy, psychological burden, resources, and awareness as relevant themes. Stakeholders agree on the importance of early diagnosis and informing the family. Dutch healthcare typically focuses on cure, rather than prevention. Barriers to cascade screening are paying an own financial contribution, limited resources for informing relatives, and privacy regulation. To benefit from predictive, personalized, and preventive medicine, the roles and responsibilities of stakeholders in genetic testing as a preventive strategy, and informing family members, need to be carefully realigned.

**Keywords:** familial hypercholesterolemia; cascade screening; sociotechnical analysis; stakeholder analysis; personalized prevention

## 1. Introduction

Familial hypercholesterolemia (FH) is one of the most common human inherited disorders, characterized by high levels of serum total cholesterol and low-density lipoprotein cholesterol (LDL-C). Two forms are characterized according to the mode of inheritance of the disease (autosomal recessive and autosomal dominant FH). Both forms lead to premature atherosclerosis and cardiovascular problems [1,2]. The autosomal recessive form is an extremely rare condition worldwide (except in the island of Sardinia, Italy), and it is caused by defects in the *LDLRAP1* gene [3]. With prevalence ranging between 1:200 and 1:500 worldwide, autosomal dominant FH is the most common form which is caused by gene mutations, most notably in the low-density lipoprotein receptor (*LDLR*) gene, or defects in genes involved in cholesterol metabolism (*APOB, PCSK9*). In this paper, we will focus on the autosomal dominant type of FH. The diagnosis of FH is based on high concentrations of LDL-C, family history of hypercholesterolemia, presence of premature coronary artery disease, and cholesterol deposition in the form of xanthomas and/or arcus senilis [4]. Genetic testing can confirm a diagnosis in about 80% of cases, and international guidelines differ on the importance of genetic testing for treatment [5,6]. Currently, FH is globally underdiagnosed and undertreated [1]. The risk of cardiovascular events can be reduced by medication via statins, and adopting a healthy lifestyle [7]. The early diagnosis and treatment initiation is critical for patients with FH. The risk of premature death from cardiovascular disease is four times greater for untreated FH patients than it is for those who do not suffer from FH [8]. Due to the autosomal dominant inheritance of this type of FH, first degree family members have a 50% chance of also carrying the same pathogenic gene variant. Genetic screening of family members allows for personalized prevention, and it is paramount to find and inform these family members in a timely manner.

An important question is how family members—who, at that point, are still considered to be healthy and feel healthy, but are nevertheless at risk—can be traced and informed in an ethically responsible and efficient manner? Newson and Humphries [8] differentiated direct and indirect strategies. In a direct approach, healthcare professionals or representatives from a screening program contact family members directly, after having obtained the addresses from the proband or index patient in whom the mutation has been detected. Another indirect option is that the proband or index patient contacts his or her family members. Newson and Humphries argue that direct contacting is efficient and ethically justifiable in certain conditions. For instance, the index could inform the family members first that he or she has had genetic testing, and that the family will be contacted soon with more information. In this way, receiving an unsolicited letter form a healthcare provider might be less of a shock. As family dynamics may differ, how best to approach the family should be discussed with the proband, who might take up a more or a less active role [9].

In several European countries, initiatives were started to identify FH patients and trace family members using various approaches. The Netherlands is among the very few countries where a systematic screening program was introduced, and proved an inspiration to other countries [10,11]. The Dutch screening started in 1994 [12], was developed into a national screening program in 2004, and was characterized by the proactive tracing, direct contacting, informing, and testing of healthy family members of an index patient. After the addresses were obtained from the index, patient family members were asked to be visited and tested at home by a nurse employed as a genetic field worker at the Foundation for Tracing Familial Hypercholesterolemia (StOEH). For the index, patient complex genetic testing was performed at the laboratory of the Amsterdam University Medical Center. Once the mutation was identified, family members were only tested for the familial mutation, which was relatively cheap. The pedigrees and mutations were registered in a database, and whenever a new index was identified, the database was checked to see if this person might be related to a known family in the database, so genetic testing could be personalized. The program was found to be cost-effective [13]. The programme had always been regarded as a project, and when it started, it was expected that most carriers would have been detected by 2010, based upon an estimated heterozygote frequency of 1:500. When evidence accrued that the heterozygote frequency was actually >1:250, it became clear that not all carriers could be found by that year. The funding was extended from 2010 to 2013. Between 2004 and 2014, 15,000 FH patients were identified [8]. During this decade, financial support was provided by the Ministry of Health, and the program was coordinated by the National Institute of Public Health and the Environment (RIVM). Though successful, the screening program ended in 2014, leaving an estimated 40,000 of the expected 70,000 mutation carriers in the Netherlands unidentified. After 2014, other actors in regular healthcare were supposed to take over, coordinated by the newly established foundation LEEFH (Dutch Expertise Centre for Inheritance Testing of Cardiovascular Diseases). The budget was reduced, and strategies to approach healthy relatives had to be reconsidered. In the regular healthcare system, official inhabitants of the Netherlands have to purchase obligatory insurance of a "basic healthcare package", for which persons with a low income receive governmental reimbursement. The insurance covers the financial costs after falling ill, and includes "indicated prevention" for persons at an individually increased risk, but not population screening and vaccination programs. The latter are typically funded from public health budgets. For individual healthcare cost, an "own risk" of 385€ (in 2018) applies for medication and hospital expenses per year, including laboratory testing. Since the ending of the publicly funded screening program in 2014, people may have to pay up to the amount of the own risk to get tested.

After ending the screening program, the yearly number of index patients identified almost halved, to about 141 in 2015. However, most notably, the number of family members identified dropped when family screenings dwindled from over 2000 to around 400 in 2015 [14,15].

Healthcare professionals were concerned and pleaded to continue the screening program, also drawing attention to the fact that less children with FH would now be identified [16]. In 2016, the Dutch Minister of Health stated that the proactive and direct approach, as it had been conducted at the time of the screening program, would not be reinstalled [17]. Though the ending of the Dutch screening was not unanticipated, a new argument surfaced. Patients should make autonomous choices in making use of healthcare or screening, and home visits were seen as too "paternalistic". In other words: the acceptability of the screening program was questioned by policymakers. FH care had to be integrated in regular healthcare, while for the tracing of family members, the government pointed to existing facilities in clinical genetics. Following standards in clinical genetics, it was stressed that the index patient is responsible for informing family members, who can then decide whether they want to make an appointment for discussing genetic testing [14,17]. Healthcare professionals can support the index by, for instance, giving family letters to the index, so he or she can distribute these to family members.

The history of the Dutch screening program and its recent abandoning of a proactive and direct approach provides us with an excellent opportunity to explore the pros and cons of various approaches to informing healthy family members on their genome. In an era of increasing possibilities for predictive, preventive, and personalized medicine, the question how to balance these pros and cons is topical.

This study explores opinions on how active healthcare professionals can or should inform (healthy) family members when a patient is diagnosed with a hereditary condition, using FH as an example. By identifying and interviewing a range of relevant stakeholders, we aim to clarify arguments for and against more proactive, direct approaches, and show varying responses to and requirements for informing family members, given a changing landscape with new regulatory restraints. For the stakeholders involved, this can contribute to a process of mutual learning and attunement of their practices. By making these arguments and choices available to an international audience, we hope to add to the international discussion on best practices in tracing and informing healthy family members on their genome.

## 2. Materials and Methods

Literature on cascade screening for FH in the Netherlands and national policy concerning the program was studied, stakeholder groups were selected, and interviews with six persons from five stakeholder groups were conducted.

The stakeholders were identified based on a conceptual model for a sociotechnical analysis. In a sociotechnical analysis the roles and arguments of different actors or stakeholders in a network are studied to understand how an innovation, such as genetic testing, becomes part of, and shapes, a new healthcare practice [18,19]. In this process, also, the conditions for use and capacities of a technology become more clearly defined (co-evolution of technology and social-ethical context). In this model, the sources of dynamics may stem from various domains, requiring stakeholders in other domains to adapt their practices. Technological innovation in the scientific domain, for instance, may challenge current practice. New findings or changes, in demand by public and patients, may require healthcare professionals to adapt the organization of services. Also, evaluation of acceptability of procedures by regulatory, advisory, and governmental agencies may provoke changes in healthcare. In our analysis, we will use this conceptual model to describe how stakeholders in The Netherlands are realigning their practices in genetic testing and informing family members in a changing healthcare landscape, after the ending of the FH screening program in 2014. In this case, changes in technology were not the source of dynamics.

After the screening program ended, the Minister argued that the field itself, meaning the stakeholders in FH care, had the responsibility to organize effective care themselves. We will therefore focus our attention to stakeholders in the healthcare and patient domain of the model, to see how they are responding to changed viewpoints in the policy domain on the acceptability of an active approach contacting family members directly, and are trying to reorganize their practices.

Based on the model in Figure 1, we identified five relevant stakeholders, and conducted five interviews in total with six persons (see Table 1): an official from the patient organization, two professionals from the official Netherlands' expertise center for familial cardiovascular disorders that coordinates the detection and care of FH patients (LEEFH), a lipidologist, a clinical geneticist, and an FH nurse consultant that informs patients and advises them on informing their family members.

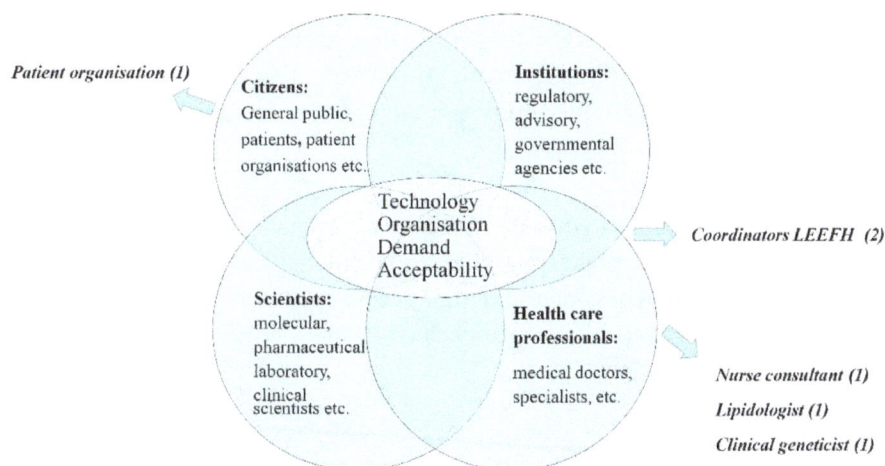

**Figure 1.** Network of stakeholders that need to be attuned in transition processes that could be initiated by dynamics in technology, organization, demand, and/or acceptability in healthcare systems (adapted from Rigter et al., 2014, [19] and Achterbergh et al., 2007, [18]).

**Table 1.** Stakeholders interviewed.

| Stakeholder | Roles in FH Screening | Abbreviation Interviews |
|---|---|---|
| Patient organization | Patient advocacy | (Patient Org.) |
| Coordinator LEEFH | Coordinating role in FH care; update database | (Coord.:1); (Coord.:2) |
| Nurse consultant | Inform about FH, make pedigree, support index with informing family by providing information | (Consult.) |
| Lipidologist | Internal medicine or vascular specialist, involved in FH diagnosis, care and treatment | (Lipid.) |
| Clinical geneticist | Genetic testing, counselling, support informing family members | (Clin. Genet.) |

The stakeholders came from three regions in the Netherlands, and included staff members of national organizations (LEEFH and patient organization) that were expected to be knowledgeable on screening policies, as well as healthcare professionals from local services in hospitals in these three regions. The clinical geneticist and lipidologist were at the senior management level and well known with local and national FH policy. The stakeholders were not representing their organizations, but were asked to reflect on informing family members given their professional experiences. A topic guide was constructed, asking about the pros and cons of different approaches to informing family members in the old screening program, the current situation, and the ideal situation, both in practical and ethical terms (see Supplementary Material S1: interview protocol stakeholder views). The interviews were semi-structured, and were held face-to-face. For LEEFH, two staff members with different functions were present at the interview, and they are listed as Coordinator 1 and 2. All authors were present during at least one interview, one author was present at all interviews (C.G.v.E.).

Respondents were informed about the research aims, and asked for consent prior to the interviews to audio record the interview, store the transcript, and use quotes. Since the consent did not include full disclosure of the transcripts, these are not provided as Supplementary Material. After the audio-recorded interviews were transcribed verbatim, the transcripts were sent to the interviewees for a member check. Thematic analysis was performed manually by two persons (C.G.v.E. and M.C.C.). The themes were inspired by the conceptual framework and established via inductive coding. The codes for two interviews were discussed until consensus was reached. The other interviews were coded based on this list by C.G.v.E. The code list is available as Supplementary Material (Table S1: Code list transcripts interviews "stakeholder views on active cascade screening for familial hypercholesterolemia 2018").

The project proposal was sent to the Ethical Review Board of VUMC, that decided that the Dutch Medical Research Involving Human Subjects Act (WMO) does not apply to the abovementioned study, and that an official approval of this study is therefore not required.

## 3. Results

When discussing the pros and cons of different approaches to informing family members, several themes became apparent: uptake, psychological burden, privacy, and autonomy (Section 3.1). In discussing the current situation or contemplating a future approach, roles and responsibilities were discussed (Section 3.2), while in addition, further needs were identified, such as raising awareness, and availability of resources (Section 3.3).

### 3.1. Pros and Cons of an Active Approach

The active approach of the former screening program was characterized by both a direct approach to contact family members after the index had given permission to do so, and the planning of visits at home or at the workplace to inform the family members, measure cholesterol and draw blood. Respondents noted the high uptake as an important benefit of the approach of the screening program.

> "We only asked them "who are your brothers and sisters?" and if it was okay, we contacted them and sent them letters … "Ok, in your family there is FH, do you want explanation?" and then within two weeks, we made a phone call to the brother asking "Did you receive this information? Is it clear? This is how the program works" and most of the time in 90% we made an appointment." (Coord.:2)

> "[Now] we can only phone, and also the nurses at the expertise centers can only phone the index patients asking them "have you talked to your brother, children?" to stimulate them. Then we send all the packages [for testing, C.G.v.E.], but then we do not get them back. If you actively approach, which is what we did, that was very, very effective". (Coord.:1)

In addition, the support for the index patient in informing family members was seen as an important advantage of the active approach. The lack of such support and the psychological burden for the index was seen an important drawback of the new system.

> "It's also emotionally very difficult for the index patient to have to tell to his brother or sister who lives far away that he has a genetic disease and it's wise to get checked and also that there are consequences for his or her children." (Coord.:1)

Policy documents mentioned paternalism as a drawback of the previous proactive and direct approach, stressing that patients should be responsible to seek healthcare autonomously. However, respondents held various opinions whether this objection was important enough to ban such direct approaches, given the otherwise substantial health gain. In weighing pros and cons, ideas of patient autonomy play an important role, such as in policy, though the ways forward envisaged by the interviewed stakeholders, based on such notions, varied.

> " ... the more autonomy the better it is, but to have autonomy you should be informed ... The best thing would be a screening program again but even if we have it back, even then, more attention would be needed for information for consenting autonomous people. We always need it, whatever system we have." (Patient Org.)

> "I think everybody is working 24 h a day, how good it is that you don't have to come to an office to get your blood drawn from 9 to 10? No, I can understand it (that the old system was seen as paternalistic C.G.v.E.) ... but my vision is completely different. I think it's very modern and I think it would be good to continue that way because then you really get your samples and you find the patients." (Coord.:1)

Privacy was seen as potentially at odds with direct contacting of family members, while also trespassing the right not to know was mentioned. As one respondent remarked:

> "It is not a reason to cut the program but this problem has always existed ... very rarely someone informed me because (they said) "I'd rather not know". The opposite happens many times." (Patient Org.)

Respondents had various ideas on modernizing the active approach. These included directly approaching family members via email addresses obtained from the index to invite the family to contact healthcare.

> "I think it's more of this time to first get this consent that you can approach these family members. I think by now most people have access to e-mail etc. So I think if we could have approached the family members directly, I would say by now you would do it by e-mail. And you will have a good e-mail about it and then you would ask the index patient: is it okay if I email this and this family member? And the index patient would say: you will receive an e-mail and they will inform you about this (FH) and if you don't want it let me know. It's true in a way that it's a bit old fashioned and not very time effective to travel in a car and visit family members." (Lipid.)

### 3.2. Roles and Responsibilities

With the termination of the screening program in 2014, stakeholders had to redefine their roles and responsibilities, given that the Minister had put the responsibility to organize effective care in their hands. In the following, we map views on the roles and responsibilities of the various stakeholders involved.

It took a while before a new coordinating organization was in operation, LEEFH. With very limited funding, they had to find and stimulate best practices. Whereas StOEH had been a centralized organization, LEEFH set up centers in various parts of the country where FH nurse consultants were installed. The way these consultants operate and the amount of time they have may differ per city, which may affect the level of support index patients have, and consequently, the uptake of cascade testing by family members.

> "So if they see that a LEEFH center is not producing enough family members they should say what is wrong how can we help or what is needed?" (Lipid.). To perform the coordinating role is difficult, as one respondent put it there is "lack of people, lack of knowledge, lack of education". (Clin. Genet.)

What remained unchanged after the end of the screening program was that patients are treated at departments of internal or vascular medicine and/or in primary care. During the screening program after genetic testing, genetic field workers of StOEH discussed tracing family members with the patient. For the treating physicians, this was perceived as a *"black hole"* (Lipid.). For those in the new system, there is an advantage in now being able to focus on the family in the care pathway:

> *"The disadvantage of the STOEH-system was that only once the pedigree was made; they didn't have any follow-up. What we do now is every time the patient is here, we check and update the pedigree, maybe new children are born or people died."* (Lipid.)

The central role of the treating physician is also underscored by the respondents from LEEFH, and this role is compared to the involvement of clinical genetics. Respondents value clinical genetics for its experience with informing the family, which might be helpful to train other professionals, or coordinate screening. However, most notably, the cost and the extra referral for the patient are seen as a drawback.

> *"Yes, we are trying also to collaborate and to learn from the expertise of the clinical geneticists: although it is not a very heavy disease and it's very easily treated, the cascade screening is difficult. It is difficult to reach the family of the index patient and we think that clinical geneticists have much more experience with that but what we are trying to do is to keep the medical care of the index patients and their families where they belong, which is the internist or a cardiologist. That's why we are making this whole network: we don't want the patient to be referred to all kinds of different stations for finding his whole family. We want to give the advice at the local out-patient clinics so that's what we are trying to do, to optimize that."* (Coord.:1)

The Minister had suggested to include clinical geneticists in FH care, as they are able to support the index patient because of their expertise in dealing with hereditary disorders. It was argued that FH could follow the model of cancer care, where the clinical geneticist would be able to directly approach family members in case this would be too burdensome for the patient [14,17]. While, in principle, clinical geneticists might directly approach family members, it is not clear if they actually do so, and how often, as the current Dutch guideline suggests that such a direct approach would only be advisable in exceptional circumstances, when the index patient is unable or unwilling to contact the family, and it is very important for the relative's health [20].

> *"We had a discussion . . . , that also in clinical genetics there is the discussion on what is the approach to the family members, what is allowed or not. In two ways, it is allowed on ethical grounds; are you allowed as a physician to contact a family member who doesn't know anything, and also financial, because the healthcare insurance companies say "you can only act when there is a disease and the patients come to you". But . . . an active approach . . . is prevention, it is not healthcare."* (Coord.:2)

Among clinical geneticists in the Netherlands, there is currently a difference of opinion, as especially in the north of the Netherlands, clinical geneticists support the idea of referring FH patients to clinical genetics. They argue cost can be contained, as the casemix will become more favorable by including more simple diagnoses, such as in the part of FH cases [21].

Respondents indicated to see the nurse consultants as ideally positioned to support the index patient, informing the family members:

> *"But I think that the role of the genetic fieldworkers or nurses . . . always [have] more time to talk with people and to inform them than doctors; the specialist or also general physicians, they don't take or have time, but nurse practitioners who do have some time . . . I think they should be more in charge in this process."* (Patient Org.)

Such nurses could be trained by clinical genetics and be connected either to the genetics department or internal medicine.

> *"I think there is some plus in having nurse practitioners coming from the area in which the disease is involved. But you can also have nurse practitioners from the genetics. It can be possible. And probably a mix would be perfect. But they should be trained."* (Clin. Genet.)

The role of the general practitioner (GP) has become more important after the screening program ended. Not only does the GP have to be aware of FH, but also discussing the risk for family members and stimulating the patient to contact these relatives has become important, as there is no organization to do so. Respondents expressed concern that GPs did not have enough knowledge, and mentioned cases of GPs not referring for genetic testing. However, experiences of collaboration differ according to region:

> "So a lot of times the GP says do it at your place [hospital] but if a patient for some reason, e.g., economical reasons, says it's too expensive in the hospital and I want to go back to my GP, we urge the GP to also check the family members." (Lipid.)

The RIVM (National Institute of Public Health and the Environment) might be given a task to set up a central organization of cascade screening for all sorts of hereditary disorders.

> "I think this cascade screening is really aiming at … living better and longer. For all these [hereditary] diseases. So in my view this is prevention. And it should be paid not from the budget of health care but by the national prevention budget. And in my view here there is a task for RIVM … it should be a national program, a screening program for genetic known diseases in which there are actionable interventions. Then we have a national program, we have a national database and it is much cheaper and, more importantly, we can also give care at a very high systematic similar level to all these people. Because one of the problems now is that carriers are informed by the GP, by this person, by that person, all kinds of persons and they tell them very different stories … If we have a centre in which all care is coordinated and information is coordinated … [They] can be factually informed and really helped during their path." (Clin. Genet.)

### 3.3. Resources and Awareness

When the cascade screening was an official program supported by the government, funding for the human resources and the DNA testing was provided from public health budgets. Now that regular healthcare has to integrate this preventive service, staff has to become available to actively support the provision of information to relatives. For counselling by internal medicine only recently has a tariff been agreed. Healthcare providers, such as lipidologists, or the nurse consultants in their department, are paid for counselling patients on informing their family members if their hospital also includes a genetics center. Clearly this raises a threshold for LEEFH centers operating in peripheral hospitals without a clinical genetics department.

A barrier for a direct approach is the fact that healthcare insurance only covers when an individual patient visits the doctor with a question. Organizing a prevention program is not covered:

> "[Health care insurance companies] have to agree that if we actively approach family members who might have FH that they are still insured although it's the health care system that approaches them instead of them … approaching the health care system with a question." (Lipid.)

> "Do they [health insurance companies] think that actively approaching FH patients or family members is insured healthcare or not. They've been too vague about it. So for me it's unsure what they mean." (Lipid.)

There is reimbursement to the individual patient for "indicated prevention" which would be requested by individuals at increased risk [22]. However, the cost of the program would not be reimbursed, unlike national screening programs.

Furthermore, the DNA test is covered by basic health insurance in the Netherlands, but the first 385€ (in 2018) of any hospital care or medication has to be paid by the individual patient, the so-called "own risk". Thus, unlike national screening programs, the own risk is a barrier for healthy individuals considering genetic testing. Hospital care is, in the Dutch situation in general, not an offer to healthy persons, but driven by questions of diseased patients. Therefore, to allow for complete reimbursement of preventive services, the healthy relative of FH patients has to be fitted into the system of "insured care".

Respondents indicated that after ending the program, an effort has to be made to make people and stakeholders, such as GPs, aware of hereditary forms of high cholesterol.

*"And an important difference between having a population screening and not having is awareness, because of ... the capacity of publishing things, so people know it exists and especially general practitioners are remembered time to time of these people and there are happening things around such a program."* (Patient Org.)

*"You should have some way to reach big groups and that would be via media, television, radio, YouTube, Facebook. Because if people read things like that, then they start thinking maybe I should get tested ... "* (Consult.)

## 4. Discussion

In this study, we explored stakeholder opinions on how active healthcare professionals can or should inform (healthy) family members when a patient is diagnosed with FH. When discussing the pros and cons of different approaches to informing family members, several themes became apparent: uptake, psychological burden, privacy, and autonomy. Interviewees strongly valued the high effectiveness of the previously adopted active approach and direct contacting. In the new indirect approach, the autonomy of family members is underscored, as relatives should seek healthcare, while privacy of family members is protected as they are only approached by the index. Respondents thought patients should make autonomous choices, but to do so, good information and awareness is needed. The new system offers little support for index patients informing their family members, and the psychological burden can weigh heavily on the index, further reducing uptake. Resources for giving information and supporting the index in the new system are reduced, while tasks are relegated to regular healthcare, and stakeholders are still finding ways to develop best practices and define their roles and responsibilities in FH care, given new regulatory restraints.

Barriers to cascade testing mentioned by the stakeholders are paying an own financial contribution, limited resources for informing relatives, and privacy regulation. LEEFH is well-positioned to discuss best practices with the range of stakeholders in the field. Discussions with Dutch healthcare insurance have recently led to dedicated funds for nurse consultants being able to counsel patients and help them inform their family [15]. If this were extended to nurses working in hospitals without clinical genetic centers, informing relatives will become more sustainable. The fact that healthy persons have to pay for a preventive service (because of the "own risk") is not yet solved. Well educated people with sufficient income might ask for FH-testing more often than people with low income and low health literacy. Thus, the current approach focusing on "own responsibility" might be less effective than the previous program, and might also increase inequity.

As for the privacy regulation, an important issue today is the different interpretation of the new General Data Protection Regulation (GDPR) in different hospitals, potentially making stakeholders reluctant to be more active. Clarity is needed on what is allowed and what not. If this is clear, more knowledge sharing among stakeholders on best practices on active approaches without direct contacting will assist in limiting this barrier. A promising practice mentioned by stakeholders was actively stimulating patients within current restraints, such as checking by phone if they succeeded in informing family members, and asking about informing the family during follow-up care.

Such options for a more active approach gained prominence during a public discussion that ensued after a Dutch BRCA family went to court [23]. In this family, a young woman got breast cancer which was found to be hereditary. The family was shocked to hear a pedigree had been made years before for another family member, but information about the mutation had not reached their branch of the family. This initiated discussion among healthcare professionals questioning what they are allowed to do in the era of new privacy laws. There is renewed discussion on the question of what the public expects of healthcare when information is available that is of relevance to them: is there a duty of care or a duty to inform? Geneticists had actually followed current guidelines, so officially, they were not to blame. However, the guidelines allow for support of the index patient, and geneticists themselves argued that they should be more active in overseeing the process of informing family members and check whether the index has been able to inform family members [24]. An initiative has started to develop new interdisciplinary guidelines on informing family members that can change the regulatory landscape and can also affect FH care.

Challenges for the future, when more predictive, personalized, and preventive possibilities arise, include mainstreaming genetics. FH care can be an example, using the strengths of clinical genetics, in training other healthcare professionals on drawing pedigrees, counselling, emotional support, support in tracing and informing family members. With the increasing numbers of older citizens in EU countries, prevention is becoming a more central theme in healthcare. Especially in conditions where genetics offers a substantial and quantifiable risk estimate, and prevention is available, these preventive services should be prioritized.

More government involvement is needed as a formally organized screening program could standardize support and information, and lead to more equitable healthcare. Many countries, such as Poland, Norway, and the UK, now develop FH care with this new vision of genetic preventive medicine. We hope that the role of stakeholders elsewhere will be described, and support the further development of predictive, personalized, and preventive services.

**Author Contributions:** Conceptualization, M.C.C. and C.G.v.E.; Methodology, C.G.v.E. and M.C.C.; Formal Analysis, C.G.v.E. and M.C.C.; Investigation, C.G.v.E., M.C.C., V.B. and P.P.; Data Curation, C.G.v.E.; Writing—Original Draft Preparation, C.G.v.E. and M.C.C.; Writing—Review & Editing, V.B. and P.P.; Visualization, P.P.; Supervision, M.C.C. and C.G.v.E.; Project Administration, C.G.v.E.

**Funding:** This research was conducted as part of the PRECeDI project (Personalized PREvention of Chronic Diseases) funded by the European Union's Horizon 2020 research and innovation program MSCA-RISE-2014: Marie Skłodowska-Curie Research and Innovation Staff Exchange (grant agreement number: 645740).

**Acknowledgments:** The authors appreciate the interviewees for their cooperation.

# References

1.  Nordestgaard, B.G.; Chapman, M.J.; Humphries, S.E.; Ginsberg, H.N.; Masana, L.; Descamps, O.S.; Wiklund, O.; Hegele, R.A.; Raal, F.J.; Defesche, J.C.; et al. Familial hypercholesterolaemia is underdiagnosed and undertreated in the general population: Guidance for clinicians to prevent coronary heart disease: Consensus statement of the European Atherosclerosis Society. *Eur. Heart J.* **2013**, *34*, 3478–3490. [CrossRef] [PubMed]

2.  Austin, M.A.; Hutter, C.M.; Zimmern, R.L.; Humphries, S.E. Familial hypercholesterolemia and coronary heart disease: A HuGE association review. *Am. J. Epidemiol.* **2004**, *160*, 421–429. [CrossRef] [PubMed]

3.  Soutar, A.K. Rare genetic causes of autosomal dominant or recessive hypercholesterolaemia. *IUBMB Life* **2010**, *62*, 125–131. [CrossRef] [PubMed]

4.  Goldberg, A.C.; Hopkins, P.N.; Toth, P.P.; Ballantyne, C.M.; Rader, D.J.; Robinson, J.G.; Daniels, S.R.; Gidding, S.S.; De Ferranti, S.D.; Ito, M.K.; et al. Familial hypercholesterolemia: Screening, diagnosis and management of pediatric and adult patients: Clinical guidance from the National Lipid Association Expert Panel on Familial Hypercholesterolemia. *J. Clin. Lipidol.* **2011**, *5*, S1–S8. [CrossRef] [PubMed]

5.  Pang, J.; Lansberg, P.J.; Watts, G.F. International developments in the care of familial hypercholesterolemia: Where now and where to next? *J. Atheroscler. Thromb.* **2016**, *23*, 505–519. [CrossRef] [PubMed]

6.  Migliara, G.; Baccolini, V.; Rosso, A.; D'Andrea, E.; Massimi, A.; Villari, P.; De Vito, C. Familial hypercholesterolemia: A systematic review of guidelines on genetic testing and patient management. *Front. Public Health* **2017**, *5*, 252. [CrossRef] [PubMed]

7.   Robinson, J.G.; Goldberg, A.C. Treatment of adults with familial hypercholesterolemia and evidence for treatment: Recommendations from the National Lipid Association Expert Panel on Familial Hypercholesterolemia. *J. Clin. Lipidol.* **2011**, *5*, S18–S29. [CrossRef] [PubMed]

8.   Carpay, M.E.M.; Van Der Horst, A.; Hoebee, B. Eindrapportage Bevolkingsonderzoek naar Familiaire Hypercholesterolemie: Organisatie en Opbrengsten—RIVM Briefrapport 2014-0152. Available online: http://www.rivm.nl/bibliotheek/rapporten/2014-0152.pdf (accessed on 10 July 2018).

9.   Newson, A.J.; Humphries, S.E. Cascade testing in familial hypercholesterolaemia: How should family members be contacted? *Eur. J. Hum. Genet.* **2005**, *13*, 401–408. [CrossRef] [PubMed]

10.  Paul, C. *Familial Hypercholesterolaemia: Identification and Management*; National Institute for Health and Care Excellence: London, UK, 2008.

11.  Rubio-Marín, P.; Michán-Doña, A.; Maraver-Delgado, J.; Arroyo-Olivares, R.; Varea, R.B.; De Isla, L.P.; Mata, P. Cascade screening program for familial hypercholesterolemia. *Endocrinol. Diabetes Nutr.* **2018**, *65*, 280–286. [CrossRef] [PubMed]

12.  Umans-Eckenhausen, M.A.; Defesche, J.C.; Sijbrands, E.J.G.; Scheerder, R.L.J.M.; Kastelein, J.J.P. Review of first 5 years of screening for familial hypercholesterolaemia in The Netherlands. *Lancet* **2001**, *357*, 165–168. [CrossRef]

13.  Pears, R.; Griffin, M.; Futema, M.; Humphries, S. Improving the cost-effectiveness equation of cascade testing for familial hypercholesterolaemia. *Curr. Opin. Lipidol.* **2015**, *26*, 162–168. [CrossRef] [PubMed]

14.  Dumay, A.C.M. Advies Opsporing Familiaire Hypercholesterolemie: RIVM-Centrum voor Bevolkingsonderzoek. Available online: http://docplayer.nl/36269614-Advies-opsporing-familiaire-hypercholesterolemie-rivm-centrum-voor-bevolkingsonderzoek.html (accessed on 28 August 2018).

15.  Louter, L.; Defesche, J.; Van Lennep, J.R. Cascade screening for familial hypercholesterolemia: Practical consequences. *Atheroscler. Suppl.* **2017**, *30*, 77–85. [CrossRef] [PubMed]

16.  Galema-Boers, J.M.; Versmissen, J.; Van Lennep, H.W.R.; Dusault-Wijkstra, J.E.; Williams, M.; Van Lennep, J.E.R. Cascade screening of familial hypercholesterolaemia must go on. *Atherosclerosis* **2015**, *242*, 415–417. [CrossRef] [PubMed]

17.  Schipper, E.I. Letter of the Minister of Health, Welfare and Sport to the House of Commons, The Hague 30 September 2016, Parliamentary Documentation 32793-239. Available online: https://www.tweedekamer.nl/kamerstukken/brieven_regering/detail?id=2016Z17909&did=2016D36825 (accessed on 30 August 2018).

18.  Achterbergh, R.; Lakeman, P.; Stemerding, D.; Moors, E.H.M.; Cornel, M.C. Implementation of preconceptional carrier screening for cystic fibrosis and haemoglobinopathies: A sociotechnical analysis. *Health Policy* **2007**, *83*, 277–286. [CrossRef] [PubMed]

19.  Rigter, T.; Henneman, L.; Broerse, J.E.W.; Shepherd, M.; Blanco, I.; Kristoffersson, U.; Cornel, M.C. Developing a framework for implementation of genetic services: Learning from examples of testing for monogenic forms of common diseases. *J. Community Genet.* **2014**, *5*, 337–347. [CrossRef] [PubMed]

20.  Menko, F.H.; Aalfs, C.M.; Henneman, L.; Stol, Y.; Wijdenes, M.; Otten, E.; Ploegmakers, M.M.; Legemaate, J.; Smets, E.M.; De Wert, G.M.; et al. Dutch society for clinical genetics. *Fam. Cancer* **2013**, *12*, 319–324. [CrossRef] [PubMed]

21.  Hoedemaekers, Y.M.; Knoers, N.; Van Langen, I. Familieonderzoek FH kan binnen de reguliere zorg. *Medisch Contact* **2014**, *43*, 2116–2118.

22.  Kroes, M.E.; Mastenbroek, C.G.; Couwenbergh, B.T.L.E.; Zan Eijndhoven, M.J.A.; Festen, C.C.S.; Rikken, F. Van Preventie Verzekerd. Available online: https://www.zorginstituutnederland.nl/publicaties/rapport/2007/07/16/van-preventie-verzekerd (accessed on 10 July 2018).

23.  Jorritsma, E.; Van Steenbergen, E. Gevaarlijke Genen: Dat Wist het Ziekenhuis. Available online: https://www.nrc.nl/nieuws/2015/08/27/gevaarlijke-genen-dat-wist-het-ziekenhuis-1527031-a449290 (accessed on 4 August 2018).

24.  Kwant, L. De Genetici Moeten Toezien op Inlichten Familie. Available online: https://www.medischcontact.nl/nieuws/laatste-nieuws/artikel/genetici-moeten-toezien-op-inlichten-familie.htm (accessed on 4 August 2018).

# 10

# Poverty Status and Childhood Asthma in White and Black Families: National Survey of Children's Health

Shervin Assari [1,2,3,*] ⓘ and Maryam Moghani Lankarani [2]

[1] Department of Psychology, University of California, Los Angeles (UCLA), Los Angeles, CA 90095, USA
[2] Department of Psychiatry, University of Michigan, Ann Arbor, MI 48104, USA; lankaranii@yahoo.com
[3] Center for Research on Ethnicity, Culture and Health, School of Public Health, University of Michigan, Ann Arbor, MI 90095, USA
* Correspondence: assari@umich.edu

**Abstract:** *Background:* Living above the poverty line reduces the risk of physical illnesses, including childhood asthma (CA). Minorities' Diminished Return theory, however, suggests that the protective effects of socioeconomic status (SES) on health are weaker for racial minorities than White families. It is unknown whether the association between SES and CA differs for White and Black families. *Aims:* Using a national sample, the current study compared Black and White families for the association between living above the poverty line and CA. *Methods:* Data came from the National Survey of Children's Health (NSCH), 2003–2004, a national telephone survey. A total of 86,537 Black or White families with children (17 years old or younger) were included in the study. This sample was composed of 76,403 White (88.29%) and 10,134 Black (11.71%) families. Family SES (living above the poverty line) was the independent variable. The outcome was CA, reported by the parent. Age, gender, and childhood obesity were the covariates. Race was conceptualized as the moderator. A number of multivariable logistic regressions were used in the pooled sample and specific to each race for data analysis. *Results:* In the pooled sample, living above the poverty line was associated with lower odds of CA. An interaction was found between race and living above the poverty line on odds of CA, indicating a smaller association for Black compared to White families. Although race-stratified logistic regressions showed negative associations between living above the poverty line and CA in both White and Black families, the magnitude of this negative association was larger for White than Black families. *Conclusions:* The health gain from living above the poverty line may be smaller for Black than White families. Due to the existing Minorities' Diminished Return, policies that merely reduce the racial gap in SES may not be sufficient in eliminating racial health disparities in the United States. Public policies must go beyond reducing poverty to address structural and environmental risk factors that disproportionately impact Blacks' health. Policies should help Black families gain health as they gain upward social mobility. As they are more likely to face societal and structural barriers, multi-level interventions are needed for the health promotion of Blacks.

**Keywords:** socioeconomic status; poverty; income; ethnic groups; Blacks; ethnicity; asthma

## 1. Introduction

The protective effects of socioeconomic status (SES) on health [1–8] are not equal across racial groups [9,10]. While high family SES, such as family income and parental education, are protective overall [11,12], and low SES, financial strain, and poverty may partially explain why racial minorities suffer from worse childhood health [13], the smaller health gain from SES among minorities may be another mechanism by which racial disparities in health exist [9,10].

According to Minorities' Diminished Return theory [9], unequal health gain from SES is a neglected mechanism behind racial health disparities [10]. Supporting this theory [9,10], considerable research has shown that SES has stronger effects on drinking patterns [14], depressive symptoms [15], suicidality [16], chronic disease [15], and mortality [17–20] for Whites than Blacks. Either due to the extra costs of upward social mobility for Blacks compared to Whites [21,22], or high levels of discrimination among Blacks [23], SES generates less health for Blacks than Whites. In some extreme examples, high SES not only does not improve health, but also becomes a risk factor for poor health of Blacks. For instance, income was positively associated with Major Depressive Disorder (MDD) among Black boys [24] and Black men [25,26]; and high education attainment is associated with a higher risk of suicide in Black women [16] and an increase in future depressive symptoms in Black men [15].

While high SES promotes health of the general population [27–29], this effect is not universal across racial groups [9,10,30–33]. Racial groups vary widely in their capacity to navigate the system and translate their SES resources to tangible health outcomes [23,34,35]. Although high SES reduces exposure to risks [27–29], these effects are unequal across various social groups [21,22,36]. That is, the very same SES indicator, such as income, generates a smaller change in purchasing power for the economically and socially disadvantaged group, compared to the privileged group [37–40]. In other words, high SES better enhances the majorities' access to goods and services, and the health [27–29,41] of Whites compared to Blacks [42]. As society treats groups by their race and skin color, the same increase in SES generates smaller leverage in material resources, human capital, and psychological assets for Blacks than Whites [43,44]. One explanation for this pattern is the extra psychological and physiological costs of upward social mobility [21–23] for Blacks [24,41], which minimize the health gain from high SES [42,45] in this population. Blacks may also have a higher risk of using high cost effortful coping for upward social mobility [46,47]. These mechanisms collectively suggest that SES may have a smaller effect on the health of Blacks compared to Whites [34,48], as the Minorities' Diminished Return hypothesis has suggested [9,10].

Childhood asthma (CA) is the leading chronic disease for children under 18 in the United States (US) [1]. Approximately seven million children suffer from asthma in the US Significant disparities in CA exist across race and socioeconomic status (SES) groups [1]. Low SES and Black families are at higher risk for CA. Prevalence of CA is 8.2%, 9.9%, and 12.2% among families with income above 200%, between 100% and 200%, and less than 100% of the federal poverty line, respectively. The risk of hospitalization, having an emergency department visit, or death from CA are all two to four times higher in Black families, compared to White families [1]. Case et al., in 2002, showed that chronic diseases such as asthma follow the social gradient in income [49].

To better understand whether Minorities' Diminished Return theory also explains some of the racial disparities in CA, we compared Black and White families for the negative association between living above the poverty line and CA. Although research has established the effects of race [50] and SES [51,52] on CA, very few studies have ever studied multiplicative effects of race and SES on CA [53]. So, it is still unknown whether it is race and SES or race or SES that cause CA disparities [54]. To generate generalizable results on the multiplicative effects of race and SES on CA, we used data from the National Survey of Children's Health (NSCH), a study with a nationally representative sample of children 18 years old or younger. In line with the Minorities' Diminished Return theory [9], we hypothesized that SES (living above the poverty line) would have a larger protective effect on CA for White compared to Black families.

## 2. Materials and Methods

### 2.1. Design and Setting

This study used a cross-sectional design. The current study used data from the NSCH (Heights Ville, MD, USA), a nationally representative study sponsored by the National Center for

Health Statistics (NCHS). NSCH was a landmark survey that generated national and state-level representative prevalence estimates for a variety of children's health indicators [55–57].

## 2.2. Ethics

The NSCH study protocol was approved by the CDC's Institutional Review Board (IRB). Adolescents' parents/legal guardians provided informed consent. Adolescents provided assent. More information on ethical aspects of the study is available [58].

## 2.3. Sampling

Similar to other national studies, such as the National Immunization Study [55–57] the NSCH sampling frame was based on the State and Local Area Integrated Telephone Survey (SLAITS) [55–57]. To briefly describe the study sampling procedure, trained interviewers called telephone numbers at random to identify households with at least one child under the age of 18. From eligible households, one child was randomly selected for the interview. The study also included an interview with the adult in the household who knew the most about the child's health and well-being. After excluding participants based on race/ethnicity criteria, our analytic sample consisted of 86,537 children who were 17 years old or younger (76,403 White (88.29%) and 10,134 Black (11.71%)).

## 2.4. Data Collection

The study conducted an overall number of 102,353 interviews. All the interviewers were completed between January 2003 and July 2004 and were performed either in English or Spanish. Trained interviewers asked parents/guardians a series of questions regarding their child's physical, emotional, and behavioral health, as well as access to health care [55–57].

## 2.5. Variables

The current study included the following variables: child race, child demographic factors (gender and age), family socioeconomic status (SES), and child health status (overweight, and CA).

*Race.* For confidentiality purposes, the NSCH collected child race as White only, African American/Black only, other races, and multiple races. The current study only included Blacks and Whites [55–57].

*Family Poverty Status (Living Above the Poverty Line).* Interviewers asked parents/guardians about household income [55–57]. Income to household size was based on the Department of Health and Human Services federal poverty guidelines [55–57]. Living above the poverty line was defined as a dichotomous variable (1 above federal poverty level or above vs. 0 less than federal poverty level) [58,59].

*Overweight.* Overweight status was a dichotomous variable calculated based on BMI which was derived from the parent's or guardian's reports on the height and weight of the child. Parents and guardians were asked the following two questions: "How tall is your child now?" and "How much does your child weigh now?"; BMI based on parent-reported height and weight strongly correlates with BMI based on direct measurements of height and weight [60,61]. BMI was calculated as weight (kilograms) divided by height (meters) squared. To define overweight status, the Centers for Disease Control and Prevention (CDC) gender- and age-specific growth charts were used [62]. BMI $\geq$ 95th percentile was considered as overweight [62–64]. We operationalized the variable as a two-level categorical variable (overweight vs. non-overweight).

*Childhood Asthma (CA).* A single item was used to measure the history of CA. Parents were asked, "Has a doctor or health professional ever told you that your child has Asthma? Responses included (0) No, (1) Yes, (6) Do not know, and (7) Refused. This self-reported measure of physician diagnosis has been used in the Panel Study of Income Dynamics (PSID), as well as the Behavioral Risk Factor Surveillance System (BRFSS) state-based telephone survey. Self-reported physician diagnoses are valid and reliable self-reported measures of lifetime asthma in both children and adults [65,66].

*2.6. Data Analysis*

*Weights.* To generate nationally representative results, the NSCH sampling weights were applied. These weights are calculated based on a base sampling weight and adjustment for multiple telephone lines per household, as well as for non-response. The weights were post-stratified so that the sum of weights for each state equals the total number of children in that state as estimated for the July 2003 US census data [55–57].

To account for the NSCH complex survey design (due to clustering, stratification, and non-response), we used Stata 13.0 (Stata Corp., College Station, TX, USA) to analyze the data. Taylor series approximation was used for the estimation of complex design-based standard errors (SE) and variance. All percentages, means, SEs, confidence intervals (CI), and $p$ values reflect the sampling weights and are thus generalizable to nationally representative estimates.

To describe our sample, we reported frequency tables (%) and means with 95% CIs. For bivariate analysis, a Spearman correlation test was used. We ran multiple logistic regression models, first in the pooled sample and then in Whites and Blacks. In the pooled sample, the first model only included the main effects of living above the poverty line, race, and covariates. The second model also included the race × living above the poverty line interaction term. In all models, family SES (living above the poverty line) was the independent variable; CA was the dependent variable; and age, gender, and overweight status were covariates. Race was the focal moderator. Adjusted Odds Ratio (OR), 95% CI, and associated $p$ values were reported. $p$ values less than 0.05 were considered significant.

## 3. Results

### 3.1. Descriptives

This analysis included 86,537 Black or White children (17 years old or younger). This sample was composed of 76,403 White (88.29%) and 10,134 Black (11.71%).

Table 1 summarizes the descriptive statistics for the pooled sample, as well as White and Black children. As this table shows, Black children were from families with a lower education and lower income, and who were at a higher risk of being overweight.

**Table 1.** Descriptive statistics in the pooled sample and by race.

| Characteristics | All ($n$ = 86,537) | Whites ($n$ = 76,403) | Blacks ($n$ = 10,134) |
|---|---|---|---|
| | % (95% CI) | % (95% CI) | % (95% CI) |
| Child Race | | | |
| White | 82.27 (81.69–82.83) | - | - |
| Black | 17.73 (17.17–18.31) | - | - |
| Child Gender | | | |
| Male | 51.08 (50.43–51.73) | 51.45 (50.77–52.13) | 49.38 (47.55–51.21) |
| Female | 48.92 (48.27–49.57) | 48.55 (47.87–49.23) | 50.62 (48.79–52.45) |
| Parental Education (High school) * | | | |
| No | 29.00 (28.37–29.63) | 26.24 (25.61–26.89) | 41.77 (39.93–43.63) |
| Yes | 71.00 (70.37–71.63) | 73.76 (73.11–74.39) | 58.23 (56.37–60.07) |
| Family Living Outside Poverty * | | | |
| No | 13.32 (12.79–13.85) | 9.58 (10.08–10.08) | 30.62 (28.86–32.45) |
| Yes | 86.68 (86.15–87.21) | 90.42 (89.92–90.89) | 69.38 (67.55–71.14) |
| Child Overweight * | | | |
| No | 75.84 (75.27–76.40) | 78.56 (77.99–79.11) | 63.23 (61.41–65.00) |
| Yes | 24.16 (23.60–24.73) | 21.44 (20.89–22.01) | 36.77 (35.00–38.59) |
| Child Asthma * | | | |
| No | 86.20 (85.74–86.65) | 87.37 (86.92–87.81) | 80.75 (79.20–82.22) |
| Yes | 13.80 (13.35–14.26) | 12.63 (12.19–13.08) | 19.25 (17.78–20.80) |
| | **Mean (CI)** | **Mean (CI)** | **Mean (CI)** |
| Child Age (Year) | 8.71 (8.65–8.77) | 8.68 (8.62–8.74) | 8.84 (8.67–9.00) |
| Income to Need Ratio * | 5.38 (5.35–5.41) | 5.70 (5.66–5.73) | 3.90 (3.82–3.99) |

\* $p < 0.05$.

## 3.2. Bivariate Correaltions

Table 2 summarizes the bivariate associations in the pooled sample. As this table shows, parent education was negatively associated with CA among children.

**Table 2.** Correlation matrix in the pooled sample ($n$ = 86,537).

| Characteristics | 1 | 2 | 3 | 4 | 5 | 6 | 7 |
|---|---|---|---|---|---|---|---|
| 1 Child Race (Blacks) | 1.00 | | | | | | |
| 2 Child Gender (Females) | 0.01 * | 1.00 | | | | | |
| 3 Child Age (Year) | −0.00 | −0.01 * | 1.00 | | | | |
| 4 Low Parental Education (Low SES) | −0.10 * | −0.00 | −0.03 | 1.00 | | | |
| 5 Living Above the Poverty Line (High SES) | 0.19 * | 0.00 | −0.03 | −0.27 * | 1.00 | | |
| 6 Childhood Overweight | 0.12 * | −0.07 * | −0.26 * | −0.09 * | 0.09 * | 1.00 | |
| 7 Childhood Asthma | 0.06 * | −0.06 * | 0.06 | −0.02 * | 0.04 | 0.04 | 1.00 |

\* $p < 0.05$.

## 3.3. Pooled Sample Logistic Regressions

Table 3 shows the results of two logistic regressions, one without interactions and one with race by SES interactions. Model 1 showed that in the pooled sample, living above the poverty line was negatively associated with odds of CA. Model 2 showed an interaction between the effects of race and poverty status on odds of CA, suggesting that the negative association between living above the poverty line on odds of CA was smaller for Black, compared to White, families (Table 3).

**Table 3.** Summary of logistic regression models in the pooled sample.

| Characteristics | Model 1 (All; $n$ = 86,537) | | | Model 2 (All; $n$ = 86,537) | | |
|---|---|---|---|---|---|---|
| | Main Effects | | | Main Effects + Interactions | | |
| | OR | 95% CI | $p$ | OR | 95% CI | $p$ |
| Living Above the Poverty Line | 0.84 ** | 0.74–0.95 | 0.008 | 0.73 *** | 0.63–0.85 | 0.001 |
| Parental Education (Low) | 0.93 | 0.85–1.02 | 0.140 | 0.95 | 0.86–1.04 | 0.271 |
| Child Race (Blacks) | 1.55 *** | 1.38–1.73 | 0.001 | 1.21 | 0.93–1.58 | 0.163 |
| Child Gender (Females) | 0.68 *** | 0.63–0.73 | 0.001 | 0.68 *** | 0.63–0.73 | 0.001 |
| Child Age (Year) | 1.04 *** | 1.03–1.05 | 0.001 | 1.04 *** | 1.03–1.05 | 0.001 |
| Childhood Overweight | 1.35 *** | 1.23–1.49 | 0.001 | 1.35 *** | 1.22–1.48 | 0.001 |
| Low Parental Education × Race | - | - | - | 0.95 | 0.75–1.19 | 0.635 |
| Living Above the Poverty Line × Race | - | - | - | 1.41 * | 1.08–1.86 | 0.013 |
| Intercept | 0.19 *** | 0.16–0.23 | 0.001 | 0.22 *** | 0.17–0.27 | 0.001 |

Outcome: Childhood Asthma, Confidence Interval (CI); \* $p < 0.05$, \*\* $p < 0.01$, \*\*\* $p < 0.001$.

## 3.4. Race Stratified Logistic Regressions

Table 4 shows the results of two logistic regressions specific to race. Model 3 and Model 4 showed a negative association between living above the poverty line (income to need ratio) and CA for White (Model 3) and Black (Model 4) children; however, the magnitude of the negative association was larger for White than Black families.

**Table 4.** Summary of logistic regression models by race.

| Characteristics | Model 3 (Whites; $n$ = 76,403) | | | Model 4 (Blacks; $n$ = 10,134) | | |
|---|---|---|---|---|---|---|
| | OR | 95% CI | $p$ | OR | 95% CI | $p$ |
| Living Above the Poverty Line | 0.73 *** | 0.63–0.84 | 0.001 | 1.05 | 0.84–1.32 | 0.679 |
| Low Parental Education | 0.94 | 0.85–1.04 | 0.242 | 0.90 | 0.74–1.11 | 0.339 |
| Child Gender (Females) | 0.66 *** | 0.61–0.72 | 0.001 | 0.73 ** | 0.60–0.89 | 0.002 |
| Child Age (Year) | 1.05 *** | 1.04–1.06 | 0.001 | 1.01 | 0.99–1.03 | 0.436 |
| Childhood Overweight | 1.36 *** | 1.22–1.51 | 0.001 | 1.28 * | 1.03–1.58 | 0.026 |
| Intercept | 0.20 *** | 0.16–0.26 | 0.001 | 0.32 *** | 0.20–0.50 | 0.001 |

Outcome: Childhood Asthma, Confidence Interval (CI); \* $p < 0.05$, \*\* $p < 0.01$, \*\*\* $p < 0.001$.

## 4. Discussion

The current study showed two findings. First, there was an association between SES and CA in the pooled sample. Second, Blacks and Whites differed in the negative association between family SES (i.e., income to need ratio) and CA. Prevalence of CA was lower for high SES Blacks and Whites; however, this association was stronger for White than Black families.

The first finding on the protective effect of poverty status against CA was in line with the epidemiology [67] and economics [49] literature that has shown a social and economic gradient in children's health. This literature was reviewed and explained by Case et al., in 2002 [49]. The second finding that the very same SES indicator (living above the poverty line) shows a stronger negative association with CA for White than Black families is similar to the results of studies on the association between family SES and self-rated health, obesity, and impulse control [68–70]. This is partly because Black families with high educational attainment have a higher risk of staying in poverty, compared to White families [71,72].

It was only recently that Minorities' Diminished Return was found to be valid in children [68,69], as most of the supporting literature has recruited adults [15,16] or older adults [34,42]. Although the exact mechanism for a smaller health gain of SES among Blacks is still unclear, these findings support the growing evidence that differential gains start early in life and are partially responsible for racial health disparities in childhood [69]. That is, smaller health effects of family SES on the health of Black children is one reason for worse health outcomes in Black children, compared to White children [68,71]. Further, the socially privileged majority group and the socially and economically disadvantaged minority group do not equally gain from the same SES resources.

In another related study, using data following 1781 youth from birth to age 15 from the Fragile Families and Child Wellbeing Study (FFCWS) [69], Black-White differences were found in the protective effect of family structure and family SES at birth on subsequent BMI at age 15. The study revealed race by family SES and race by family structure interactions on BMI, indicating smaller effects for Blacks compared to Whites. Race by gender stratified regressions showed the most consistent patterns of associations between family SES and future BMI for male and female Whites. Family SES and structure at birth did not protect Black males or Black females against obesity 15 years later. The study was one of the first to show that the Minorities' Diminished Return theory also holds for youth [69].

The results of this study should be interpreted with caution. Our results do not suggest that Blacks are unable to efficiently use their available SES resources or turn their SES resources into tangible health outcomes. This argument has been used to blame, marginalize, and stigmatize Blacks for a low chance of upward social mobility. Despite having historically been victims of slavery, racism, and discrimination [73], their socioeconomic status and poverty has been wrongly attributed to their culture [74]. Instead, it is the social structure, segregation, and structural racism that are responsible for Minorities' Diminished Return [9,10]. Black families face disproportionately higher rates of societal and structural barriers in their lives that may hinder their ability to gain health from any SES resource that becomes available to them. The current US social system fails Blacks by charging them extra psychological and physiological costs to climb the social ladder. In a race-aware society, the process of upward social mobility is associated with more social, psychological, and physiological costs for Blacks than Whites [21,22]. The current US system is designed to maximize the gain of the privileged group even if it may cause only minimum gains for other social groups [9,10]. This offers rationale for why the US is experiencing a stubbornly high Black-White economic gap.

The easy-to-identify trait of Black race in the US has facilitated activities that systematically force Blacks into worse environments than Whites of their same SES. These forces outside the Black community in real estate, private and public facilities, and professional services can act with virtual impunity despite efforts to control them [54,75–77]. Sometimes they are "unconscious behaviors" of people and institutions exercising some power or professional "gate-keeping", which exacerbates segregation and discrimination [78–80]. In others, they are conscious and are defended as protection against "reverse racism" [81–83].

SES may not similarly enhance the environment for Whites and Blacks, thus high SES Black families may be at a higher risk of environmental exposures to allergens, tobacco smoke, and indoor and outdoor air pollution. Other mechanisms, such as smoking, that may be more cultural than structural, may be involved. Research has shown that education has smaller protective effects against smoking [33], which may increase the risk of CA [84]. These mechanisms should be explored in future research.

One reason why SES may fail to show strong effects for Blacks is that high SES Blacks face high levels of interpersonal and instructional aspirations. Black families who seek new opportunities are forced to fight societal barriers that increase the costs of moving up the social ladder. One example of this is the effect of discrimination on reduced health gains that commonly follow high SES [15]. We argue that in the presence of racism and discrimination, and in a race–and–color–aware society, high aspirations may not be protective but detrimental to Blacks' health. This is in line with the recent research suggesting that high SES may be a vulnerability factor for Black families [23,24], a finding which is replicated for adults [23] and adolescents [24]. Of course, we are not suggesting that Blacks should not have high aspirations. Instead, we argue that upward social mobility should not be associated with extra costs for minority groups, and assert that all groups should benefit equally from climbing the social ladder [21,22].

The finding on the overall protective effect of family SES against odds CA is in line previous studies on the protective effects of high SES against a wide range of health outcomes [69,85–89]. Low SES is a root cause of illness, and CA is not an exception to this general rule [1]. Several state-of-the-art studies have shown the well-established link between SES and health [2–7,90].

However, this SES gain is smaller for Blacks, a pattern that is not limited to childhood [9,10]. A study showed that education better changes the drinking habits of Whites than Blacks in older adults [42]. In the Health and Retirement Study (HRS), high income was associated with low BMI for White women and Black women, but not for White men and Black men. High educational attainment was also associated with higher physical activity and sleep quality for White men, White women, and Black women, but not Black men [34]. Among adults, education [18], employment [91], neighborhood quality [92], and social contacts [93] generate a smaller gain in life expectancy for Blacks than for Whites. All these findings are in concert and support the Minorities' Diminished Return theory of the systematically smaller health gain of SES for Blacks than Whites [16,18,34,94].

*Limitations*

Our study had a few methodological limitations. As the study used a cross-sectional design, causal conclusions are not plausible. Despite the temporal ambiguity of exposure (current poverty level) and outcome (lifetime CA prevalence), it is more plausible to conceptualize poor SES as a cause and CA as an outcome. Although CA may contribute to or be followed by greater family poverty, CA is often preceded by abysmal inner-city conditions [41,95–97]. This study measured CA using self-reported data. Although self-reported data are valid to measure CA [65,66], the diagnosis of CA not being confirmed to meet NHLBI or other society guidelines (bronchodilator response, etc.) is a major limitation. The study is at risk of omitted confounders. We, however, controlled for the effects of obesity which is linked to SES, as well as CA medications, particularly preventive inhaled corticosteroids [98]. This study is prone to bias due to non-classical measurement error. The poverty line is endogenous, as families have some control over what their income is (through what job they choose and how many hours they work). Overall, the poverty line is not the best SES measure as it does not adjust for cost of living, and families with the same poverty status may face different levels of financial hardship depending on the part of the country. Given that many federal and state anti-poverty programs are tied to income, there may be asymmetric bunching (with many families just below, but very few just above). To address this problem, future research may use a "donut" specification, as explained by Barreca, et al., in 2011 [99]. This approach drops families within 10% or 20% of the poverty line, to reduce measurement bias [99]. In the current study, we did not have income values but levels, so we could not use "donut" specification. In addition, the study did not collect data on parents' race. The results may differ for Black and White children with White and non-White parents. This study was limited to Blacks and Whites only. Future research should test if other minority groups such as Hispanics, Indian Americans, immigrants, sexual minorities, and other minority groups also gain less from their positive SES indicators. As shown in Table 4, the ORs for Blacks were not statistically significant. This may be partially due to the imbalanced sample sizes between Blacks and Whites. Although the NSCH data set contained variables for Hispanic ethnicity, the sample size of Hispanic Blacks was very small. So, we could not model the differences between Hispanic Whites and Hispanic Blacks. As a result, we limited our sample to non-Hispanic White and non-Hispanic Blacks. More research is also needed on the role of other ethnic groups, regions, and neighborhoods on these relationships. Future research should replicate the findings reported here among other marginalized groups, such as immigrants. Third, all the study measures were those at an individual level. There is a need for future research on contextual factors that surround Black and White families across SES levels. We also do not know if these findings hold for other SES indicators such as family structure, household size, employment, and wealth. The data were old (13 years old). The results should be replicated using other similar data sets such as PSID, NHANES, NHIS, or BRFSS. Research may also try to replicate these findings for educational attainment and other SES measures. Despite these limitations, this is one of the first studies to explore Black-White variation in the link between SES and CA.

## 5. Conclusions

In the United States, the negative association between living above the poverty line and CA is smaller for Black families compared to their White counterparts. Future research should use longitudinal data to establish causation between SES and asthma by race. The role of structural racism, interpersonal discrimination, and societal barriers in these patterns should be explored. Public and economic policy solutions should go beyond equalizing SES and eliminate Minorities' Diminished Return from SES, which is a neglected contributor to racial health disparities in the US Policy solutions to health disparities require jointly addressing race and SES, as race and SES do not operate independently.

**Author Contributions:** S.A. designed and performed the current analysis. M.M.L. drafted the paper and contributed to the interpretation of the findings. Both authors contributed to the revisions and confirmed the final version of the paper.

**Funding:** This current research received no external funding.

**Acknowledgments:** The National Survey of Children's Health (NSCH) was funded by the United States Department of Health and Human Services, Health Resources and Services Administration, and Maternal and Child Health Bureau. Shervin Assari is supported by the Heinz C. Prechter Bipolar Research Fund and the Richard Tam Foundation at the University of Michigan. Shervin Assari is also supported by the UCLA BRITE Center.

## References

1.  American Lung Association (ALA). Socioeconomic and Racial Asthma Disparities in Asthma. Available online: www.lung.org/local-content/illinois/documents/socioeconomic-asthma-disparities.pdf (accessed on 1 April 2018).
2.  Mirowsky, J.; Ross, C.E. *Education, Social Status, and Health*; Aldine de Gruyter: New York, NY, USA, 2003.
3.  Bowen, M.E.; González, H.M. Childhood socioeconomic position and disability in later life: Results of the health and retirement study. *Am. J. Public Health* **2010**, *100*, S197–S203. [CrossRef] [PubMed]
4.  Herd, P.; Goesling, B.; House, J.S. Socioeconomic position and health: The differential effects of education versus income on the onset versus progression of health problems. *J. Health Soc. Behav.* **2007**, *48*, 223–238. [CrossRef] [PubMed]

5. Kim, J. Intercohort trends in the relationship between education and health: Examining physical impairment and depressive symptomatology. *J. Aging Health* **2008**, *20*, 671–693. [CrossRef] [PubMed]

6. Van de Mheen, H.; Stronks, K.; Looman, C.W.N.; Mackenbach, J.P. Does childhood socioeconomic status influence adult health through behavioural factors? *Int. J. Epidemiol.* **1998**, *27*, 431–437. [CrossRef] [PubMed]

7. Leopold, L.; Engelhardt, H. Education and physical health trajectories in old age. Evidence from the Survey of Health, Ageing and Retirement in Europe (SHARE). *Int. J. Public Health* **2013**, *58*, 23–31. [CrossRef] [PubMed]

8. Johnson-Lawrence, V.D.; Griffith, D.M.; Watkins, D.C. The effects of race, ethnicity and mood/anxiety disorders on the chronic physical health conditions of men from a national sample. *Am. J. Men's Health* **2013**, *7*, 58S–67S. [CrossRef] [PubMed]

9. Assari, S. Unequal gain of equal resources across racial groups. *Int. J. Health Policy Manag.* **2017**, *6*. [CrossRef] [PubMed]

10. Assari, S. Health Disparities Due to Minorities Diminished Return: Policy Solutions. *Soc. Issues Policy Rev.* **2018**, *12*, 112–145. [CrossRef]

11. Alaimo, K.; Olson, C.M.; Frongillo, E.A., Jr.; Briefel, R.R. Food insufficiency, family income, and health in US preschool and school-aged children. *Am. J. Public Health* **2001**, *91*, 781–786. [PubMed]

12. Shah, C.P.; Kahan, M.; Krauser, J. The health of children of low-income families. *Can. Med. Assoc. J.* **1987**, *137*, 485–490.

13. Chen, E. Why socioeconomic status affects the health of children: A psychosocial perspective. *Curr. Dir. Psychol. Sci.* **2004**, *13*, 112–115. [CrossRef]

14. Hummer, R.A.; Lariscy, J.T. Educational attainment and adult mortality. In *International Handbook of Adult Mortality*; Springer: Berlin, Germany, 2011; pp. 241–261.

15. Assari, S. Combined Racial and Gender Differences in the Long-Term Predictive Role of Education on Depressive Symptoms and Chronic Medical Conditions. *J. Racial Ethn. Health Disparities* **2016**. [CrossRef] [PubMed]

16. Assari, S. Ethnic and Gender Differences in Additive Effects of Socio-economics, Psychiatric Disorders, and Subjective Religiosity on Suicidal Ideation among Blacks. *Int. J. Prev. Med.* **2015**, *6*. [CrossRef] [PubMed]

17. Hayward, M.D.; Hummer, R.A.; Sasson, I. Trends and group differences in the association between educational attainment and US adult mortality: Implications for understanding education's causal influence. *Soc. Sci. Med.* **2015**, *127*, 8–18. [CrossRef] [PubMed]

18. Assari, S.; Lankarani, M.M. Race and Urbanity Alter the Protective Effect of Education but not Income on Mortality. *Front. Public Health* **2016**, *4*. [CrossRef] [PubMed]

19. Backlund, E.; Sorlie, P.D.; Johnson, N.J. A comparison of the relationships of education and income with mortality: The National Longitudinal Mortality Study. *Soc. Sci. Med.* **1999**, *49*, 1373–1384. [CrossRef]

20. Everett, B.G.; Rehkopf, D.H.; Rogers, R.G. The Nonlinear Relationship between Education and Mortality: An Examination of Cohort, Race/Ethnic, and Gender Differences. *Popul. Res. Policy Rev.* **2013**, *32*, 893–917. [CrossRef] [PubMed]

21. Fuller-Rowell, T.E.; Doan, S.N. The social costs of academic success across ethnic groups. *Child Dev.* **2010**, *81*, 1696–1713. [CrossRef] [PubMed]

22. Fuller-Rowell, T.E.; Curtis, D.S.; Doan, S.N.; Coe, C.L. Racial disparities in the health benefits of educational attainment: A study of inflammatory trajectories among African American and white adults. *Psychosom. Med.* **2015**, *77*, 33–40. [CrossRef] [PubMed]

23. Hudson, D.L.; Bullard, K.M.; Neighbors, H.W.; Geronimus, A.T.; Yang, J.; Jackson, J.S. Are benefits conferred with greater socioeconomic position undermined by racial discrimination among African American men? *J. Mens Health* **2012**, *9*, 127–136. [CrossRef] [PubMed]

24. Assari, S.; Caldwell, C.H. High Risk of Depression in High-Income African American Boys. *J. Racial Ethn. Health Disparities* **2017**. [CrossRef] [PubMed]

25. Hudson, D.L.; Neighbors, H.W.; Geronimus, A.T.; Jackson, J.S. The relationship between socioeconomic position and depression among a US nationally representative sample of African Americans. *Soc. Psychiatry Psychiatr. Epidemiol.* **2012**, *47*, 373–381. [CrossRef] [PubMed]

26. Assari, S.; Caldwell, C.H. Social determinants of perceived discrimination among black youth: Intersection of ethnicity and gender. *Children* **2018**, *5*, 24. [CrossRef] [PubMed]

27. Phelan, J.C.; Link, B.G.; Tehranifar, P. Social conditions as fundamental causes of health inequalities: Theory, evidence, and policy implications. *J. Health Soc. Behav.* **2010**, *51*, S28–S40. [CrossRef] [PubMed]

28. Link, B.G.; Phelan, J. Social conditions as fundamental causes of health inequalities. *Handbook Med. Sociol.* **2010**, *2010*, 3–17.

29. Link, B.; Phelan, J. Social conditions as fundamental causes of disease. *J. Health Soc. Behav.* **1995**, *36*, 80–94. [CrossRef]

30. Assari, S. Social Determinants of Depression: The Intersections of Race, Gender, and Socioeconomic Status. *Brain Sci.* **2017**, *7*, 156. [CrossRef] [PubMed]

31. Assari, S. Socioeconomic Status and Self-Rated Oral Health; Diminished Return among Hispanic Whites. *Dent. J.* **2018**, *6*, 11. [CrossRef] [PubMed]

32. Assari, S. High Income Protects Whites but Not African Americans against Risk of Depression. *Healthcare* **2018**, *6*, 37. [CrossRef] [PubMed]

33. Assari, S.; Mistry, R. Educational Attainment and Smoking Status in a National Sample of American Adults; Evidence for the Blacks' Diminished Return. *Int. J. Environ. Res. Public Health* **2018**, *15*, 763. [CrossRef] [PubMed]

34. Assari, S.; Nikahd, A.; Malekahmadi, M.R.; Lankarani, M.M.; Zamanian, H. Race by Gender Group Differences in the Protective Effects of Socioeconomic Factors against Sustained Health Problems across Five Domains. *J. Racial Ethn. Health Disparities* **2016**. [CrossRef] [PubMed]

35. Hudson, D.L. Race, Socioeconomic Position and Depression: The Mental Health Costs of Upward Mobility. Doctoral Dissertation, The University of Michigan, Ann Arbor, MI, USA, 2009.

36. Keil, J.E.; Sutherland, S.E.; Knapp, R.G.; Tyroler, H.A. Does equal socioeconomic status in black and white men mean equal risk of mortality? *Am. J. Public Health* **1992**, *82*, 1133–1136. [CrossRef] [PubMed]

37. Cooper, R.S. Health and the social status of blacks in the United States. *Ann. Epidemiol.* **1993**, *3*, 137–144. [CrossRef]

38. Williams, D.R.; Collins, C. Racial residential segregation: A fundamental cause of racial disparities in health. *Public Health Rep.* **2001**, *116*, 404–416. [CrossRef]

39. Williams, D.R.; Yu, Y.; Jackson, J.S.; Anderson, N.B. Racial differences in physical and mental health: Socio-economic status, stress and discrimination. *J. Health Psychol.* **1997**, *2*, 335–351. [CrossRef] [PubMed]

40. Williams, D.R.; Neighbors, H.W.; Jackson, J.S. Racial/ethnic discrimination and health: Findings from community studies. *Am. J. Public Health* **2003**, *93*, 200–208. [CrossRef] [PubMed]

41. Brunello, G.; Fort, M.; Schneeweis, N.; Winter-Ebmer, R. The Causal Effect of Education on Health: What Is the Role of Health Behaviors? *Health Econ.* **2016**, *25*, 314–336. [CrossRef] [PubMed]

42. Assari, S.; Lankarani, M.M. Education and Alcohol Consumption among Older Americans; Black-White Differences. *Front. Public Health* **2016**, *4*, 67. [CrossRef] [PubMed]

43. Juhn, Y.J.; Beebe, T.J.; Finnie, D.M.; Sloan, J.; Wheeler, P.H.; Yawn, B.; Williams, A.R. Development and initial testing of a new socioeconomic status measure based on housing data. *J. Urban Health* **2011**, *88*, 933–944. [CrossRef] [PubMed]

44. Ross, C.E.; Wu, C.L. The links between education and health. *Am. Social. Rev.* **1995**, *60*, 719–745. [CrossRef]

45. Montez, J.K.; Hummer, R.A.; Hayward, M.D. Educational attainment and adult mortality in the United States: A systematic analysis of functional form. *Demography* **2012**, *49*, 315–336. [CrossRef] [PubMed]

46. Tyson, K.; Darity, W., Jr.; Castellino, D.R. It's not "a black thing": Understanding the burden of acting white and other dilemmas of high achievement. *Am. Sociol. Rev.* **2005**, *70*, 582–605. [CrossRef]

47. Neighbors, H.W.; Njai, R.; Jackson, J.S. Race, ethnicity, John Henryism, and depressive symptoms: The national survey of American life adult reinterview. *Res. Hum. Dev.* **2007**, *4*, 71–87. [CrossRef]

48. Montez, J.K.; Hummer, R.A.; Hayward, M.D.; Woo, H.; Rogers, R.G. Trends in the educational gradient of US adult mortality from 1986 through 2006 by race, gender, and age group. *Res. Aging* **2011**, *33*, 145–171. [CrossRef] [PubMed]

49. Case, A.; Darren, L.; Christina, P. Economic Status and Health in Childhood: The Origins of the Gradient. *Am. Econ. Rev.* **2002**, *92*, 1308–1334. [CrossRef] [PubMed]

50. Pearlman, D.N.; Zierler, S.; Meersman, S.; Kim, H.K.; Viner-Brown, S.I.; Caron, C. Race disparities in childhood asthma: Does where you live matter? *J. Natl. Med. Assoc.* **2006**, *98*, 239–247. [PubMed]

51. Thakur, N.; Oh, S.S.; Nguyen, E.A.; Martin, M.; Roth, L.A.; Galanter, J.; Gignoux, C.R.; Eng, C.; Davis, A.; Meade, K.; et al. Socioeconomic status and childhood asthma in urban minority youths. The GALA II and SAGE II studies. *Am. J. Respir. Crit. Care Med.* **2013**, *188*, 1202–1209. [CrossRef] [PubMed]

52. Carroll, K. Socioeconomic status, race/ethnicity, and asthma in youth. *Am. J. Respir. Crit. Care Med.* **2013**, *188*, 1180–1181. [CrossRef] [PubMed]

53. Smith, L.A.; Hatcher-Ross, J.L.; Wertheimer, R.; Kahn, R.S. Rethinking race/ethnicity, income; and childhood asthma: Racial/ethnic disparities concentrated among the very poor. *Public Health Rep.* **2005**, *120*, 109–116. [CrossRef] [PubMed]

54. Feagin, J.R. Excluding blacks and others from housing: The foundation of white racism. *Cityscape* **1999**, *4*, 79–91.

55. Blumberg, S.J.; Foster, E.B.; Frasier, A.M.; Satorius, J.; Skalland, B.J.; Nysse-Carris, K.L.; Morrison, H.M.; Chowdhury, S.R.; Connor, K.S. Design and operation of the National Survey of Children's Health, 2007. *Vital Health Stat.* **2012**, *55*, 1–149.

56. Van Dyck, P.; Kogan, M.D.; Heppel, D.; Blumberg, S.J.; Cynamon, M.L.; Newacheck, P.W. The National Survey of Children's Health: A new data resource. *Matern Child Health J.* **2004**, *8*, 183–188. [CrossRef] [PubMed]

57. Bramlett, M.D.; Blumberg, S.J. Family structure and children's physical and mental health. *Health Aff.* **2007**, *26*, 549–558. [CrossRef] [PubMed]

58. National Survey of Children's Health. CATI Instrument. Available online: https://ftp.cdc.gov/pub/health_statistics/nchs/slaits/nsch07/1a_Survey_Instrument_English/NSCH_Questionnaire_052109.pdf (accessed on 1 April 2018).

59. Wallace, S.P.; Padilla-Frausto, D.I.; Smith, S.E. Older adults need twice the federal poverty level to make ends meet in California. *Policy Brief UCLA Cent Health Policy Res.* **2010**, *8*, 1–8.

60. Spencer, E.A.; Appleby, P.N.; Davey, G.K.; Key, T.J. Validity of self-reported height and weight in 4808 EPIC-Oxford participants. *Public Health Nutr.* **2002**, *5*, 561–565. [CrossRef] [PubMed]

61. Stewart, A.L. The reliability and validity of self-reported weight and height. *J. Chronic Dis.* **1982**, *35*, 295–309. [CrossRef]

62. Taylor, A.W.; Dal Grande, E.; Gill, T.K.; Chittleborough, C.R.; Wilson, D.H.; Adams, R.J. How valid are self-reported height and weight? A comparison between CATI self-report and clinic measurements using a large cohort study. *Aust. N. Z. J. Public Health* **2006**, *30*, 238–246. [CrossRef] [PubMed]

63. Lang, I.A.; Kipping, R.R.; Jago, R.; Lawlor, D.A. Variation in childhood and adolescent obesity prevalence defined by international and country-specific criteria in England and the United States. *Eur. J. Clin. Nutr.* **2011**, *65*, 143–150. [CrossRef] [PubMed]

64. Dumith, S.C.; FariasJúnior, J.C. Overweight and obesity in children and adolescents: Comparison of three classification criteria based on body mass index. *Rev. Panam. Salud Publ.* **2010**, *28*, 30–35. [CrossRef]

65. Valerio, M.A.; Andreski, P.M.; Schoeni, R.F.; McGonagle, K.A. Examining the association between childhood asthma and parent and grandparent asthma status: Implications for practice. *Clin. Pediatr.* **2010**, *49*, 535–541. [CrossRef] [PubMed]

66. Bhan, N.; Glymour, M.M.; Kawachi, I.; Subramanian, S.V. Childhood adversity and asthma prevalence: Evidence from 10 US states (2009–2011). *BMJ Open Respir. Res.* **2014**. [CrossRef] [PubMed]

67. Victorino, C.C.; Gauthier, A.H. The social determinants of child health: Variations across health outcomes—A population-based cross-sectional analysis. *BMC Pediatr.* **2009**, *9*, 53. [CrossRef] [PubMed]

68. Assari, S.; Caldwell, C.H.; Mincy, R. Family Socioeconomic Status at Birth and Youth Impulsivity at Age 15; Blacks' Diminished Return. *Children* **2018**, *5*, 58. [CrossRef] [PubMed]

69. Assari, S.; Thomas, A.; Caldwell, C.H.; Mincy, R.B. Blacks' Diminished Health Return of Family Structure and Socioeconomic Status; 15 Years of Follow-up of a National Urban Sample of Youth. *J. Urban Health* **2018**, *95*, 21–35. [CrossRef] [PubMed]

70. Assari, S.; Caldwell, C.H.; Mincy, R.B. Maternal Educational Attainment at Birth Promotes Future Self-Rated Health of White but Not Black Youth: A 15-Year Cohort of a National Sample. *J. Clin. Med.* **2018**, *7*, 93. [CrossRef] [PubMed]

71. Assari, S. Parental Education Better Helps White than Black Families Escape Poverty: National Survey of Children's Health. *Economies* **2018**, *6*, 30. [CrossRef]

72.  Assari, S. Diminished Economic Return of Socioeconomic Status for Black Families. *Soc. Sci.* **2018**, *7*, 74. [CrossRef]

73.  Adler, N.E.; Stewart, J. Reducing obesity: Motivating action while not blaming the victim. *Milbank Q.* **2009**, *87*, 49–70. [CrossRef] [PubMed]

74.  Jones, R.K.; Luo, Y. The culture of poverty and African-American culture: An empirical assessment. *Sociol. Perspect.* **1999**, *42*, 439–458. [CrossRef]

75.  Johnson, J.H.; Parnell, A.; Joyner, A.M.; Christman, C.J.; Marsh, B. Racial apartheid in a small North Carolina town. *Rev. Black Political Econ.* **2004**, *31*, 89–107. [CrossRef]

76.  Bass, S. Policing space, policing race: Social control imperatives and police discretionary decisions. *Soc. Justice* **2001**, *28*, 156–176.

77.  Goldberg, D.T. The new segregation. *Race Soc.* **1998**, *1*, 15–32. [CrossRef]

78.  Sewell, A.A.; Jefferson, K.A.; Lee, H. Living under surveillance: Gender, psychological distress, and stop-question-and-frisk policing in New York City. *Soc. Sci. Med.* **2016**, *159*, 1–13. [CrossRef] [PubMed]

79.  Pearce, D.M. Gatekeepers and homeseekers: Institutional patterns in racial steering. *Soc. Probl.* **1979**, *26*, 325–342. [CrossRef]

80.  Sewell, A.A. Opening the Black Box of Segregation: Real Estate and Racial Health Disparities. In *Race and Real Estate*; Oxford University Press: Oxford, UK, 2015.

81.  Burley, D. White racial reasoning: Rational racism in the perceptions of white males. *Hum. Soc.* **2005**, *29*, 116–125. [CrossRef]

82.  Norton, M.I.; Sommers, S.R. Whites see racism as a zero-sum game that they are now losing. *Perspect. Psychol. Sci.* **2011**, *6*, 215–218. [CrossRef] [PubMed]

83.  Chang, R.S. Reverse Racism: Affirmative Action, the Family, and the Dream that is America. *Hastings Const. Law Q.* **1995**, *23*, 1115.

84.  Farber, H.J.; Knowles, S.B.; Brown, N.L.; Caine, L.; Luna, V.; Qian, Y.; Lavori, P.; Wilson, S.R. Secondhand tobacco smoke in children with asthma: Sources of and parental perceptions about exposure in children and parental readiness to change. *Chest* **2008**, *133*, 1367–1374. [CrossRef] [PubMed]

85.  Marmot, M.; Allen, J.J. Social determinants of health equity. *Am. J. Public Health* **2014**. [CrossRef] [PubMed]

86.  Sobal, J.; Stunkard, A.J. Socioeconomic status and obesity: A review of the literature. *Psychol. Bull.* **1989**, *105*, 260–275. [CrossRef] [PubMed]

87.  McLaren, L. Socioeconomic status and obesity. *Epidemiol. Rev.* **2007**, *29*, 29–48. [CrossRef] [PubMed]

88.  Ben-Shlomo, Y.; Kuh, D. A life course approach to chronic disease epidemiology: Conceptual models, empirical challenges and interdisciplinary perspectives. *Int. J. Epidemiol.* **2002**, *31*, 285–293. [CrossRef] [PubMed]

89.  Ogden, C.L.; Lamb, M.M.; Carroll, M.D.; Flegal, K.M. Obesity and socioeconomic status in adults: United States 1988–1994 and 2005–2008. Available online: https://www.cdc.gov/nchs/data/databriefs/db50.pdf (accessed on 1 April 2018).

90.  Lynch, J.; Smith, G.D. A life course approach to chronic disease epidemiology. *Ann. Rev. Public Health* **2005**, *26*, 1–35. [CrossRef] [PubMed]

91.  Assari, S. Life Expectancy Gain Due to Employment Status Depends on Race, Gender, Education, and Their Intersections. *J. Racial Ethn. Health Disparities* **2017**. [CrossRef] [PubMed]

92.  Assari, S.; Caldwell, C.H. Neighborhood Safety and Major Depressive Disorder in a National Sample of Black Youth; Gender by Ethnic Differences. *Children* **2017**, *4*, 14. [CrossRef] [PubMed]

93.  Assari, S. Whites but Not Blacks Gain Life Expectancy from Social Contacts. *Behav. Sci.* **2017**, *7*, 68. [CrossRef] [PubMed]

94.  Assari, S. The link between mental health and obesity: Role of individual and contextual factors. *Int. J. Prev. Med.* **2014**, *5*, 247–249. [PubMed]

95.  Andresen, E.M.; Malmgren, J.A.; Carter, W.B.; Patrick, D.L. Screening for depression in well older adults: Evaluation of a short form of the CES-D (Center for Epidemiologic Studies Depression Scale). *Am. J. Prev. Med.* **1994**, *10*, 77–84. [CrossRef]

96.  Antonakis, J.; Bendahan, S.; Jacquart, P.; Lalive, R. On making causal claims: A review and recommendations. *Leadersh. Q.* **2010**, *21*, 1086–1120. [CrossRef]

97.  Dawid, A.P.; Faigman, D.L.; Fienberg, S.E. Fitting science into legal contexts: Assessing effects of causes or causes of effects? *Sociol. Methods Res.* **2014**, *43*, 359–390. [CrossRef]

98. Scholtens, S.; Wijga, A.H.; Seidell, J.C.; Brunekreef, B.; de Jongste, J.C.; Gehring, U.; Smit, H.A. Overweight and changes in weight status during childhood in relation to asthma symptoms at 8 years of age. *J. Allergy Clin. Immunol.* **2009**, *123*, 1312–1318. [CrossRef] [PubMed]

99. Barreca, A.I.; Guldi, M.; Lindo, J.M.; Waddell, G.R. Saving babies? Revisiting the effect of very low birth weight classification. *Q. J. Econ.* **2011**, *126*, 2117–2123. [CrossRef] [PubMed]

# 11

# Long-Term Melatonin Therapy for Adolescents and Young Adults with Chronic Sleep Onset Insomnia and Late Melatonin Onset: Evaluation of Sleep Quality, Chronotype, and Lifestyle Factors Compared to Age-Related Randomly Selected Population Cohorts

Tom C. Zwart [1,2] ⓘ, Marcel G. Smits [3,4], Toine C.G. Egberts [2,5], Carin M.A. Rademaker [5] and Ingeborg M. van Geijlswijk [1,2,*]

[1]  Faculty of Veterinary Medicine, Pharmacy Department, Utrecht University, Utrecht 3584 CM, The Netherlands; tomczwart@gmail.com

[2]  Utrecht Institute for Pharmaceutical Sciences (UIPS), Department of Pharmacoepidemiology and Clinical Pharmacology, Faculty of Science, Utrecht University, Utrecht 3584 CG, The Netherlands; A.C.G.Egberts@uu.nl

[3]  Department of Sleep-wake disorders and Chronobiology, Gelderse Vallei Hospital, Ede 6716 RP, The Netherlands; smitsm@zgv.nl

[4]  Governor Kremers Centre, Maastricht University, Maastricht 6229 GR, The Netherlands

[5]  Department of Clinical Pharmacy, Division of Laboratory and Pharmacy, University Medical Centre Utrecht, Utrecht 3584 CX, The Netherlands; C.Rademaker@umcutrecht.nl

*   Correspondence: i.m.vangeijlswijk@uu.nl

**Abstract:** The extent of continuance of melatonin therapy initiated in pre-pubertal children with chronic sleep onset insomnia (CSOI) was investigated in young adult life. Sleep timing, sleep quality, adverse events, reasons for cessation of therapy, and patient characteristics with regard to therapy regimen, chronotype and lifestyle factors possibly influencing sleeping behavior were assessed. With an online survey using questionnaires (Pittsburgh Sleep Quality Index, Insomnia Severity Index, Morningness-Eveningness Questionnaire, and Munich Chronotype Questionnaire), outcomes were measured and compared with age-related controls. These controls were extracted from published epidemiological research programs applying the same questionnaires. At the moment of the survey, melatonin was still continued by 27.3% of the patients, with a mean treatment duration of 10.8 years. The overall average treatment duration was 7.1 years. Sleep quality of both discontinued and persistent melatonin users did not deviate from controls. Sleep timing and chronotype scores indicated evening type preference in all responders. Adverse events were scarce but the perceived timing of pubertal development suggested a tendency towards delayed puberty in former and current users of melatonin. This study may underestimate the number of children that are able to stop using melatonin due to the response rate (47.8%) and appeal for continuing users. Sleep timing parameters were based on self-reported estimates. Control populations were predominantly students and were of varying nationalities. The statistical power of this study is low due to the limited sample size. Melatonin therapy sustained for 7.1 years does not result in substantial deviations of sleep quality as compared to controls and appears to be safe. The evening type preference suggests a causal relation with CSOI. This study shows that ten years after initiation of treatment with melatonin for CSOI, approximately 75% of the patients will have normal sleep quality without medication.

**Keywords:** melatonin; children; CSOI; long-term; efficacy; safety

## 1. Introduction

Since the introduction of melatonin as a treatment option for children with chronic sleep onset insomnia (CSOI), efficacy issues and safety concerns have been debated. Recently, the publication of clinical recommendations [1] and guidelines [2] for the use of melatonin in children renewed this debate on safety [3,4]. Melatonin is widely used as an over-the-counter (OTC) dietary food supplement in Europe and the USA. Many healthcare workers and parents perceive the absence of adverse events reports as confirmation that melatonin is safe. However, others remain skeptical as information on the effectiveness and safety of long-term melatonin therapy is still limited. Although studies in small populations over limited periods of time have shown persistent effectiveness on sleep timing and no alarming adverse effects [5–8], more data on melatonin therapy over longer periods of time are needed to confirm these findings and to answer the question of what patient characteristics may predict duration of melatonin therapy.

The current study comprises an evaluation of a group of Dutch adolescents and young adults who started melatonin therapy during early childhood for CSOI 9–12 years ago. Primary objectives are (1) to evaluate (dis)continuance of melatonin therapy, actual sleep timing and actual sleep quality on average ten years after treatment initiation, and (2) to investigate the occurrence of adverse events and reasons for melatonin cessation. Secondary objectives are to assess patient characteristics with regard to (1) treatment features and attitudes, (2) chronotype and (3) lifestyle factors that might interfere with endogenous and exogenous melatonin pharmacokinetics, thereby possibly affecting effectiveness of melatonin therapy, long-term treatment outcomes, and the need for continuance of therapy. This study compares former and persistent melatonin users to age-related controls.

## 2. Materials and Methods

### 2.1. Study Design

All 69 children that finished the melatonin dose finding (Meldos) trial [9], which was conducted between February 2004 and May 2007, were invited to participate in this follow-up study. The study consisted of an electronic, online survey with questions regarding demographics, melatonin therapy features and attitudes, timing of puberty development, lifestyle factors and four validated international questionnaires evaluating sleep timing, sleep quality and chronotype. Last known home addresses of all Meldos participants were provided by Gelderse Vallei Hospital Ede and additional contact information of participants' parents was available from the Meldos trial and a previous follow-up study [7]. All eligible participants were contacted by telephone, e-mail, postal mail or Facebook. Respondents who agreed to participate in the study were sent an e-mail containing a personal, unique web link providing them access to our online questionnaire. The study protocol was categorized as research not subjected to the Medical Research Involving Human Subjects Act by the Medical Ethics Committee of the University Medical Center Utrecht (UMCU) and approved by the local Research Assessment Committee (BCWO) of the Gelderse Vallei Hospital Ede, both located in The Netherlands. The study was registered in the Netherlands Trial Registry (NTR5930).

### 2.2. Participants

All 69 former participants of the Meldos trial [9] were eligible to participate in this second long-term evaluation. The Meldos trial included children diagnosed with CSOI, aged 6–12, who did not respond to sleep hygiene measures and suffered from sleep onset insomnia for more than four nights per week for more than one year. Sleep onset insomnia was defined as sleep onset later than 20:30 for children aged 6, and for older children 15 min later per year until the age of 12 (22:00) and average sleep onset latency (SOL) exceeding 30 min. Exclusion criteria were CSOI due to psychiatric or pedagogic problems, known intellectual disability, pervasive developmental disorder, chronic pain, known disturbed hepatic or renal function, epilepsy, prior use of melatonin, and use of stimulants, neuroleptics, benzodiazepines, clonidine, antidepressants, hypnotics or beta-blockers within 4 weeks before enrolment.

### 2.3. Control Population

To evaluate the effects of long-term melatonin use in our patient group, and to identify characteristics of patients diagnosed with chronic sleep onset insomnia at a young age, we compared our study group (N = 33) with results found in epidemiological research programs applying the same questionnaires. These populations represent the "normal" population in late 10 s and early 20 s, and vary from N = 154 for the PSQI questionnaire to N = 9500 for smoking habits in the Dutch National Drug Monitoring.

### 2.4. Questionnaire

The questionnaire consisted of eight parts to assess the various aspects regarding patient characteristics, therapy effectiveness, and safety associated with melatonin treatment.

### 2.5. Patient Characteristics

#### 2.5.1. Demographics and Melatonin Use

Gender, age, weight, length, marital status, offspring and highest level of education were registered. Melatonin treatment features and attitudes were evaluated by assessing (dis)continuation of melatonin use, treatment duration, current dose, therapy habits like temporary discontinuation of therapy (drug holidays) and reasons for final cessation of therapy.

#### 2.5.2. Chronotype

Chronotype was assessed with the Kerkhof version of the Morningness-Eveningness Questionnaire (MEQ) and a Dutch version of the Munich Chronotype Questionnaire (MCTQ). The MEQ is a nineteen item, self-administered questionnaire which differentiates between morning- and evening type, first published by Horne & Östberg in 1976 [10,11]. It has been validated in various languages and populations and is widely used for chronotype evaluation [12]. In 1984, a Dutch shortened version of the MEQ was published by Kerkhof [13]. The Kerkhof MEQ consists of seven items, five of which are scored on a 1–4 scale. The remaining questions are scored on a time scale. Total score ranges from 7–31, which is interpreted as follows: '7–10' = definitely evening type, '11–14' = moderate evening type, '15–21' = neither type, '22–25' = moderate morning type and '26–31' = definitely morning type. It was validated in a population consisting of mainly students (N = 275) with an average age of 22.7 years [13]. The Kerkhof MEQ was implemented in our questionnaire since it is simpler than the original MEQ and has shown comparable validity [10,13].

The MCTQ evaluates sleep timing on both working- and non-working days with regard to bedtime, time till lights out, SOL, wake time and time till rise [14]. The MCTQ has been validated with sleep logs, actimetry, Dim Light Melatonin Onset (DLMO) and the MEQ and has shown high correlations [15–17]. In this study, a Dutch version of the MCTQ was used which is available on the Ludwig Maximilian University München website [18]. With the results of the MCTQ the midpoint between sleep onset time (SOT) and wake-up time is calculated, which is defined as midsleep on free days (MSF) [19]. The MSF is strongly correlated with DLMO and is an indicator for chronotype [14,20]. Additionally, the MSF was corrected for workday derived sleep debt resulting in the MSFSC, as described by Roenneberg et al. in 2004 [21].

#### 2.5.3. Lifestyle Factors

Smoking habits were evaluated with three items from the smoking section of the Dutch Health Survey (DHS) 2014 [22]. Current smoking status (smoker versus non-smoker), type of tobacco product and smoking frequency were assessed.

Average daily caffeine consumption was evaluated with three food frequency questions on the average daily consumption of coffee, tea and caffeinated energy drinks over the past twelve months. These food frequency data were multiplied with the caffeine content of a standardized portion of the respective beverage types, as adopted from the Netherlands Nutrition Centre [23].

The use of electronic devices at bedtime was evaluated with three questionnaire items: (1) whether the participant owned a smartphone or tablet, (2) whether the device was brought into the bedroom at bedtime and (3) how often it was used after lights out. Options for the latter question were 'never', 'less than half of the time', 'more than half of the time' or 'always'.

### 2.6. Therapy Effectiveness

### 2.6.1. Sleep Quality

Sleep quality was examined with the Pittsburgh Sleep Quality Index (PSQI), adapted for the Dutch population as provided by eProvide®. The PSQI is a self-rated nineteen item questionnaire to assess sleep quality and sleep disturbances over the past month [24]. It addresses seven items of sleep: subjective sleep quality, SOL, sleep duration, habitual sleep efficiency, sleep disturbances, use of sleep medication and daytime dysfunction. Each item is weighted on a 0–3 scale. Item scores are summed up to yield the global PSQI score which ranges from 0–21, higher scores indicating worse sleep quality. A cut-off value of greater than five is defined to distinguish between good and poor sleepers.

Insomnia severity was evaluated with the Insomnia Severity Index (ISI), adapted for the Dutch population as provided by eProvide®. The ISI encompasses a self-rated, seven item questionnaire to determine the participants' perception of his or her insomnia severity [25,26]. The ISI evaluates subjective symptoms and consequences of insomnia over the past two weeks in seven items of insomnia: severity of sleep onset and sleep maintenance difficulties, satisfaction with the current sleep pattern, interference with daily functioning, noticeability of impairment attributed to the sleep problem and the degree of distress or concern caused by the sleep problem. Items are scored on a five-point scale from 0 (none) to 4 (very severe), which are summed to a total score of 0–28. Total ISI-score is interpreted as follows: '0–7' = no clinically significant insomnia, '8–14' = subthreshold insomnia, '15–21' = moderate insomnia, '22–28' = severe insomnia.

### 2.6.2. Sleep Timing

Sleep timing, bedtime, time till lights out, SOL, wake up time and time till rise after wake up were assessed with the MCTQ. With these parameters SOT, rise time (RT) and total sleep time (TST) were calculated.

### 2.6.3. Safety

Occurrence of therapy associated adverse events like headaches (explicitly solicited) or other adverse events, occurrence of rebound sleep disturbances after (temporary) cessation of therapy, the use of co-medication and perceived timing of pubertal development, were evaluated. Perceived pubertal timing was evaluated with one questionnaire item, by which participants were asked to indicate whether they felt their timing of pubertal development was any earlier or later than most other boys or girls of the same age. Options were 'much earlier', 'somewhat earlier', 'about the same', 'somewhat later' or 'much later'. This questionnaire item was derived from the Puberty Development Scale (PDS) [27].

### 2.7. Statistical Analysis

All data were analyzed in IBM SPSS Statistics 23. Independent sample T-tests were performed in Microsoft Excel 2016. Data on sleep timing, MEQ, PSQI, ISI and lifestyle factors were missing from one participant from the group that had discontinued therapy, this group is referred to as the melatonin treatment discontinuation (STOP) group. Data on occurrence of headache were missing from seven participants from the STOP group. Due to the low number of the persistent users—this group is referred to as the melatonin treatment continuation (CONT) group—statistical analysis was performed for the comparison of young adults using melatonin during their childhood (this study = STOP+CONT) versus the randomly selected age-related population in several cohort studies. Differences within this study between STOP and CONT group are limited to descriptive analysis.

## 3. Results

### 3.1. Patient Characteristics

33 of the 69 former Meldos participants responded (response rate: 47.8%), 32 of which were complete. One responder did not complete the ISI, PSQI, MEQ and MCTQ questionnaires. Nine respondents (27.3%) still used melatonin after an average treatment duration of 10.8 years: CONT group. Twenty-four respondents (72.7%) had discontinued therapy: STOP group. The pattern of melatonin continuation, discontinuation and non-response during the Meldos trial, the first long-term evaluation (Meldos LT1) and the current study (Meldos LT2) are schematically depicted in Figure 1.

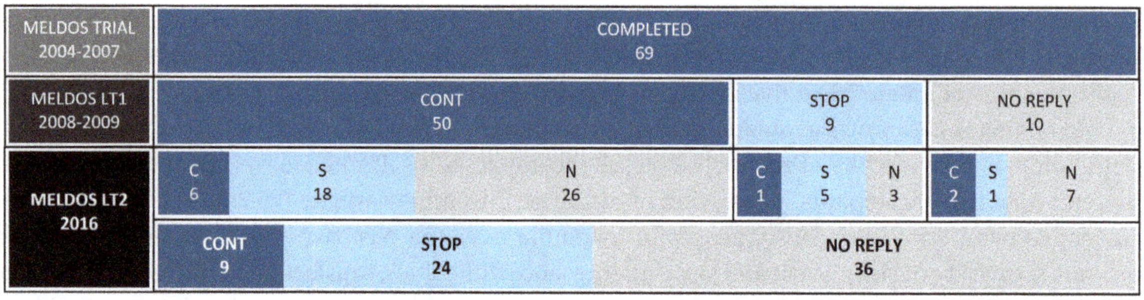

**Figure 1.** Melatonin continuation, melatonin discontinuation and non-response during the Meldos trial, the Meldos LT1 and the Meldos LT2. CONT/C: continuation; STOP/S: discontinuation; N: no reply.

The melatonin treatment continuation over the years of the 33 participants of the current study is schematically depicted in Figure 2.

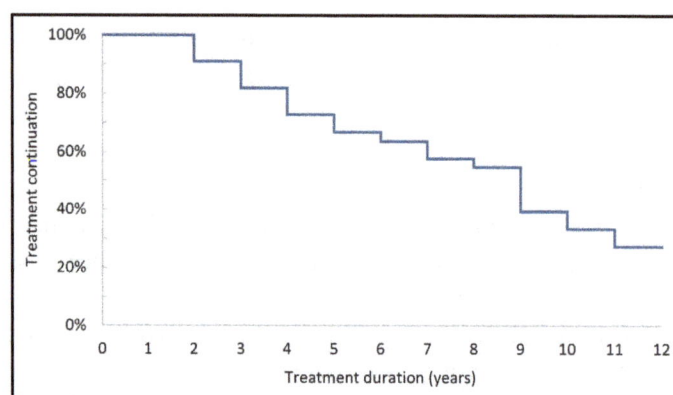

**Figure 2.** Melatonin treatment continuation of the 33 participants over the years.

Demographics and treatment features in the total population and specified to the CONT and STOP groups are shown in Table 1. With regard to education, responses indicating higher professional, pre-university and university education were combined and designated as 'high education level'. Responses indicating secondary and lower vocational education and elementary school as highest achieved education level were combined and designated as 'low education level'.

**Table 1.** Demographics and treatment features of the total population (this study) and the CONT and STOP groups.

|  |  | This Study | CONT | STOP |
|---|---|---|---|---|
| N |  | 33 | 9 | 24 |
| Males |  | 14 (42.4%) | 2 (22.2%) | 12 (50.0%) |
| Age (years) | Mean | 19.6 | 20.3 | 19.4 |
|  | Range | 16.7 to 23.2 | 17.6 to 21.9 | 16.7 to 23.2 |
|  | SD | 1.9 | 1.5 | 2.0 |
| TD (years) | Mean | 7.1 | 10.8 | 5.7 |
|  | Range | 1.0 to 11.9 | 9.6 to 11.9 | 1.0 to 10.9 |
|  | SD | 3.5 | 0.8 | 3.2 |
| Dose (mg) | Mean | n/a | 2.9 | n/a |
|  | Range | n/a | 0.5 to 5.0 | n/a |
|  | SD | n/a | 1.6 | n/a |
| TOA (hh:mm) | Mean | n/a | 21:46 | n/a |
|  | Range | n/a | 19:00 to 23:00 | n/a |
|  | SD | n/a | 1:06 | n/a |
| BMI (kg/m$^2$) | Mean | 21.2 | 23.1 | 20.5 |
|  | Range | 17.0 to 29.8 | 19.0 to 29.8 | 17.0 to 26.6 |
|  | SD | 2.7 | 3.3 | 2.1 |
| Education level | High | 21 (63.6%) | 7 (77.8%) | 14 (58.3%) |
|  | Low | 12 (36.4%) | 2 (22.2%) | 10 (41.7%) |
| Relationship | Yes | 11 (33.3%) | 1 (11.1%) | 10 (41.2%) |
|  | No | 22 (66.7%) | 8 (88.9%) | 14 (58.8%) |
| Offspring | Yes | 1 (3.0%) | 0 (0.0%) | 1 (4.2%) |
|  | No | 32 (97.0%) | 9 (100.0%) | 23 (95.8%) |

TD: treatment duration, TOA: time of administration, BMI: body mass index.

In the CONT group, four participants had temporarily (>6 months) discontinued therapy, but indicated to have restarted since. Five interrupted therapy during holidays and three skipped medication on a weekly basis during weekends. Reasons for interruption were a delayed sleep rhythm during holidays and weekends and checking the need for continuance of therapy. In the STOP group, twenty-one participants indicated to have adopted a delayed sleep rhythm and no longer needed melatonin to fall asleep at the desired (later) bedtime. Two reported unsatisfactory effects on sleep timing as the reason for discontinuation, and one participant did not remember the reason for discontinuation.

### 3.2. Chronotype

Timing of midsleep on work (MSW) and free (MSF) days of this study were compared to data from Zavada et al., who reported on sleep timing in a population of 1342 Dutch students aged under 25 [16]. To facilitate comparison to the controls, Kerkhof MEQ scores were converted into Horne-Östberg MEQ scores. The Horne-Östberg MEQ score ranges from 16–86, with categories '16–30' = definitely evening type, '31–41' = moderate evening type, '42–58' = neither type, '59–69' = moderate morning type and '70–86' = definitely morning type [10]. Mean Horne-Östberg MEQ score of our total population was compared to data from Zavada et al. [16].

Results for MSW, MSF and MEQ score comparisons are depicted in Figure 3.

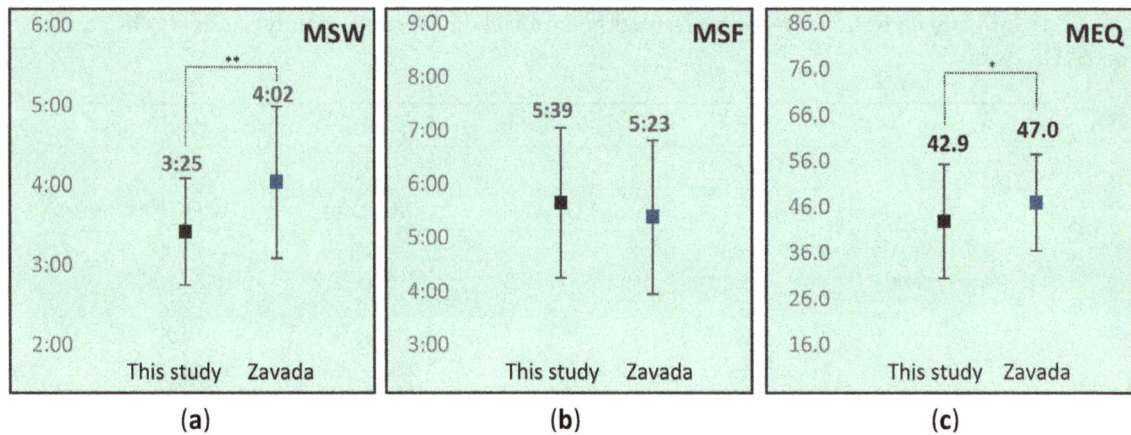

**Figure 3.** Comparison of mean midsleep on work days (MSW) (**a**), midsleep free days (MSF) (**b**) and Morningness-Eveningness Questionnaire MEQ (**c**) score between this study (N = 32) and data from Zavada et al. (N = 1342) [16]. MSW and MSF in hh:mm. Whiskers represent standard deviations. * $p < 0.05$; ** $p < 0.01$.

As is depicted in Figure 3, MSW score, and mean MEQ score of the total population in this study were statistically significant lower than that of controls in the Zavada study, indicating a preference towards eveningness in our population as compared to controls. MSF scores did not differ from the population of 1342 Dutch students.

Results for this study group with regard to self-rated morningness-eveningness (M/E-ness), as derived from Kerkhof MEQ question item 7, were compared to data from the National Sleep Survey (NSS) 2016. The NSS 2016 reported on the sleep timing of a population of 1372 Dutch students aged 21.7 [28]. Results are depicted in Figure 4. In the control population 61% rated their selves as neither morning nor evening type, as compared to this study population only 15.6%. In this study 81.3% could be categorized as eveningness type, in the control population this was 32%.

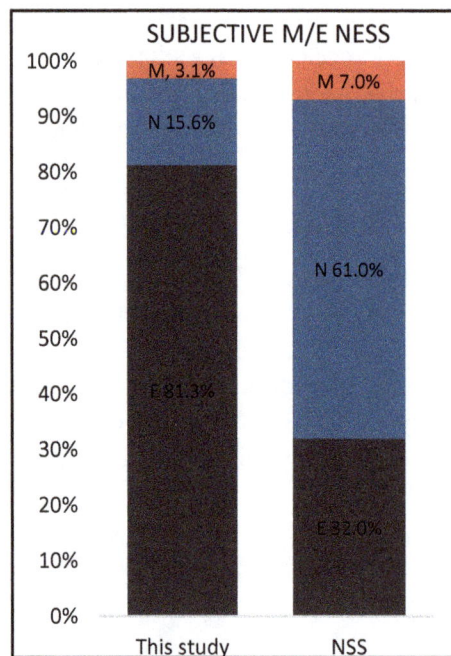

**Figure 4.** Self-rated morningness-eveningness (M/E-ness) from this study (N = 32) and data from the NSS 2016 (N = 1372) [28]. M: morning type; N: neither type; E: evening type.

### 3.3. Lifestyle Factors

Cigarette smoking prevalence in this study was compared to data from the Netherlands National Drug Monitor (NDM) 2015 report, which reported on smoking prevalence of Dutch 16–20 old's. 23% of this age group reported to smoke now and again (N = 9500), compared to this study 6 persons, 18.2% [29].

Estimated mean daily caffeine consumption over the past twelve months of this study group was compared to data from the European Food Safety Authority (EFSA) 2015 report on the safety of caffeine, which reported on mean daily caffeine intake in a population of 1142 Dutch adolescents aged 10–17, being 69.5 mg/day [30]. Mean caffeine consumption, was 78.3 mg/day for this study group.

All respondents possessed a smartphone or tablet and all but one (96.9%), brought the device into the bedroom at bedtime. Results on the use of electronic devices were compared to data from Fossum et al., who reported the use of electronic devices at bedtime at least once a week in a population of 532 Norwegian students aged 22.9 on average was 94.7% [31]. The results of that study refer to the use of any type of electronic device at bedtime (television, computer, gaming console, tablet, mobile phone or audio player), while results from this study refer specifically to the use of a smartphone or tablet at bedtime.

### 3.4. Therapy Effectiveness

#### 3.4.1. Sleep Quality

PSQI and ISI scores from the CONT and STOP group combined were compared to data from control populations. PSQI scores were compared to data from John et al., who reported on the PSQI scores of a population of 154 Dutch students aged 20.6 on average [32]. ISI scores were compared to data from Gerber et al. [33], who reported on the ISI scores of a population of 862 Swiss students with a mean age of 24.7 years. Results from these comparisons are depicted in Figure 5.

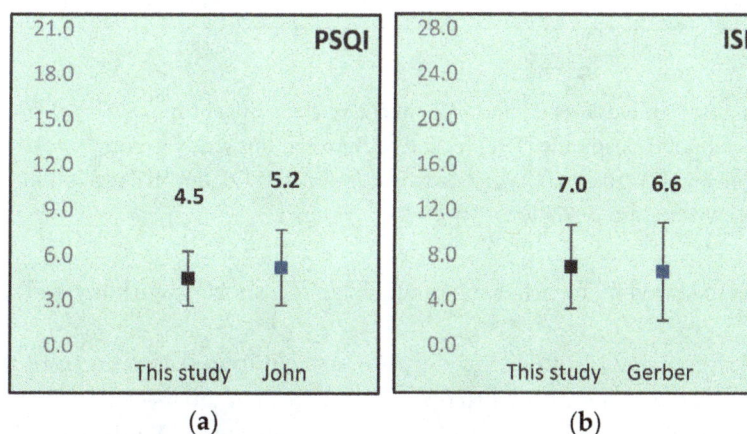

**Figure 5.** Comparison of mean Pittsburgh Sleep Quality Index (PSQI) (**a**) and Insomnia Severity Index (ISI) (**b**) scores of this study (N = 32) and data from control populations (PSQI: N = 154 [32], ISI: N = 862 [33]). Whiskers represent standard deviations.

Overall, no differences between the population in this study and age related controls were found for PSQI or ISI scores. The CONT group showed a tendency towards higher mean PSQI and ISI scores than the STOP group (data not shown). Participants with PSQI scores greater than 5 were designated as 'poor sleepers' PSQI scores greater than 7 were considered 'possible insomniacs'. This study group included poor sleepers and no possible insomniacs. Participants with ISI scores 8–14 are considered 'subthreshold insomnia'. This study group included nine (28.1%) subthreshold insomniacs and no moderate insomniacs, the pathologic PSQI and ISI scores coincide for seven participants, two participants have only one pathologic score.

### 3.4.2. Sleep Timing

The SOTs, RTs and TSTs for both work- and free days of this study were compared to data from Zavada et al. [16]. Results of these comparisons are depicted in Figure 6.

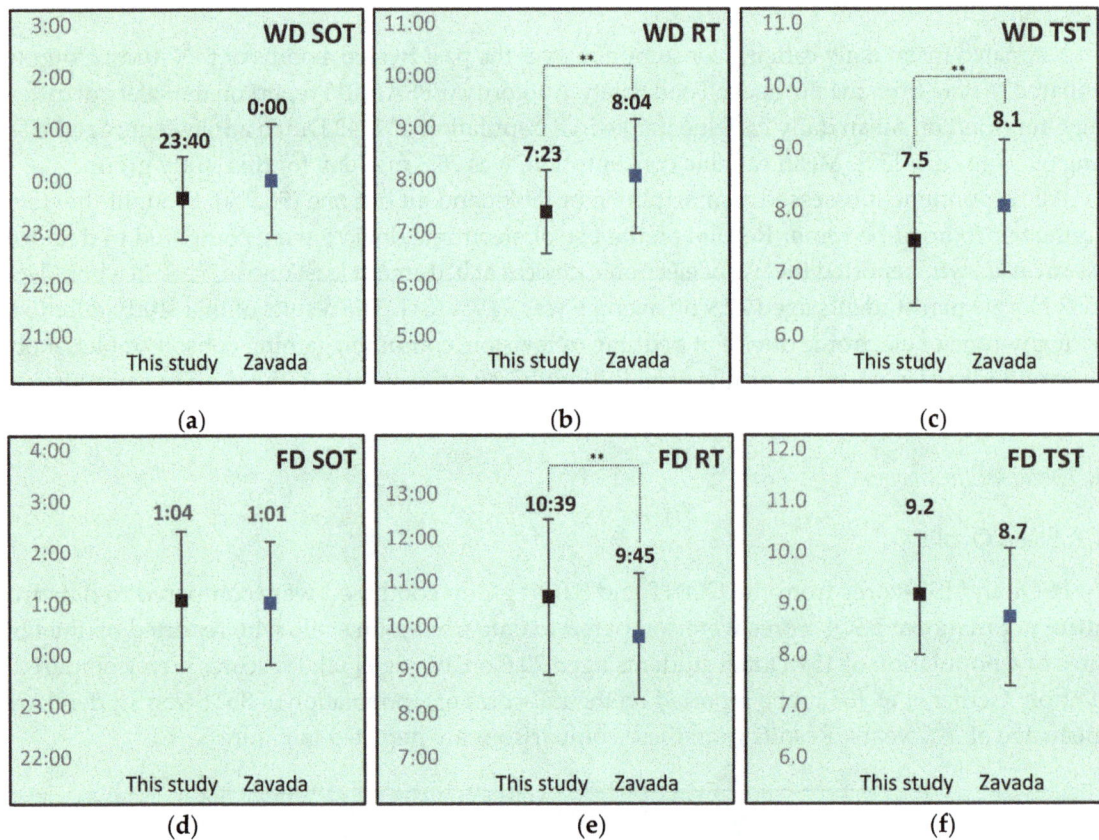

**Figure 6.** Comparison of work- (**a–c**) and free (**d–f**) day sleep onset time (SOT) (**a**) and (**d**), rise time (RT) (**b**) and (**e**) and total sleep time (TST) (**c**) and (**f**) between this study group (N = 32) and data from Zavada et al. (N = 1342) [16]. WD: work day; FD: free day. SOT and RT in hh:mm. TST in hours. Whiskers represent standard deviations. * $p < 0.05$; ** $p < 0.01$.

This study group showed an earlier mean workday RT, shorter workday TST, and later free day RT than controls.

SOL was also determined in this study group, and compared to data from the NSS 2016 [28]. In the current study, 14 (43.7%) indicated to need over 20 min to fall asleep, mean sleep onset latency (SOL) was 34.7 min. During the previous study 16 (27.1%) reported SOLs of over 20 min, with a mean SOL of 35.1 min [7]. The mean SOL from the NSS 2016 (N = 1372) was 26.0 min [28].

### 3.5. Safety

### 3.5.1. Adverse Effects

The questionnaire on occurrence of adverse events in was answered by 26 participants in this study. Outcomes on headache and nausea at start were comparable to the previous long-term study, with one third reporting a headache once a month or more, two third seldom or never [7]. One participant reported restless legs and drowsiness.

Eleven participants (39.3%) experienced sleeping difficulties following (temporary) discontinuation. Thirteen participants (39.4%) used co-medication including budesonide, desloratadine, fluticasone, levocetirizine, mebeverine, methylphenidate, miconazole, oral contraceptives, risperidone, ropinirole and salbutamol.

### 3.5.2. Pubertal Timing

With regard to perceived pubertal timing, two participants filled in the option 'much earlier'. For statistical reasons, the answers 'much earlier' and 'somewhat earlier' were combined and designated as 'earlier'. This is also applicable for the option 'much later' (N = 1), this answer was combined with the option 'somewhat later' and the combination designated as 'later'. Results were compared with data from Bratberg et al., who reported on perceived pubertal timing in a population of 8951 Norwegian adolescents and young adults aged 13–19 [34]. In the supplementary material, Bratberg et al. stratified pubertal timing results into two age groups: 13–15 and 16–19 year olds. The pubertal timing results of the group of 16–19 year olds (N = 4058) was compared to the Meldos participants. 31.3% of the participants experienced their pubertal timing as late while controls in Bratberg's study 17.0% denounced their pubertal timing late. Results are depicted in Figure 7.

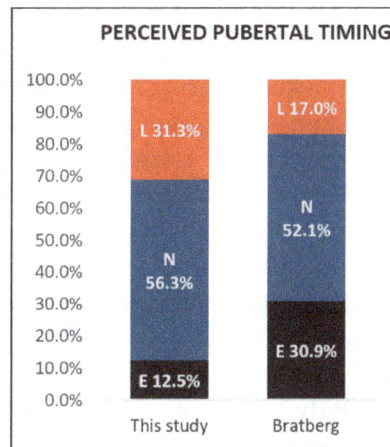

**Figure 7.** Perceived pubertal timing in this study and from Bratberg et al. (N = 4058) [34]. L: later; N: normal; E; earlier.

## 4. Discussion

Of 33 responders, 27.3% (N = 9) still used melatonin after an average treatment duration of 10.8 years. Participants show sleep quality which does not deviate from controls aged 20.6 [32], and comparable insomnia severity as compared to controls. These findings suggest sleep quality and insomnia severity of these former problem sleepers have generally normalized over time possibly facilitated by adopting a postponed sleeping rhythm, whereupon the misalignment of biological and social timing during (pre) puberty is resolved [35]. The problem sleepers in the continuation group use melatonin at higher doses than the other five participants in this group, 3, 4 and twice 5 mg, versus 0.5, 1, 2 and twice 3 mg, without deviations with respect to timing of administration, co-medication or lifestyle factors compared to the other participants from the CONT group. As high melatonin doses may result in spill-over effects [36], the applied melatonin doses might have been too high in these participants, resulting in poor sleep quality and insomnia. SOL from both groups did not deviate from Dutch controls aged 21.7 which suggests the SOL of our population generally normalized since early childhood. 31.3% of the participants experienced their pubertal timing as late which is a larger proportion than the 17.0% of controls in Bratberg's study that denounced their pubertal timing as late.

Chronotype MEQ score of this study population was significantly lower than seen in controls aged <25. Assessment of subjective M/E-ness showed a distinctively large presence of self-reported evening types in our population as compared to Dutch students aged 21.7 [16]. These findings suggest an inclination to the evening type in our population, suggestive for a causal relationship with CSOI.

Smoking has been associated with sleep disturbance, resulting in shorter TSTs, longer SOLs and worse sleep quality (higher PSQI scores) for current smokers than former and never smokers [37,38]. On the other hand, fatigue resulting from sleep difficulties and poor sleep quality might stimulate smoking [39]. Additionally, late chronotypes are more often habitual smokers than normal or early chronotypes [40]. Interestingly, smoking prevalence in this study group, which showed an inclination to the late chronotype, was comparable to controls aged 16–20. Caffeine consumption in this study group was comparable to the consumption in a cohort study in Dutch adolescents aged 10–18. Problem sleepers could be prone to consume more caffeine in an attempt to compensate for their daytime sleepiness. Caffeine consumption is associated with sleeping difficulties in adolescents and young adults (shorter sleep duration and increased SOL and wake time after sleep onset), this could add to their sleeping difficulties [41]. Late chronotype is associated with a higher caffeine consumption [40,42] but not in this study group. Combined with the smoking habits observation we speculate that this study group, despite the eveningness preferences, might be more aware of favorable attitudes with regard to healthy sleep conduct. In respect of the use of electronic devices at bedtime, this study group did not seem to deviate from controls aged 22.8 [31].

Tobacco smoke [43–45] and caffeine [46,47] interfere with CYP1A2 metabolism thus effecting endogenous and exogenous melatonin levels and light emitted from electronic devices suppresses endogenous melatonin levels [48–50]. Smoking and higher consumption of caffeine might enhance the need for continuance of therapy, or at least do not support ending therapy.

Perceived pubertal timing was at about the same time as that of their peers for 50% of our population. These results are consistent with data from controls aged 16–19. The percentage of our population that indicated their timing of pubertal onset occurred later than that of their peers suggested an inclination towards delayed timing of pubertal development. However, one should be careful when interpreting these results, as perceived pubertal timing is only indicative of and not directly related to the actual timing of pubertal development [51]. Also, perceptions about pubertal timing results are known to be dependent on the age of assessment and to vary during maturation [51,52].

Sleep timing parameters of this study group showed earlier RTs and shorter TSTs on work days, and later RTs and longer TSTs on free days than controls aged <25. The combination of short workday TSTs, long free day TSTs and late free day RTs might indicate compensation of workday derived sleep debt, a phenomenon typical for the late chronotype [14,53]. As our population indeed showed an inclination to the evening chronotype, these results were consistent with this.

During the previous long-term evaluation, Van Geijlswijk et al. reported a mean bedtime of 20:54 (SD 0:44) and mean TST of 9.6 h (SD 0.85) [7]. In the current study, mean bedtime and TST were 23:40 (SD 1:08) and 8.3 h (SD 0.85) respectively. The decline seen in TST with respect to the previous long-term evaluation was consistent with our expectations, as sleep duration gradually decreases in the transition from childhood to adolescence and into early adulthood [54,55]. This decrease in TST during maturation is mainly assigned to later bedtimes and not earlier RTs, which corresponds with our findings. SOL from this study groups did not deviate from Dutch controls aged 21.7 which suggests the SOL of our population had generally normalized (lowered) since early childhood. This finding is in contrast to normative age-related SOL transitions, as SOL generally remains stable during early maturation and (moderately) increases with age after reaching full adulthood [56]. However, these normative age-related SOL transition might not directly apply to our population because of their history of CSOI. During the previous study, SOL was registered as "20 min or shorter" (SOL unspecified) or "longer than 20 min" (SOL specified) [7]. 43 (72.9%) indicated to sleep within 20 min or less, whereas 16 (27.1%) reported SOLs of over 20 min. Mean SOL in the latter group was 35.1 min. In the current study, 14 (43.7%) indicated to need over 20 min to fall asleep, mean SOL was 34.7 min. These results suggest SOL to have generally remained stable since the previous follow-up study.

Consistent with results from the previous long-term evaluation, adverse events were scarce and seemed to be of acceptable nature. Occurrence of headache was comparable between both study groups and not higher than the prevalence of headache amongst various European countries (50%), as reported by Stovner et al. [57]. Reported co-medication included ropinirole, which is authorized for the treatment of restless legs syndrome. As restless legs syndrome has been reported as an adverse effect of melatonin [58], the use of ropinirole might indicate the occurrence of an unreported adverse event here, which however could not be substantiated.

*Strenghts and Limitations*

This study is, to our knowledge, the first to evaluate the effectiveness and safety of pediatric melatonin therapy over more than a decade. Combining information from treatment initiation and outcomes during early childhood and continuance through adolescence and into early adulthood is unique and renders this study very valuable. However, several methodological limitations of the study must be addressed. First, an overestimation of the percentage of melatonin continuation might have occurred, as former participants who still use melatonin could have been more willing to participate in this study than those who discontinued melatonin. This might have resulted in a higher response rate amongst melatonin users as compared to non-users, and, therefore, result in an underestimation of children that are able to stop using melatonin. Secondly, sleep timing parameters were based on self-reported estimates instead of objectively measured with for instance polysomnography or actimetry. Another aspect to be taken into account is that the implemented control populations consisted mainly of students. Student populations deviate from the general population with respect to education level and social obligations and might therefore not be ideal to function as control populations in general. However, as 63.6% of our population was enrolled in or had completed higher education, our population was actually quite closely related to student populations with respect to education level and social obligations. Furthermore, some student populations used for comparison originated from Norway and Switzerland. These populations may deviate from their age-related Dutch peers with respect to sleep habits, which could have influenced some of our findings. And lastly, statistical power of the study was low due to the limited sample size and occurrence of recall bias as a result of the implementation of various retrospective question items could not be ruled out.

## 5. Conclusions

We found that of the children with sleep onset problems related to delayed endogenous melatonin onset treated with exogenous melatonin initiated before the age of twelve, 27% continue melatonin therapy into adulthood. Participants did not show deviations from age-related controls with regard to sleep quality, indicating sleep quality to have normalized over time. In our population the number of the evening chronotype as compared to controls of the same age is significantly higher, suggesting a causal relation with CSOI. More participants perceived pubertal timing as late as compared to controls of the same age. To which extent these subjective results indicate an actual delay in onset of puberty as a result of melatonin treatment in early childhood is inconclusive. Participants in this study showed shorter total sleep time during workdays and more compensation for workday-derived sleep debt during weekends, which is attributable to the prevailing eveningness preference.

A total 36 of the 69 children prescribed melatonin did not respond to our call. The distribution of STOP and CONT could be different in the non-responders. Our study may underestimate the number of children that are able to stop using melatonin. Sleep timing parameters were based on self-reported estimates. Control populations were predominantly students with varying nationalities. These populations may deviate from our age-related study population. The statistical power of the study was low due to the limited sample size and occurrence of recall bias as a result of the implementation of various retrospective question items cannot be ruled out.

In conclusion, long-term melatonin therapy appeared to be safe after an average of 7.1 years treatment based on data from this limited population. The results of this study indicate that approximately 75% of the children with CSOI who are treated with melatonin will have normal sleep quality without medication ten years later.

**Author Contributions:** T.Z., M.S., T.E., C.R. and I.G. conceived and designed the experiments; T.Z. performed the experiments; T.Z. and I.G. analyzed the data; M.S. contributed materials/analysis tools; T.Z. and I.G. wrote the paper.

# References

1.  Bruni, O.; Alonso-Alconada, D.; Besag, F.; Biran, V.; Braam, W.; Cortese, S.; Moavero, R.; Parisi, P.; Smits, M.; Heijden, K.V.D.; et al. Current role of melatonin in pediatric neurology: Clinical recommendations. *Eur. J. Paediatr. Neurol.* **2015**, *19*, 122–133. [CrossRef] [PubMed]
2.  Auger, R.R.; Burgess, H.J.; Emens, J.S.; Deriy, L.V.; Thomas, S.M.; Sharkey, K.M. Clinical Practice Guideline for the Treatment of Intrinsic Circadian Rhythm Sleep-Wake Disorders: Advanced Sleep-Wake Phase Disorder (ASWPD), Delayed Sleep-Wake Phase Disorder (DSWPD), Non-24-Hour Sleep-Wake Rhythm Disorder (N24SWD), and Irregular Sleep-Wake Rhythm Disorder (ISWRD). An Update for 2015: An American Academy of Sleep Medicine Clinical Practice Guideline. *J. Clin. Sleep Med.* **2015**, *11*, 1199–1236. [CrossRef] [PubMed]
3.  Kennaway, D.J. Paediatric use of melatonin. *Eur. J. Paediatr. Neurol.* **2015**, *19*, 489–490. [CrossRef] [PubMed]
4.  Bruni, O.; Alonso-Alconada, D.; Besag, F.; Biran, V.; Braam, W.; Cortese, S.; Moavero, R.; Parisi, P.; Smits, M.; Heijden, K.V.D.; et al. Paediatric use of melatonin (Author reply to D. J. Kennaway). *Eur. J. Paediatr. Neurol.* **2015**, *19*, 491–493. [CrossRef] [PubMed]
5.  Carr, R.; Wasdell, M.B.; Hamilton, D.; Weiss, M.D.; Freeman, R.D.; Tai, J.; Rietveld, W.J.; Jan, J.E. Long-term effectiveness outcome of melatonin therapy in children with treatment-resistant circadian rhythm sleep disorders. *J. Pineal Res.* **2007**, *43*, 351–359. [CrossRef] [PubMed]
6.  Hoebert, M.; van der Heijden, K.B.; van Geijlswijk, I.M.; Smits, M.G. Long-term follow-up of melatonin treatment in children with ADHD and chronic sleep onset insomnia. *J. Pineal Res.* **2009**, *47*, 1–7. [CrossRef] [PubMed]
7.  Van Geijlswijk, I.M.; Mol, R.H.; Egberts, T.C.; Smits, M.G. Evaluation of sleep, puberty and mental health in children with long-term melatonin treatment for chronic idiopathic childhood sleep onset insomnia. *Psychopharmacology* **2011**, *216*, 111–120. [CrossRef] [PubMed]
8.  Van Geijlswijk, I.M.; Korzilius, H.P.; Smits, M.G. The use of exogenous melatonin in delayed sleep phase disorder: A meta-analysis. *Sleep* **2010**, *33*, 1605–1614. [CrossRef] [PubMed]
9.  Van Geijlswijk, I.M.; van der Heijden, K.B.; Egberts, A.C.; Korzilius, H.P.; Smits, M.G. Dose finding of melatonin for chronic idiopathic childhood sleep onset insomnia: An RCT. *Psychopharmacology* **2010**, *212*, 379–391. [CrossRef] [PubMed]
10. Horne, J.A.; Ostberg, O. A self assessment questionnaire to determine Morningness Eveningness in human circadian rhythms. *Int. J. Chronobiol.* **1976**, *4*, 97–110. [PubMed]
11. Hofstra, W.A.; Gordijn, M.C.M.; Van Hemert-Van Der Poel, J.C.; Van Der Palen, J.; De Weerd, A.W. Chronotypes and subjective sleep parameters in epilepsy patients: A large questionnaire study. *Chronobiol. Int.* **2010**, *27*, 1271–1286. [CrossRef] [PubMed]
12. Di Milia, L.; Adan, A.; Natale, V.; Randler, C. Reviewing the psychometric properties of contemporary circadian typology measures. *Chronobiol. Int.* **2013**, *30*, 1261–1271. [CrossRef] [PubMed]
13. Kerkhof, G. A Dutch questionnaire for the selection of morning and evening types (in Dutch). *Ned. Tijdschr. Psychol.* **1984**, *39*, 281–294.
14. Roenneberg, T.; Wirz-Justice, A.; Merrow, M. Life between Clocks: Daily Temporal Patterns of Human Chronotypes. *J. Biol. Rhythm.* **2003**, *18*, 80–90. [CrossRef] [PubMed]
15. Roenneberg, T.; Kuehnle, T.; Juda, M.; Kantermann, T.; Allebrandt, K.; Gordijn, M.; Merrow, M. Epidemiology of the human circadian clock. *Sleep Med. Rev.* **2007**, *11*, 429–438. [CrossRef] [PubMed]
16. Zavada, A.; Gordijn, M.C.; Beersma, D.G.; Daan, S.; Roenneberg, T. Comparison of the Munich Chronotype Questionnaire with the Horne-Ostberg's Morningness-Eveningness Score. *Chronobiol. Int.* **2005**, *22*, 267–278. [CrossRef] [PubMed]
17. Kantermann, T.; Sung, H.; Burgess, H.J. Comparing the Morningness-Eveningness Questionnaire and Munich ChronoType Questionnaire to the Dim Light Melatonin Onset. *J. Biol. Rhythm.* **2015**, *30*, 449–453. [CrossRef] [PubMed]

18. LMU, M. Munich Chronotype Questionnaire. Available online: https://www.bioinfo.mpg.de/mctq/core_work_life/core/introduction.jsp?language=dut (accessed on 24 March 2016).

19. Kühnle, T. *Quantitative Analysis of Human Chronotypes*; Ludwig Maximilian University München: München, Germany, 2006.

20. Terman, J.S.; Terman, M.; Lo, E.S.; Cooper, T.B. Circadian time of morning light administration and therapeutic response in winter depression. *Arch. Gen. Psychiatry* **2001**, *58*, 69–75. [CrossRef] [PubMed]

21. Roenneberg, T.; Kuehnle, T.; Pramstaller, P.P.; Ricken, J.; Havel, M.; Guth, A.; Merrow, M. A marker for the end of adolescence. *Curr. Biol.* **2004**, *14*, R1038–R1039. [CrossRef] [PubMed]

22. Wingen, M. Health Survey Questionnaire. 2014. Available online: https://www.cbs.nl/nl-nl/onze-diensten/methoden/onderzoeksomschrijvingen/aanvullende%20onderzoeksbeschrijvingen/vragenlijsten-gezondheidsenquete-vanaf-2014 (accessed on 1 March 2018).

23. Netherlands Nutrition Centre Factsheet Caffeine. Available online: http://www.voedingscentrum.nl/Assets/Uploads/voedingscentrum/Documents/Professionals/Pers/Factsheets/English/factsheet%20Cafeine%20engelse%20versie%20vormgeving%20def%20LR.pdf (accessed on 26 July 2016).

24. Buysse, D.J.; Reynolds III, C.F.; Monk, T.H.; Berman, S.R.; Kupfer, D.J. The Pittsburgh sleep quality index: A new instrument for psychiatric practice and research. *Psychiatry Res.* **1989**, *28*, 193–213. [CrossRef]

25. Morin, C. *Insomnia: Psychological Assessment and Management*; Guilford: New York, NY, USA, 1993.

26. Bastien, C.H.; Vallières, A.; Morin, C.M. Validation of the Insomnia Severity Index as an outcome measure for insomnia research. *Sleep Med.* **2001**, *2*, 297–307. [CrossRef]

27. Petersen, A.C.; Crockett, L.; Richards, M.; Boxer, A. A self-report measure of pubertal status: Reliability, validity, and initial norms. *J. Youth Adolesc.* **1988**, *17*, 117–133. [CrossRef] [PubMed]

28. Van der Heijden, K.B.; Hamburger, H. Dutch Society for Sleep-Wake Research National Sleep Survey 2016: Sleep and Studying. 2016. Available online: www.nswo.nl/userfiles/files/PersberichtNSWO2016.pdf (accessed on 1 March 2018).

29. Van Laar, M.W.; Van Ooyen-Houben, M.M.J.; Cruts, A.A.N.; Meijer, R.F.; Croes, E.A.; Ketelaars, A.P.M.; Van der Pol, P.M. Trimbos Institute, Netherlands Institute of Mental Health and Addiction National Drug Monitor: Annual Update 2015. 2016. Available online: https://assets.trimbos.nl/docs/24dd30ba-464f-4dcd-a740-20ac058d310b.pdf (accessed on 1 March 2018).

30. European Food Safety Authority (EFSA) Scientific Opinion on the Safety of Caffeine. 2015. Available online: http://onlinelibrary.wiley.com/doi/10.2903/j.efsa.2015.4102/epdf (accessed on 1 March 2018).

31. Fossum, I.N.; Nordnes, L.T.; Storemark, S.S.; Bjorvatn, B.; Pallesen, S. The association between use of electronic media in bed before going to sleep and insomnia symptoms, daytime sleepiness, morningness, and chronotype. *Behav. Sleep Med.* **2014**, *12*, 343–357. [CrossRef] [PubMed]

32. John, K.M.; Van den Berg, J.F. Chronotype, sleep quality and depressive symptoms: A cross-sectional study among Dutch students. *Annu. Proc. NSWO* **2014**, *25*, 64–67.

33. Gerber, M.; Lang, C.; Lemola, S.; Colledge, F.; Kalak, N.; Holsboer-Trachsler, E.; Puhse, U.; Brand, S. Validation of the German version of the insomnia severity index in adolescents, young adults and adult workers: Results from three cross-sectional studies. *BMC Psychiatry* **2016**, *16*, 174. [CrossRef] [PubMed]

34. Bratberg, G.H.; Nilsen, T.I.; Holmen, T.L.; Vatten, L.J. Perceived pubertal timing, pubertal status and the prevalence of alcohol drinking and cigarette smoking in early and late adolescence: A population based study of 8950 Norwegian boys and girls. *Acta Paediatr.* **2007**, *96*, 292–295. [CrossRef] [PubMed]

35. Martin, J.S.; Gaudreault, M.M.; Perron, M.; Laberge, L. Chronotype, Light Exposure, Sleep, and Daytime Functioning in High School Students Attending Morning or Afternoon School Shifts: An Actigraphic Study. *J. Biol. Rhythm.* **2016**, *31*, 205–217. [CrossRef] [PubMed]

36. Braam, W.; van Geijlswijk, I.; Keijzer, H.; Smits, M.G.; Didden, R.; Curfs, L.M. Loss of response to melatonin treatment is associated with slow melatonin metabolism. *J. Intellect. Disabil. Res.* **2010**, *54*, 547–555. [CrossRef] [PubMed]

37. McNamara, J.P.; Wang, J.; Holiday, D.B.; Warren, J.Y.; Paradoa, M.; Balkhi, A.M.; Fernandez-Baca, J.; McCrae, C.S. Sleep disturbances associated with cigarette smoking. *Psychol. Health Med.* **2014**, *19*, 410–419. [CrossRef] [PubMed]

38. Cohrs, S.; Rodenbeck, A.; Riemann, D.; Szagun, B.; Jaehne, A.; Brinkmeyer, J.; Grunder, G.; Wienker, T.; Diaz-Lacava, A.; Mobascher, A.; et al. Impaired sleep quality and sleep duration in smokers-results from the German Multicenter Study on Nicotine Dependence. *Addict. Biol.* **2014**, *19*, 486–496. [CrossRef] [PubMed]

39. Clark, A.J.; Salo, P.; Lange, T.; Jennum, P.; Virtanen, M.; Pentti, J.; Kivimaki, M.; Vahtera, J.; Rod, N.H. Onset of impaired sleep as a predictor of change in health-related behaviours; analysing observational data as a series of non-randomized pseudo-trials. *Int. J. Epidemiol.* **2015**, *44*, 1027–1037. [CrossRef] [PubMed]

40. Wittmann, M.; Dinich, J.; Merrow, M.; Roenneberg, T. Social jetlag: Misalignment of biological and social time. *Chronobiol. Int.* **2006**, *23*, 497–509. [CrossRef] [PubMed]

41. Owens, J.; Au, R.; Carskadon, M.; Millman, R.; Wolfson, A.; Braverman, P.K.; Adelman, W.P.; Breuner, C.C.; Levine, D.A.; Marcell, A.V.; et al. Insufficient sleep in adolescents and young adults: An update on causes and consequences. *Pediatrics* **2014**, *134*, e921–e932. [CrossRef] [PubMed]

42. Taylor, D.J.; Clay, K.C.; Bramoweth, A.D.; Sethi, K.; Roane, B.M. Circadian phase preference in college students: Relationships with psychological functioning and academics. *Chronobiol. Int.* **2011**, *28*, 541–547. [CrossRef] [PubMed]

43. Ozguner, F.; Koyu, A.; Cesur, G. Active smoking causes oxidative stress and decreases blood melatonin levels. *Toxicol. Ind. Health* **2005**, *21*, 21–26. [CrossRef] [PubMed]

44. Ursing, C.; Wikner, J.; Brismar, K.; Rojdmark, S. Caffeine raises the serum melatonin level in healthy subjects: An indication of melatonin metabolism by cytochrome P450(CYP)1A2. *J. Endocrinol. Investig.* **2003**, *26*, 403–406. [CrossRef] [PubMed]

45. Ogilvie, B.W.; Torres, R.; Dressman, M.A.; Kramer, W.G.; Baroldi, P. Clinical assessment of drug-drug interactions of tasimelteon, a novel dual melatonin receptor agonist. *J. Clin. Pharmacol.* **2015**, *55*, 1004–1011. [CrossRef] [PubMed]

46. Hartter, S.; Nordmark, A.; Rose, D.M.; Bertilsson, L.; Tybring, G.; Laine, K. Effects of caffeine intake on the pharmacokinetics of melatonin, a probe drug for CYP1A2 activity. *Br. J. Clin. Pharmacol.* **2003**, *56*, 679–682. [CrossRef] [PubMed]

47. Ursing, C.; von Bahr, C.; Brismar, K.; Rojdmark, S. Influence of cigarette smoking on melatonin levels in man. *Eur. J. Clin. Pharmacol.* **2005**, *61*, 197–201. [CrossRef] [PubMed]

48. Lemola, S.; Perkinson-Gloor, N.; Brand, S.; Dewald-Kaufmann, J.F.; Grob, A. Adolescents' electronic media use at night, sleep disturbance, and depressive symptoms in the smartphone age. *J. Youth Adolesc.* **2015**, *44*, 405–418. [CrossRef] [PubMed]

49. Falbe, J.; Davison, K.K.; Franckle, R.L.; Ganter, C.; Gortmaker, S.L.; Smith, L.; Land, T.; Taveras, E.M. Sleep duration, restfulness, and screens in the sleep environment. *Pediatrics* **2015**, *135*, e367–e375. [CrossRef] [PubMed]

50. Wood, B.; Rea, M.S.; Plitnick, B.; Figueiro, M.G. Light level and duration of exposure determine the impact of self-luminous tablets on melatonin suppression. *Appl. Ergon.* **2013**, *44*, 237–240. [CrossRef] [PubMed]

51. Dubas, J.S.; Graber, J.A.; Petersen, A.C. A Longitudinal Investigation of Adolescents' Changing Perceptions of Pubertal Timing. *Dev. Psychol.* **1991**, *27*, 580–586. [CrossRef]

52. Cance, J.D.; Ennett, S.T.; Morgan-Lopez, A.A.; Foshee, V.A. The Stability of Perceived Pubertal Timing Across Adolescence. *J. Youth Adolesc.* **2012**, *41*, 764–775. [CrossRef] [PubMed]

53. Vitale, J.A.; Roveda, E.; Montaruli, A.; Galasso, L.; Weydahl, A.; Caumo, A.; Carandente, F. Chronotype influences activity circadian rhythm and sleep: Differences in sleep quality between weekdays and weekend. *Chronobiol. Int.* **2015**, *32*, 405–415. [CrossRef] [PubMed]

54. Iglowstein, I.; Jenni, O.G.; Molinari, L.; Largo, R.H. Sleep duration from infancy to adolescence: Reference values and generational trends. *Pediatrics* **2003**, *111*, 302–307. [CrossRef] [PubMed]

55. Hayley, A.C.; Skogen, J.C.; Overland, S.; Wold, B.; Williams, L.J.; Kennedy, G.A.; Sivertsen, B. Trajectories and stability of self-reported short sleep duration from adolescence to adulthood. *J. Sleep Res.* **2015**, *24*, 621–628. [CrossRef] [PubMed]

56. Ohayon, M.M.; Carskadon, M.A.; Guilleminault, C.; Vitiello, M.V. Meta-analysis of quantitative sleep parameters from childhood to old age in healthy individuals: Developing normative sleep values across the human lifespan. *Sleep* **2004**, *27*, 1255–1273. [CrossRef] [PubMed]

57. Stovner, L.J.; Andree, C. Prevalence of headache in Europe: A review for the Eurolight project. *J. Headache Pain* **2010**, *11*, 289–299. [CrossRef] [PubMed]

58. Anonymous. European Medicines Agency (EMA) Circadin: EPAR—Product Information. 2009. Available online: http://www.cma.europa.eu/docs/en_GB/document_library/EPAR_-_Product_Information/human/000695/WC500026811.pdf (accessed on 1 March 2018).

# 12

# Health-Related Quality of Life after Pediatric Severe Sepsis

**Prachi Syngal** [1] **and John S. Giuliano Jr.** [2,*]

[1]  Pediatric Intensive Care Medicine, Yale-New Haven Children's Hospital, New Haven, CT 06520, USA;
prachi.syngal@yale.edu

[2]  Department of Pediatrics, Section Critical Care Medicine, Yale University School of Medicine,
New Haven, CT 06520, USA

*   Correspondence: john.giuliano@yale.edu

**Abstract:** Background: Pediatric severe sepsis is a public health problem with significant morbidities in those who survive. In this article, we aim to present an overview of the important studies highlighting the limited data available pertaining to long-term outcomes of survivors of pediatric severe sepsis. Materials and Methods: A review of literature available was conducted using PUBMED/Medline on pediatric severe sepsis outcomes. Long-term outcomes and health-related quality of life (HRQL) following severe sepsis was defined as any outcome occurring after discharge from the hospital following an episode of severe sepsis which affected either the survivor or the survivor's family members. Results: Many children are discharged with worse clinical and functional outcomes, depending on their diagnosis, treatments received, psychological effects, and the impact of their illness on their parents. Additionally, they utilize healthcare services more than their peers and are often readmitted soon after discharge. However, pediatric HRQL studies with worthwhile outcome measures are limited and the current data on pediatric sepsis is mainly retrospective. Conclusions: There is significant and longstanding morbidity seen in children and their families following a severe sepsis illness. Further prospective data are required to study the long-term outcomes of sepsis in the pediatric population.

**Keywords:** HRQL; morbidity; social impact; readmissions; septic shock

## 1. Introduction

Pediatric severe sepsis remains a burdensome public health problem. More than 42,000 children develop severe sepsis each year in the United States alone, and 4400 of these children die [1]. In 1995, Watson et al. reported an incidence of 0.56 cases per 1000 children per year in children under 19 years of age in the US, with the highest mortality noted among neonates [2]. Hartmen et al. showed a steady increase by 81% in the prevalence of sepsis from 1995 to 2005. However, they noted a decline in case fatalities from 10.3 to 8.9% [3]. Unfortunately, these studies may have underestimated the true mortality rate in children with severe sepsis, as they were mostly retrospective studies based on diagnosis codes. Knowing this, an international multicentered prospective point prevalence study was conducted which showed a severe sepsis point prevalence of 8.2% and an increased mortality rate of 25% [1]. Justifiably, most pediatric studies focus on interventions to reduce mortality from sepsis, but emerging data suggest that late outcomes after severe sepsis survival are poor. Morbidity in children following severe sepsis is now similar to that in critically ill adults [1]. In a large prospective trial from European Childhood Life-threatening Disease Study (EUCLIDS) conducted in 52 pediatric intensive care units (PICUs) over seven European countries from July 2012 to January 2016, the authors reported an overall disability rate of 31%, among which 24% was reported in previously healthy children on discharge [4]. Disability was defined as a Pediatric Overall Performance Category (POPC) scale >1, need for skin graft, amputation, or hearing loss. Two other studies showed similar data with disability rates of 28–34% [1,5]. However, recovery remains a long process, with many still feeling effects on their physical, social, emotional, and school functioning for months to years after discharge [6]. Taken collectively, many of these domains form the framework for health-related quality of life (HRQL), simply defined as child's or parent's perceived physical and mental health over time. This narrative review focuses on the long-term outcomes following discharge after severe sepsis in children.

## 2. Materials and Methods

This paper consists of a narrative review highlighting key literature available on pediatric severe sepsis outcomes. Studies were identified using electronic databases. Searches were performed in April and May 2018 on PUBMED/Medline. Retrieval of the data was limited to ages 0 to 18 years and to publications in English. Adult literature was included when data on certain topics were absent in children. Index terminology was used, employing Medical Subject Heading (MeSH) along with appropriate keywords. Keywords used for the literature search included: pediatrics, severe sepsis, health-related quality of life (HRQL), pediatric intensive care unit (PICU), morbidity, long-term outcomes, disability, mortality, epidemiology of sepsis, social impact, readmissions, and septic shock. The keywords were generated via synonyms and consulting the existing literature. Titles and abstracts were reviewed for relevance with full articles downloaded when appropriate. Our search identified around 50 articles. Articles not meeting the inclusion criteria were excluded during the review process, resulting in 33 eligible articles. Studies included in the review were publications on pediatric critical illness outcomes, studies on pediatric severe sepsis, and articles on pediatric and adult HRQL. Long-term outcomes and HRQL following severe sepsis were defined as any outcome occurring after hospital discharge from the hospital following an episode of severe sepsis which affected either the survivor or the survivor's family members.

## 3. Results

Many studies investigating pediatric intensive care outcomes have shown that though most survivors had normal functioning, a significant number of children suffered from substantial psychosocial, physical, and neurocognitive deficits [7–11]. As mentioned above, a recent prospective severe sepsis point prevalence study described morbidity outcomes which lend themselves to future outcome research. The Sepsis Prevalence, OUtcomes, and Therapies (SPROUT) study was conducted over 5 days throughout 2013–2014 at 128 sites in 26 countries and described a pediatric severe sepsis point prevalence of 8.2% and mortality of 25% [1]. Of the survivors, 17% exhibited new moderate to severe functional disability compared to their admission baseline functioning, with mild disability defined as any increase in Pediatric Overall Performance Category (POPC) and moderate disability defined as a discharge POPC score ≥3 and an increase of POPC by ≥1 from baseline [1]. Since these scores were calculated at discharge, almost one in six pediatric severe sepsis survivors were discharged with more disabilities than when they were admitted. It is not clear when these patients return to their pre-admission quality of life, if at all. Farris et al. also described similar results in their review of 384 children who survived severe sepsis by examining the data from the RESOLVE trial (REsearching severe Sepsis and Organ dysfunction in children: a gLobal perspectiVE) [5]. The trial was conducted from November 2002 to April 2005 in 104 study sites in 18 countries. Functional outcome was scored based on POPC score, where poor functional outcome or significant decline in functional status was defined as a POPC score ≥3 and an increase from baseline when measured at discharge or 28 days after trial enrollment. They noted that 34% of survivors exhibited a decline in their functional status at 28 days, as their POPC scores deteriorated one point from the pre-illness score. Moreover, 18% of survivors had poor POPC outcome with a significant decline in their functional status [5]. These results are not unique to pediatrics. Studies examining severe sepsis outcomes in older populations were independently associated with substantial and persistent new cognitive impairment and functional disability among survivors [12].

Children who survive critical illness may develop new or worse neuropsychological functioning as well. A prospective case control study in school-aged children with meningoencephalitis, sepsis, and other disorders followed children for 3–6 months following ICU discharge was performed by Als et al. in 2007 to 2010 [13,14]. The teachers of the survivors described declines in academic performance and neuropsychological testing revealed significant deficiencies while attempting memory tasks when compared to healthy controls [14]. Risk factors for worse neuropsychological impairment were: younger aged children, lower socioeconomic class, and the development of seizures during their admission. Another study conducted to explore neuropsychological outcomes in children admitted to the PICU further investigated problems with memory and found that pattern recognition memory, commonly mapped to the temporal lobe, was most affected in the septic group. These findings suggest that there may be organic changes to the pediatric brain following an episode of severe sepsis [15]. Unfortunately, this is only speculation and future testing to is needed determine its validity. As demonstrated by Rees et al. in 2004, post-traumatic stress disorder (PTSD) was also found to be higher by 21% in severe sepsis survivors within 6–12 months after the PICU discharge, as compared to children discharged from the general ward [16].

The concept of quality of life has seen considerable growth in the past decade. Most of the studies employ the World health Organization's (WHO) definition of health as their conceptual basis. In 1948, WHO defined health as "a state of complete physical, mental, and social well-being; not merely the absence of disease" [17]. Quality of life has been defined as "an individual's perception of their position in life, in the context of the culture, environment and value systems in which they live, and in relation to their goals, expectations, standards and concerns". In pediatric literature, researchers have noted the importance of a child's developmental age and family's impact on HRQL [6,17]. Multiple pediatric HRQL tools are available and, despite a lack of consensus on which HRQL tool is best suited for pediatric critical care clinical trials, some key determinants of poor HRQL outcomes in children have been identified. Multiple studies have shown that children with a diagnosis of severe sepsis, especially if the central nervous system was involved, had lower HRQL compared to age-matched peers also admitted to a pediatric intensive care unit (PICU) [5,14]. Others have also shown that this HRQL derangement can last for years [18,19]. Buysee et al. studied patients who survived meningococcal septic shock (MSS) between the years 1988 and 2001 to evaluate the association of MSS patients and different long-term outcomes. They reported a significant association with problem behavior, hence long-term low HRQL based on low emotional and behavioral problem scales up to 2 years after discharge from the pediatric intensive care unit. A lower association was noted with adverse physical outcomes. In addition to physical ailments affecting pediatric HRQL, psychological and social/family determinants also were shown to play an important role in a child's healing process [6]. Asperberro et al. performed a focused review on studies from 1980 to 2015 and identified key determinants in predicting poor HRQL, including reason for PICU admission (sepsis, meningoencephalitis, trauma), antecedent illness (chronic comorbid conditions), treatments received (prolonged cardiopulmonary resuscitation, long-stay patients, invasive technology), psychological outcomes (post-traumatic stress disorder, parent anxiety/depression), and social and environmental characteristics (low socioeconomic status, parental education and functioning) [6]. A higher level of parental and family stress has been shown to slow down a child's recovery from the illness, thereby negatively affecting the HRQL.

Besides lower neuropsychological and functional outcomes following an admission for severe sepsis, these children also utilize healthcare more than their peers [2,20]. In a retrospective cohort study conducted in Washington from 1990–2004, nearly half (47%) of pediatric patients formerly admitted with severe sepsis were readmitted at least once, with many readmitted multiple times. These readmissions were typically soon after discharge (median 3 months, IQR 2 days to 14 years) and 85% of these readmissions were emergent [12]. A multivariate regression analysis reported that young age (<1 year), hematologic or neurologic organ dysfunction, bloodstream or cardiovascular infections, and several other comorbidities were independently associated with subsequent readmission [12].

A PTSD diagnosis is significantly more common in families with a child previously admitted to the PICU as well. In a retrospective cohort study conducted in a London teaching hospital from 1998 to 2000, Rees et al. showed that PTSD was 20 times higher in parents of children admitted to the PICU compared to parents of children admitted to the general wards [16]. Other studies have found deteriorating physical health in parents and caregivers of pediatric critical illness survivors compared with adult peers [21–25]. Parents were reported to have physical symptoms such as: numbness, malaise, fatigue, headaches, and irritability. Further, stress-related symptoms such as headache, low energy, and anxiety were reported along with deleterious effects on family health behaviors such as sleep and eating patterns [15,26]. Poor parental coping coupled with decreased levels of patient functioning following PICU discharge only worsen the possibility of these patients returning to their pre-illness state.

Moreover, children are dependent on their families for their physical, emotional, and social needs. Parents of critically ill survivors may have psychological sequelae affecting their own HRQL. A reduction in parental physical and psychosocial well-being has consistently predicted problematic psychological adjustment in the child [22]. The aforementioned studies are summarized in Table 1.

**Table 1.** Long-term outcomes after pediatric severe sepsis.

| Long-Term Outcome | Study | Measurement Tool | Result |
| --- | --- | --- | --- |
| Functional outcome | Weiss 2015 [1] Farris 2013 [5] | POPC score $\geq$3 and increase in score at 28 days after trial | 28–34% of patients had worse POPC scores at discharge |
| Neuropsychological function | Als 2013 [14] Rees 2004 [16] | Cambridge Neuropsychological Test Automated Battery, the Children's Memory Scale, the Abbreviated Scale of Intelligence or Wilde Range Intelligence Test PTSD Scale for Children (CAPS-C), the Impact of Event Scale, Strengths and Difficulties Questionnaire, Birleson Depression Scale, Revised Children's Manifest Anxiety Scale, Child Somatization Inventory | Decreased neuropsychological function 3–6 months following hospital discharge; 21% of children with symptoms of PTSD |
| Healthcare cost | Watson 2003 [2] Czaja 2009 [12] | Mean length of stay, mean cost, readmissions | Increase of 1.3 million hospital days and $1.97 billion; 50% with additional hospital admission |
| Impact on family | Board 2004 [15] Rees 2004 [16] Drotar 1997 [22] Klassen 2007 [24] Pochard 2001 [25] Noyes 1999 [26] | Parental Stressor Scale, General Health Questionnaire, Beck Depression Inventory, Hospital Anxiety and Depression Scale | 27% higher rate of PTSD, worsening physical health, mental health, and negative social interactions; prevalence of anxiety and depression was 69.1% and 35.4%, respectively |

Long-term outcomes after pediatric severe sepsis. PTSD: post-traumatic stress disorder; POPC: Pediatric Overall Performance Category.

## 4. Discussion

As mentioned above, HRQL in children is influenced by factors such as the ability to keep up with developmentally appropriate activities and participate in peer group activities [6]. Unfortunately, the vast majority of HRQL literature has focused on the adult patient population. Since the pediatric brain shows more plasticity than their adult counterparts, early intervention may allow children to reach their pre-illness levels of functioning sooner [5]. As described earlier, pediatric HRQL may be more complex since the patient's family well-being is also deeply impacted [27]. In a study conducted over a period of 5 years, Carnevale found that parent-child bonding strengthened soon after admission to the PICU. Unfortunately, this relationship could become detrimental with more profound critical illness, as some parents devoted so much attention to their critically ill child that they ignored all other responsibilities [28]. Many other studies have also reported similar relationships between the severity of illness and negative family social impact [29–31].

Many pediatric HRQL tools have been developed, but only a few are considered worthwhile outcome measures [6,32,33]. More than 30 generic and 60 disease-specific HRQL tools have been developed for the pediatric population in the last 20 years [34]. Commonly used tools include the Child Health and Illness Profile (CHIP), the KIDSCREEN-52, the KINDL, and the Pediatric Quality of Life Inventory (PedsQL). Even though these instruments were constructed based on the notion of health, each tool does not measure the same aspect of a child's health. For example, PedsQL is the shortest of the tools and focuses on physical, emotional, social, and school functioning. KIDSCREEN-52 includes financial resources and autonomy domains. CHIP includes aspects that are related to a child's future health, such as resiliency and risk avoidance. Importantly, parent proxy report provides unique information and is required when the child is too young to comprehend and report the HRQL tools or unable to act due to physical, psychological, or cognitive problems [34]. Certain factors should be considered when selecting an HRQL measure. Asperberro compiled a list of six factors: psychometric properties of the tool, sensitivity of the tool to changes in time after an intervention, interpretability of the HRQL tool, response burden and other demands placed on the respondent completing the instrument, mode of administration (whether self-report or proxy version), and adaptability of the instrument to be translated to a population different from the original population for which the tool was the first devised [6]. In addition, an adequate pediatric HRQL tool should be able to evaluate a child's ability to return to their baseline physical, emotional, cognitive, and social health while considering influences from their family and environment [27]. Additionally, it should be able to take into consideration the developmental changes a child experiences over time [17].

As described, prospective data on pediatric long-term outcomes, specifically following severe sepsis, are limited. Many of the epidemiological studies on pediatric sepsis previously discussed are based on retrospective case identification and have reported limited data about long-term, out-of-hospital outcomes [1]. It should be noted that these study designs may be susceptible to recall and selection bias. The few studies that have attempted to prospectively examine long-term outcomes have been largely observational. To date, there have not been any studies focusing on management strategies to improve long-term outcomes in critically ill children with severe sepsis. This area of research is greatly needed. As a result, there are currently no specific guidelines for the follow-up or management of pediatric severe sepsis survivors.

## 5. Conclusions

In conclusion, the short-term outcomes in children following an admission for severe sepsis appear to be poor. Multiple studies have provided data on pediatric long-term outcomes, including HRQL, but assessment tools vary, making meaningful comparisons difficult. Prospective, long-term outcome studies, which may include quality improvement initiatives, are needed to determine modifiable risk factors as mortality from severe sepsis improves but morbidity worsens.

**Author Contributions:** P.S. performed the primary research and manuscript development. J.S.G.J. performed secondary research and manuscript editing.

**Funding:** The authors received no financial support for this article.

## References

1.    Weiss, S.L.; Fitzgerald, J.C.; Pappachan, J.; Wheeler, D.; Jaramillo-Bustamante, J.C.; Salloo, A.; Singhi, S.C.; Erickson, S.; Roy, J.A.; Bush, J.L.; et al. Global epidemiology of pediatric severe sepsis: The sepsis prevalence, outcomes, and therapies study. *Am. J. Respir. Crit. Care Med.* **2015**, *191*, 1147–1157. [CrossRef] [PubMed]

2.    Watson, R.S.; Carcillo, J.A.; Linde-Zwirble, W.T.; Clermont, G.; Lidicker, J.; Angus, D.C. The epidemiology of severe sepsis in children in the United States. *Am. J. Respir. Crit. Care Med.* **2003**, *167*, 695–701. [CrossRef] [PubMed]

3.    Hartman, M.E.; Linde-Zwirble, W.T.; Angus, D.C.; Watson, R.S. Trends in the epidemiology of pediatric severe sepsis. *Pediatr. Crit. Care Med.* **2013**, *14*, 686–693. [CrossRef] [PubMed]

4.    Boeddha, N.P.; Schlapbach, L.J.; Driessen, G.J.; Herberg, J.A.; Rivero-Calle, I.; Cebey-Lopez, M.; Klobassa, D.S.; Philipsen, R.; de Groot, R.; Inwald, D.P.; et al. Mortality and morbidity in community-acquired sepsis in European pediatric intensive care units: A prospective cohort study from the European Childhood Life-threatening Infectious Disease Study (EUCLIDS). *Crit. Care* **2018**, *22*, 143. [CrossRef] [PubMed]

5.    Farris, R.W.; Weiss, N.S.; Zimmerman, J.J. Functional outcomes in pediatric severe sepsis: Further analysis of the researching severe sepsis and organ dysfunction in children: A global perspective trial. *Pediatr. Crit. Care Med.* **2013**, *14*, 835–842. [CrossRef] [PubMed]

6.    Aspesberro, F.; Mangione-Smith, R.; Zimmerman, J.J. Health-related quality of life following pediatric critical illness. *Intensive Care Med.* **2015**, *41*, 1235–1246. [CrossRef] [PubMed]

7.    Colville, G.; Kerry, S.; Pierce, C. Children's factual and delusional memories of intensive care. *Am. J. Respir. Crit. Care Med.* **2008**, *177*, 976–982. [CrossRef] [PubMed]

8.    Colville, G.A.; Pierce, C.M. Children's self-reported quality of life after intensive care treatment. *Pediatr. Crit. Care Med.* **2013**, *14*, e85–e92. [CrossRef] [PubMed]

9.    Conlon, N.P.; Breatnach, C.; O'Hare, B.P.; Mannion, D.W.; Lyons, B.J. Health-related quality of life after prolonged pediatric intensive care unit stay. *Pediatr. Crit. Care Med.* **2009**, *10*, 41–44. [CrossRef] [PubMed]

10.   Knoester, H.; Grootenhuis, M.A.; Bos, A.P. Outcome of paediatric intensive care survivors. *Eur. J. Pediatr.* **2007**, *166*, 1119–1128. [CrossRef] [PubMed]

11.   Morrison, A.L.; Gillis, J.; O'Connell, A.J.; Schell, D.N.; Dossetor, D.R.; Mellis, C. Quality of life of survivors of pediatric intensive care. *Pediatr. Crit. Care Med.* **2002**, *3*, 1–5. [CrossRef] [PubMed]

12.   Czaja, A.S.; Zimmerman, J.J.; Nathens, A.B. Readmission and late mortality after pediatric severe sepsis. *Pediatrics* **2009**, *123*, 849–857. [CrossRef] [PubMed]

13.   Als, L.C.; Tennant, A.; Nadel, S.; Cooper, M.; Pierce, C.M.; Garralda, M.E. Persistence of Neuropsychological Deficits Following Pediatric Critical Illness. *Crit. Care Med.* **2015**, *43*, e312–e315. [CrossRef] [PubMed]

14.   Als, L.C.; Nadel, S.; Cooper, M.; Pierce, C.M.; Sahakian, B.J.; Garralda, M.E. Neuropsychologic function three to six months following admission to the PICU with meningoencephalitis, sepsis, and other disorders: A prospective study of school-aged children. *Crit. Care Med.* **2013**, *41*, 1094–1103. [CrossRef] [PubMed]

15.   Board, R. Father stress during a child's critical care hospitalization. *J. Pediatr. Health Care* **2004**, *18*, 244–249. [PubMed]

16.   Rees, G.; Gledhill, J.; Garralda, M.E.; Nadel, S. Psychiatric outcome following paediatric intensive care unit (PICU) admission: A cohort study. *Intensive Care Med.* **2004**, *30*, 1607–1614. [CrossRef] [PubMed]

17.   Bradlyn, A.S.; Varni, J.W.; Hinds, P.S. Assessing Health-Related Quality of Life in end-of-Life Care for Children and Adolescents. In *When Children Die: Improving Palliative and End-of-Life Care for Children and Their Families*; National Academies Press (US): Washington, DC, USA, 2003.

18.   Buysse, C.M.; Raat, H.; Hazelzet, J.A.; Hop, W.C.; Maliepaard, M.; Joosten, K.F. Surviving meningococcal septic shock: Health consequences and quality of life in children and their parents up to 2 years after pediatric intensive care unit discharge. *Crit. Care Med.* **2008**, *36*, 596–602. [CrossRef] [PubMed]

19.   Buysse, C.M.; Vermunt, L.C.; Raat, H.; Hazelzet, J.A.; Hop, W.C.; Utens, E.M.; Joosten, K.F. Surviving meningococcal septic shock in childhood: Long-term overall outcome and the effect on health-related quality of life. *Crit. Care* **2010**, *14*, R124. [CrossRef] [PubMed]

20.   Watson, R.S.; Carcillo, J.A. Scope and epidemiology of pediatric sepsis. *Pediatr. Crit. Care Med.* **2005**, *6* (Suppl. 3), S3–S5. [CrossRef] [PubMed]

21.   Daniels, D.; Moos, R.H.; Billings, A.G.; Miller, J.J., 3rd. Psychosocial risk and resistance factors among children with chronic illness, healthy siblings, and healthy controls. *J. Abnorm. Child Psychol.* **1987**, *15*, 295–308. [CrossRef] [PubMed]

22.   Drotar, D. Relating parent and family functioning to the psychological adjustment of children with chronic health conditions: What have we learned? What do we need to know? *J. Pediatr. Psychol.* **1997**, *22*, 149–165. [PubMed]

23.  Jessop, D.J.; Riessman, C.K.; Stein, R.E. Chronic childhood illness and maternal mental health. *J. Dev. Behav. Pediatr.* **1988**, *9*, 147–156. [CrossRef] [PubMed]

24.  Klassen, A.; Raina, P.; Reineking, S.; Dix, D.; Pritchard, S.; O'Donnell, M. Developing a literature base to understand the caregiving experience of parents of children with cancer: A systematic review of factors related to parental health and well-being. *Support. Care Cancer* **2007**, *15*, 807–818. [CrossRef] [PubMed]

25.  Pochard, F.; Azoulay, E.; Chevret, S.; Lemaire, F.; Hubert, P.; Canoui, P.; Grassin, M.; Zittoun, R.; le Gall, J.R.; Dhainaut, J.F.; et al. Symptoms of anxiety and depression in family members of intensive care unit patients: Ethical hypothesis regarding decision-making capacity. *Crit. Care Med.* **2001**, *29*, 1893–1897. [CrossRef] [PubMed]

26.  Noyes, J. The impact of knowing your child is critically ill: A qualitative study of mothers' experiences. *J. Adv. Nurs.* **1999**, *29*, 427–435. [CrossRef] [PubMed]

27.  Shudy, M.; de Almeida, M.L.; Ly, S.; Landon, C.; Groft, S.; Jenkins, T.L.; Nicholson, C.E. Impact of pediatric critical illness and injury on families: A systematic literature review. *Pediatrics* **2006**, *118* (Suppl. 3), S203–S218. [CrossRef] [PubMed]

28.  Carnevale, F.A. Striving to recapture our previous life: The experience of families with critically ill children. *Off. J. Can. Assoc. Crit. Care Nurs.* **1999**, *10*, 16–22. [PubMed]

29.  Graves, J.K.; Ware, M.E. Parents' and health professionals' perceptions concerning parental stress during a child's hospitalization. *Child. Health Care* **1990**, *19*, 37–42. [CrossRef] [PubMed]

30.  Sparacino, P.S.; Tong, E.M.; Messias, D.K.; Foote, D.; Chesla, C.A.; Gilliss, C.L. The dilemmas of parents of adolescents and young adults with congenital heart disease. *Heart Lung* **1997**, *26*, 187–195. [CrossRef]

31.  Wade, S.L.; Taylor, H.G.; Drotar, D.; Stancin, T.; Yeates, K.O. Family burden and adaptation during the initial year after traumatic brain injury in children. *Pediatrics* **1998**, *102 Pt 1*, 110–116. [CrossRef]

32.  Jardine, J.; Glinianaia, S.V.; McConachie, H.; Embleton, N.D.; Rankin, J. Self-reported quality of life of young children with conditions from early infancy: A systematic review. *Pediatrics* **2014**, *134*, e1129–e1148. [CrossRef] [PubMed]

33.  Watson, R.S.; Choong, K.; Colville, G.; Crow, S.; Dervan, L.A.; Hopkins, R.O.; Knoester, H.; Pollack, M.M.; Rennick, J.; Curley, M.A.Q. Life after Critical Illness in Children-Toward an Understanding of Pediatric Post-intensive Care Syndrome. *J. Pediatr.* **2018**, *198*, 16–24. [CrossRef] [PubMed]

34.  Kenzik, K.M.; Tuli, S.Y.; Revicki, D.A.; Shenkman, E.A.; Huang, I.C. Comparison of 4 Pediatric Health-Related Quality-of-Life Instruments: A Study on a Medicaid Population. *Med. Decis. Mak.* **2014**, *34*, 590–602. [CrossRef] [PubMed]

# 13

# Pain and Pain Medication among Older People with Intellectual Disabilities in Comparison with the General Population

Anna Axmon [1] (iD), Gerd Ahlström [2,*] (iD) and Hans Westergren [2,3] (iD)

[1]  Division of Occupational and Environmental Medicine, Department of Laboratory Medicine,
     Lund University, SE-221 00 Lund, Sweden; anna.axmon@med.lu.se
[2]  Department of Health Sciences, Lund University, SE-221 00 Lund, Sweden; hans.westergren@med.lu.se
[3]  Department of Pain rehabilitation, Skane University hospital, 222 85 Lund, Sweden
*   Correspondence: gerd.ahlstrom@med.lu.se

**Abstract:** Little is known about pain and pain treatment among people with intellectual disabilities (IDs). We aimed to describe pain and pain medications among older people with ID compared to the general population. Data on diagnoses and prescriptions were collected from national registers for the period between 2006 and 2012 for 7936 people with an ID and a referent cohort from the general population. IDs were associated with a decreased risk of being diagnosed with headaches, musculoskeletal pain, and pain related to the circulatory and respiratory systems, but they were associated with increased risk of being diagnosed with pain related to the urinary system. Among men, IDs were associated with an increased risk of being diagnosed with visceral pain. People with IDs were more likely to be prescribed paracetamol and fentanyl regardless of the type of pain but were less likely to be prescribed COX(1+2) and COX2 inhibitors and weak opioids. Healthcare staff and caregivers must be made aware of signs of pain among people with IDs who may not be able to communicate it themselves. Further research is needed to investigate whether people with IDs are prescribed paracetamol rather than other pain drugs due to physicians trying to avoid polypharmacy or if there are other reasons not to prescribe a greater range of pain treatments.

**Keywords:** cognitive dysfunction; fentanyl; headache; musculoskeletal pain; paracetamol; visceral pain

## 1. Introduction

The International Association for the Study of Pain (IASP) defines pain as "an unpleasant sensory and emotional experience associated with actual or potential tissue damage or described in terms of such damage" [1,2]. When the pain persists for more than three months [3] and develops into chronicity, several known co-morbidities may occur, such as psychiatric co-morbidity [4,5], sleep disturbance, cognitive and neurological dysfunction, pain sensitization [6], increased disability [7], and an increased risk for falls [8]. The diagnosis and treatment of both acute and chronic pain states are highly dependent of a patient's ability to communicate both what aggravates and what alleviates their symptoms [9–11]. Moreover, chronic pain is a well-known burden for society with large effects on well-being [12]. However, in spite of having been addressed in previous decades, many issues regarding the individual and societal burdens of pain remain unsolved [13]. Moreover, studies have indicated that chronic pain often goes untreated [7,12,14]. Even so, the increase in prescription of strong opioids for chronic pain has added over-use and side-effects on top of the pain problem for many patients [15].

Although the problem of pain among people with intellectual disabilities (IDs) has been identified in some studies [16–18], the literature is sparse. However, in clinical settings, it has been reported that pain often goes undetected and undertreated in this group [19–21]. As defined by the IASP, pain is an experience that needs to be communicated by the patient to surrounding people in order for the patient to get adequate help, and people with IDs may not be able to provide self-reports of pain [22,23], even when the person possesses verbal skills [24]. Therefore, the identification of pain among them often relies on reports from caregivers. However, caregivers have been found to underestimate the prevalence of pain among people with IDs [20], possibly due to the misconception that the pain threshold among non-communicating people with IDs is high [25].

As in the general population, pain is associated with limitations to daily functioning, emotional well-being, and quality of life among people with IDs [17]. From a societal point of view, pain among people with IDs is a significant factor affecting the number of consultations to general practitioners' practices [26]. A further problem is that the symptoms of chronic pain may mimic the deterioration of a patients' general symptomatology, especially regarding psychiatric symptoms or symptoms of cognitive dysfunction [27,28]. Therefore, there are incentives on both individual and financial levels to ensure proper pain management among people with IDs.

In the general population, there is an emerging body of knowledge on pain in the aging population which indicates a general increase in chronic pain for all individuals as they become older [4,29–31] and helps to identify a range of treatment options for pain among older people [32,33]. However, even though the life expectancy of people with IDs has increased over recent decades [34] and the number of older people with IDs is increasing rapidly [35], research on pain and pain treatment in this vulnerable group has been scarce. We have previously reported that, although people with IDs have a high prescription rate for a range of drugs, they are less likely than the general population to use prescription drugs for pain management [36]. Moreover, for some drugs, prescription patterns were shown to differ between men and women. However, these data were not linked to information on the diagnosis of pain, and therefore, whether the lower prescription of drugs for pain management was due to a lower prevalence of pain diagnoses remains unknown.

Therefore, the aim of the present study was to describe diagnoses of pain and the prescription patterns of pain medications among older people with IDs in comparison to their age-peers in the general population.

## 2. Materials and Methods

### 2.1. Registers

In Sweden, people with IDs and/or an autism spectrum disorder (ASD) may apply to their municipality for support and service to manage their daily living. These are regulated in the Act Concerning Support and Service for Persons with Certain Functional Impairment (Swedish abbreviation LSS). There are eight different measures of support available for adults: counselling, personal assistance, companion service, contact person, relief service in the home (for informal caregivers), short-time stay away from home (to relieve informal caregivers), special housing, and occupation at daily activities centers. The municipality reports all such support and service to the Swedish National Board of Health and Welfare, and the information is stored in the so called *LSS register*, which was established in 2004. This register contains information about all types of support and services provided. Data are available on the types and amounts of support, the municipality providing the support, and the identification of the person receiving the support. However, although a diagnosis of either ID or ASD is required to receive the support, there is no information regarding any diagnoses recorded in the register.

*The Swedish National Patient Register* contains information on all inpatient and outpatient specialist visits. For each visit, one primary and up to 21 secondary diagnoses are recorded and coded according to the International Statistical Classification of Diseases and Related Health Problems, 10th Revision (ICD-10). The visit is recorded at discharge, i.e., ongoing hospitalizations are not included in the register. Moreover, the register does not cover visits to primary care.

*The Swedish Prescribed Drug Register* was established in July 2005 and contains information on all dispensed prescribed drugs in Sweden, which corresponded to 84% of all drugs sold [37]. Drugs are recorded according to the Anatomic Therapeutic Chemical (ATC) classification system [38]. The ATC system classifies drugs on three levels. The first level comprises a letter and indicates the anatomical main group. For example, drugs with first level "M" are active on the musculoskeletal system. The second level (two digits) indicates the therapeutic subgroup, e.g., muscle relaxant. Information is then added at each level so that the fifth level indicates the chemical substance in the drug.

## 2.2. Study Cohorts

From the LSS register, we obtained information on all people who were at least 55 years old and alive at the end of 2012 and who had received at least one measure of support during that year, regardless of which type of support. We used such support as a proxy for having an ID, and therefore, the 7936 people identified comprised the ID cohort. By using the Swedish Register of the Total Population, Statistics Sweden provided us with a referent cohort (gPop cohort) from the general population, including one-to-one matching by sex and year of birth. Each cohort comprised 3609 (45%) women and 4327 (55%) men. The mean age of participants on 31 December 2012 was 64 years (55–96 years).

## 2.3. Pain

Through the National Patient Register, we collected information for all people in the two study cohorts for the period between 2006 and 2012 and identified visits with at least one diagnosis of pain. Pain diagnoses were categorized as headaches (G43: migraine; G44: other headache syndromes; R51: headache), musculoskeletal pain (M00–M25: arthropathies; M40–M54: dorsopathies; M75: shoulder lesions; M75: enthesopathies of lower limb, excluding the foot; M77: other enthesopathies; M79: other soft tissue disorders, not elsewhere classified), pain related to the circulatory and respiratory systems (R00–R09), visceral pain (pain related to the digestive system and abdomen, R10–R19), and pain related to the urinary system (R30–R39). The National Patient Register contains no information on whether the pain is acute or chronic and we could not, therefore, distinguish between these two types of pain.

## 2.4. Pain Medication

Through the Prescribed Drug Register, we collected information on dispensed drugs for pain treatment between 2006 and 2012. The drug groups considered were COX(1+2) inhibitors (NSAIDs (Nonsteroidal Anti-inflammatory Drugs), M01A) excluding COX2 inhibitors and glucosamine, COX2 inhibitors (M01AH01, M01AH05), paracetamols (N02BE01, N02BE51, N02BE71), strong opioids (morphine (N02AA01, N02AA51, N02AG01), oxycodone (N02AA05, N02AJ17-19), ketobemidone (N02AB01), pethidine (N02AB02), buprenorphine (N02AE01), tapentadol (N02AX06), and fentanyl (N02AB03)), weak opioids (codeine (N02AJ06-09, N02AA59, N02AA79), dextropropoxyphene (N02AC04), and tramadol (N02AX02, N02AJ13, N02AJ15), drugs used for treating migraines except dihydroergotamin (N02CC01-07, N06AX01), antiepileptics used for treating pain (gabapentin (N02AX12), pregabalin (N03AX16), lamotrigine (N03AX09), and topiramate (N03AX11)), tricyclic antidepressants used for treating pain (amitriptyline (N06AA09) and nortriptyline (N06AA10)), and selective serotonin-norepinephrine reuptake inhibitors (SNRIs) used for the treatment of pain (duloxetine (N06AX21) and venlafaxine (N06AX16)). Since fentanyl plaster is used for non-cancer pain in some institutions [39], its use is controversial. As such, we performed separate analyses for fentanyl.

## 2.5. Ethics Approval

Approval was obtained from the Regional Ethical Review Board in Lund (No. 2013/15). The National Board of Health and Welfare and Statistics Sweden performed a separate secrecy review in 2014 before providing access to the data. All analyses were performed using anonymized datasets. The authors assert that all procedures contributing to this work complied with the ethical standards of the relevant national and institutional committees on human experimentation and with the Helsinki Declaration of 1975, which was revised in 2008.

## 2.6. Statistics

Analyses of dichotomous outcomes were performed using generalized linear models (GLM) by estimating relative risks (RRs) with 95% confidence intervals (CIs). For drugs with the main indication being depression (tricyclic antidepressants and SNRIs) or epilepsy (antiepileptics), we performed sensitivity analyses in which all people with at least one diagnosis of depression (F32 and F33 in ICD-10) or epilepsy (G40 and G41), respectively, were excluded.

All analyses were performed using IBM SPSS Statistics version 23.0 (International Business Machines Corporation (IBM), Armonk, NY, USA). Analyses were only performed when both groups were comprised of more than five individuals. A two-sided $p$-value below 0.05 was considered statistically significant.

## 3. Results

### 3.1. Pain

There was a total of 4625 pain diagnoses (whereof 3109 (67%) were primary diagnoses) in the ID cohort and 6294 (4009 (64%) primary) in the gPop cohort. At visits where pain was a secondary diagnosis, the five most common primary diagnoses in the ID cohort were epilepsy (G40), unspecified mental retardation (F79), pneumonia, organism unspecified (J18), fracture of femur (S72), and non-insulin dependent diabetes mellitus (E11). In the gPop cohort, the five most common primary diagnoses were other medical care (Z51), atrial fibrillation and flutter (I48), non-insulin dependent diabetes mellitus (E11), chronic ischemic heart disease (I25), and angina pectoris (I20).

Musculoskeletal pain was the most common pain diagnosis in both cohorts even though, among people with IDs, visceral pain was also recorded for a large fraction of the cohort (see Table 1). The patterns were similar when stratified by sex. People in the ID cohort were twice as likely as those in the gPop cohort to have had a diagnosis of pain related to the urinary system during the study period (see Figure 1). Among men, but not women, having an ID was associated with an increased risk of having a diagnosis of visceral pain. People with IDs were less likely to have had diagnoses of headache, musculoskeletal pain, or pain related to the circulatory or respiratory system.

**Table 1.** Number of people with different pain diagnoses in a group of 7936 older people (3609 women and 4327 men) with intellectual disabilities (ID) and a referent cohort from the general population (gPop), one-to-one matched by sex and year of birth.

| Type of Pain | gPop | | | Intellectual Disabilities (ID) | | |
|---|---|---|---|---|---|---|
| | Women | Men | Total | Women | Men | Total |
| | n (%) | n (%) | n (%) | n (%) | n (%) | n (%) |
| Headaches | 106 (2.9) | 71 (1.6) | 177 (2.2) | 53 (1.5) | 42 (1.0) | 95 (1.2) |
| Musculoskeletal pain | 868 (24.1) | 835 (19.3) | 1703 (21.5) | 537 (14.9) | 480 (11.1) | 1017 (12.8) |
| Pain related to the circulatory and respiratory systems | 381 (10.6) | 380 (8.8) | 761 (9.6) | 206 (5.7) | 251 (5.8) | 457 (5.8) |
| Visceral pain | 422 (11.7) | 292 (6.7) | 714 (9.0) | 407 (11.3) | 454 (10.5) | 861 (10.8) |
| Pain related to the urinary system | 33 (0.9) | 89 (2.1) | 122 (1.5) | 62 (1.7) | 184 (4.3) | 246 (3.1) |

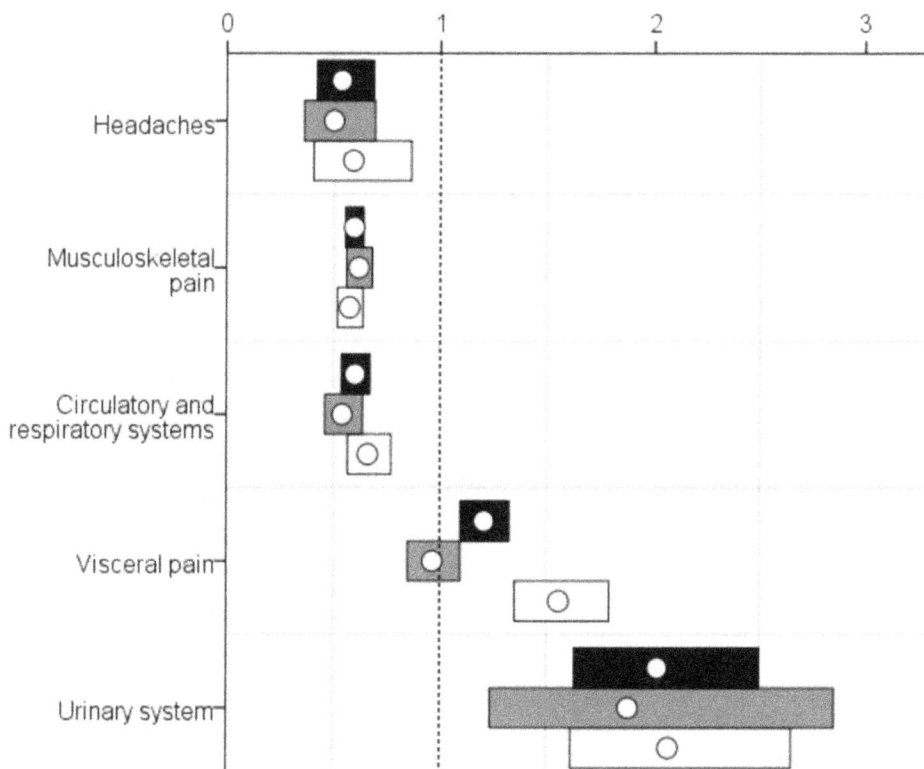

**Figure 1.** Relative risks (RRs; white dots) with 95% confidence intervals (CIs; bars; black = all, grey = women, white = men) for different pain diagnoses among 7936 older people with intellectual disabilities vs. a random sample from the general population, one-to-one matched by sex and year of birth. Dotted line indicates RR = 1, i.e., CIs not crossing indicate statistically significant RRs.

### 3.2. Pain Medication

People with IDs were more likely than those in the gPop cohort to be prescribed paracetamol for all investigated types of pain diagnoses (see Table 2 and Figure 2). There was, however, a pattern of less prescription of COX(1+2) and COX2 inhibitors as well as for weak opioids associated with ID cohort affiliation.

When excluding those with a diagnosis of epilepsy from the analyses concerning the prescription of antiepileptics, the risk of prescription in the ID cohort decreased (see Table 3). However, the results for prescribing tricyclic antidepressants and SNRIs remained similar when restricting the analyses to those without a diagnosis of depression.

In the ID cohort, 99 people (1.2%) had at least one prescription of fentanyl compared with 47 (0.6%) in the gPop cohort. Among those diagnosed with musculoskeletal pain, 37 people (4%) in the ID cohort and 27 (2%) in the gPop cohort had been prescribed fentanyl (RR 2.30, 95% CI 1.41–3.75). The corresponding numbers for those with pain related to the circulatory and respiratory systems were five (1%) and 15 people (2%; RR 0.56, 0.20–1.52), respectively; for visceral pain, there were 24 (3%) and 13 people (2%; RR 1.53, 0.79–2.99), respectively; and for pain related to the urinary system, there were seven (3%) and five people (4%; RR 0.69, 0.23–2.14), respectively. Less than five people had a prescription of fentanyl and a diagnosis of headaches.

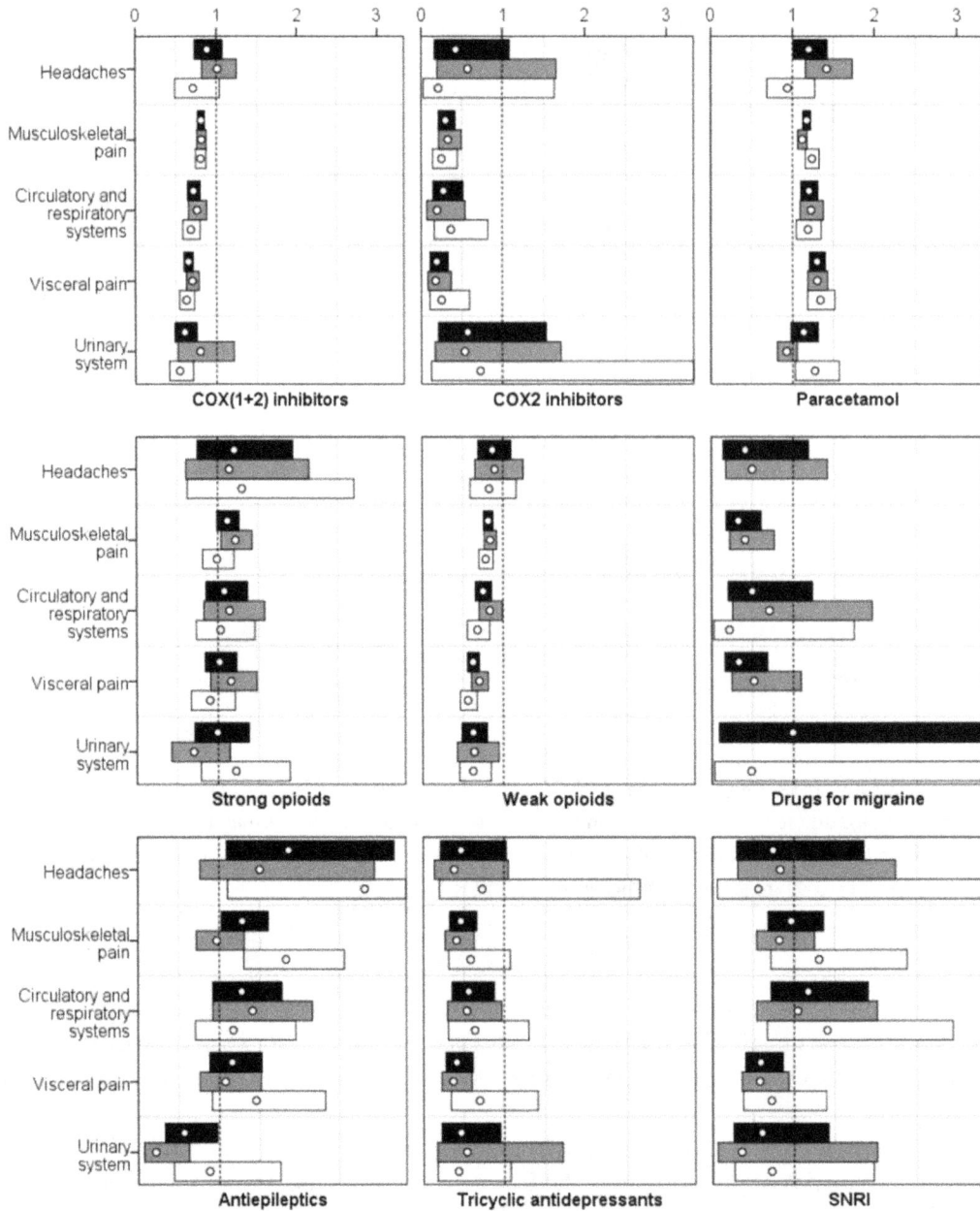

**Figure 2.** Relative risks (RRs; white dots) with 95% confidence intervals (CIs; bars; black = all, grey = women, white = men) for the prescription of pain medication among 7936 older people with intellectual disabilities vs. a random sample from the general population, one-to-one matched by sex and year of birth, stratified by pain diagnosis. The dotted line indicates RR = 1, i.e., CIs not crossing indicate statistically significant RRs.

**Table 2.** Number of people with prescriptions of different pain medications in a group of 7936 older people (3609 women and 4327 men) with intellectual disabilities (IDs) and a referent cohort from the general population (gPop), one-to-one matched by sex and year of birth, stratified by pain diagnosis.

| Type of Medication | gPop | | | ID | | |
|---|---|---|---|---|---|---|
| | Women | Men | Total | Women | Men | Total |
| | n (%) | n (%) | n (%) | n (%) | n (%) | n (%) |
| **Headaches** | | | | | | |
| COX(1+2) inhibitors | 75 (71) | 45 (63) | 120 (68) | 38 (72) | 19 (45) | 57 (60) |
| COX2 inhibitors | 14 (13) | 8 (11) | 22 (12) | 4 (8) | 1 (2) | 5 (5) |
| Paracetamol | 62 (58) | 45 (63) | 107 (60) | 44 (83) | 25 (60) | 69 (73) |
| Strong opioids | 21 (20) | 13 (18) | 34 (19) | 12 (23) | 10 (24) | 22 (23) |
| Weak opioids | 58 (55) | 45 (63) | 103 (58) | 26 (49) | 22 (52) | 48 (51) |
| Drugs for migraine | 16 (15) | 2 (3) | 18 (10) | 4 (8) | 0 (0) | 4 (4) |
| Antiepileptics | 16 (15) | 6 (8) | 22 (12) | 12 (23) | 10 (24) | 22 (23) |
| Tricyclic antidepressants | 21 (20) | 7 (10) | 28 (16) | 4 (8) | 3 (7) | 7 (7) |
| SNRI (Serotonin-norepinephrine reuptake inhibitor) | 12 (11) | 3 (4) | 15 (8) | 5 (9) | 1 (2) | 6 (6) |
| **Musculoskeletal Pain** | | | | | | |
| COX(1+2) inhibitors | 694 (80) | 637 (76) | 1331 (78) | 350 (65) | 295 (61) | 645 (63) |
| COX2 inhibitors | 128 (15) | 90 (11) | 218 (13) | 26 (5) | 13 (3) | 39 (4) |
| Paracetamol | 664 (76) | 536 (64) | 1200 (70) | 460 (86) | 382 (80) | 842 (83) |
| Strong opioids | 248 (29) | 211 (25) | 459 (27) | 187 (35) | 120 (25) | 307 (30) |
| Weak opioids | 548 (63) | 482 (58) | 1030 (60) | 284 (53) | 216 (45) | 500 (49) |
| Drugs for migraine | 47 (5) | 14 (2) | 61 (4) | 12 (2) | 0 (0) | 12 (1) |
| Antiepileptics | 100 (12) | 59 (7) | 159 (9) | 60 (11) | 62 (13) | 122 (12) |
| Tricyclic antidepressants | 99 (11) | 39 (5) | 138 (8) | 25 (5) | 13 (3) | 38 (4) |
| SNRI | 61 (7) | 24 (3) | 85 (5) | 31 (6) | 18 (4) | 49 (5) |
| **Pain Related to the Circulatory and Respiratory Systems** | | | | | | |
| COX(1+2) inhibitors | 263 (69) | 250 (66) | 513 (67) | 108 (52) | 113 (45) | 221 (48) |
| COX2 inhibitors | 38 (10) | 29 (8) | 67 (9) | 4 (2) | 7 (3) | 11 (2) |
| Paracetamol | 229 (60) | 210 (55) | 439 (58) | 152 (74) | 165 (66) | 317 (69) |
| Strong opioids | 76 (20) | 66 (17) | 142 (19) | 47 (23) | 45 (18) | 92 (20) |
| Weak opioids | 207 (54) | 186 (49) | 393 (52) | 93 (45) | 83 (33) | 176 (39) |
| Drugs for migraine | 13 (3) | 7 (2) | 20 (3) | 5 (2) | 1 (0) | 6 (1) |
| Antiepileptics | 42 (11) | 31 (8) | 73 (10) | 32 (16) | 24 (10) | 56 (12) |
| Tricyclic antidepressants | 45 (12) | 24 (6) | 69 (9) | 13 (6) | 10 (4) | 23 (5) |
| SNRI | 23 (6) | 14 (4) | 37 (5) | 13 (6) | 13 (5) | 26 (6) |
| **Visceral Pain** | | | | | | |
| COX(1+2) inhibitors | 314 (74) | 182 (62) | 496 (69) | 213 (52) | 178 (39) | 391 (45) |
| COX2 inhibitors | 47 (11) | 18 (6) | 65 (9) | 8 (2) | 7 (2) | 15 (2) |
| Paracetamol | 254 (60) | 154 (53) | 408 (57) | 319 (78) | 321 (71) | 640 (74) |
| Strong opioids | 93 (22) | 60 (21) | 153 (21) | 104 (26) | 84 (19) | 188 (22) |
| Weak opioids | 177 (42) | 99 (34) | 276 (39) | 129 (32) | 95 (21) | 224 (26) |
| Drugs for migraine | 20 (5) | 5 (2) | 25 (4) | 10 (2) | 0 (0) | 10 (1) |
| Antiepileptics | 55 (13) | 23 (8) | 78 (11) | 57 (14) | 52 (11) | 109 (13) |
| Tricyclic antidepressants | 57 (14) | 14 (5) | 71 (10) | 20 (5) | 15 (3) | 35 (4) |
| SNRI | 43 (10) | 16 (5) | 59 (8) | 24 (6) | 18 (4) | 42 (5) |
| **Pain Related to the Urinary System** | | | | | | |
| COX(1+2) inhibitors | 18 (55) | 54 (61) | 72 (59) | 27 (44) | 61 (33) | 88 (36) |
| COX2 inhibitors | 5 (15) | 2 (2) | 7 (6) | 5 (8) | 3 (2) | 8 (3) |
| Paracetamol | 31 (94) | 49 (55) | 80 (66) | 54 (87) | 129 (70) | 183 (74) |
| Strong opioids | 16 (48) | 21 (24) | 37 (30) | 21 (34) | 53 (29) | 74 (30) |
| Weak opioids | 17 (52) | 37 (42) | 54 (44) | 22 (35) | 42 (23) | 64 (26) |
| Drugs for migraine | 0 (0) | 1 (1) | 1 (1) | 1 (2) | 1 (1) | 2 (1) |
| Antiepileptics | 10 (30) | 11 (12) | 21 (17) | 4 (6) | 20 (11) | 24 (10) |
| Tricyclic antidepressants | 5 (15) | 9 (10) | 14 (11) | 5 (8) | 8 (4) | 13 (5) |
| SNRI | 3 (9) | 6 (7) | 9 (7) | 2 (3) | 9 (5) | 11 (4) |

**Table 3.** Relative risks with 95% confidence intervals for the prescription of pain medication among 7936 older people with intellectual disabilities vs. a random sample from the general population, one-to-one matched by sex and year of birth, stratified by pain diagnosis.

| Type of Pain | No Epilepsy | No Depression | |
|---|---|---|---|
| | Antiepileptics | Tricyclic Antidepressants | SNRI |
| Headaches | 1.16 (0.56–2.40) | 0.52 (0.22–1.22) | 0.40 (0.09–1.76) |
| Musculoskeletal pain | 0.90 (0.68–1.20) | 0.44 (0.30–0.66) | 0.80 (0.50–1.26) |
| Pain related to the circulatory and respiratory systems | 0.92 (0.62–1.38) | 0.44 (0.25–0.77) | 0.99 (0.46–2.11) |
| Visceral pain | 0.81 (0.58–1.13) | 0.34 (0.22–0.53) | 0.63 (0.37–1.05) |
| Pain related to the urinary system | 0.37 (0.18–0.75) | 0.47 (0.21–1.04) | 0.70 (0.20–2.43) |

## 4. Discussion

People in the ID cohort were more likely to be diagnosed with visceral pain or pain related to the urinary system. They were less likely to be diagnosed with headaches, musculoskeletal pain, or pain related to the circulatory or respiratory systems. Regardless of the type of pain, people with IDs were more likely to be prescribed paracetamol and fentanyl but were less likely to have a prescription for COX(1+2), COX2 inhibitors, weak opioids, drugs for migraine, or tricyclic antidepressants. Even though no differences were recorded between the groups for strong opioids in general, fentanyl was prescribed to twice as many people in the ID group.

When further interpreting the results from the present study, there are some potential weaknesses that need to be considered. First, using support intended for people with ID or ASD as a proxy for having an ID may have caused a dilution of the ID cohort with people with ASD but without an ID. However, among those with a diagnosis of ID and/or ASD recorded in the patient register during the study period, only 14% had ASD without an ID. Therefore, the effect of such misclassification should be minor.

Second, the national patient register does not contain information on visits to primary care. Therefore, the numbers presented in this study cannot be used to estimate the prevalence of pain among people with IDs. Moreover, in Sweden, specialist care, as a rule, requires a referral from primary care. If people with IDs differ in terms of chance of getting a referral to specialist care, this may bias the comparisons made between the ID and the gPop cohort.

Third, although the drug prescription register comprises data on all prescribed drugs dispensed at all pharmacies in Sweden, it does not contain information about over-the-counter-drugs or drugs provided to patients in inpatient care. However, among the drugs investigated in the present study, only paracetamol can be purchased without a prescription, and the interference of over-the-counter purchases should, therefore, be minor.

There are no biological or physiological reasons why patterns or the occurrence of pain would differ among people with IDs and those without IDs. Rather, we believe that the differences found between the two cohorts with respect to pain diagnoses are caused by other factors related to the individual, the caregivers, and the health care system. Diagnoses of pain are established through verbal communication between healthcare staff and the patient, physical examination, and laboratory tests (including radiology). It is, therefore, not surprising that, compared with their age peers in the general population, older people with IDs were less likely to get a diagnosis of headaches, musculoskeletal pain, or pain related to the circulatory and respiratory systems since they may not be able to report these symptoms. However, visceral pain and pain related to the urinary system are easier for the caregivers and healthcare staff to identify from bowel function, the appearance of urine, fever, local irritation, bacterial cultures, and other laboratory tests. This may explain why these types of pain are more common among people with IDs than in the general population.

Even in patients with full cognitive and physical function, diagnosing chronic pain is difficult. The recommendation is to assess patients with complex chronic pain in specialized pain rehabilitation teams consisting of pain physicians, physiotherapists, psychologists, and if needed, social workers and occupational therapists [40]. However, according to the clinical experience of the authors, people with IDs seldom have access to such teams and when they do, it is unlikely that team members with specialties other than developmental disorders will have sufficient knowledge and experience to provide care adapted to their special needs.

The pattern of differences in pain diagnoses between people with IDs and the general population was similar among men and women with the exception of visceral pain. In this study, having an ID was associated with an increased risk of diagnosis among men but not among women. This seemed to be driven by a low risk for visceral pain among women with IDs compared with women in the general population. There is a link between ovarian function and visceral pain [41,42]. Women with IDs are known to have earlier menopause than women in the general population. Therefore, even though the women in the two cohorts in the present study were of the same age (due to matching), the proportion of post-menopausal women was most likely higher in the ID cohort. Therefore, a possible explanation for the similarity in visceral pain diagnoses among older women with ID and the general population could be that one risk factor for such pain (i.e., being pre-menopausal) was less prevalent.

The recommended treatments for chronic pain are physiotherapy, Cognitive Behavioral Therapy (CBT), or Acceptance Commitment Therapy (ACT), either in individualized or in specialized pain rehabilitation programs [43,44]. Pharmacological treatment is also used but ideally as a "door-opener" to reduce pain symptoms [45]. Even so, the prescription of drugs for treating pain was common in both the ID and the gPop cohorts.

There was a pattern of increased prescription of paracetamol for people with IDs, regardless of pain diagnosis. In contrast, people with pain in the general population were more likely to have a prescription of a variety of pain treatments, such as COX(1+2) and COX2 inhibitors and weak opioids. There may be several reasons for this discrepancy among the two cohorts. People with IDs have an increased risk of polypharmacy compared to people without IDs [46]. Therefore, the choice to prescribe paracetamol may be based on a desire to not increase an already high number of drugs used by a person. The difference in the prescription of paracetamol could also be explained by a higher number of over-the-counter purchases in the general population than among people with IDs who may not have the same opportunity to visit pharmacies. Another potential explanation could be that there are financial considerations when prescribing paracetamol. In Sweden, prescribed drugs are subsidized by the state such that a single individual will never have to pay more than a set amount for prescribed drugs during a 12-month period. Therefore, it cannot be ruled out that physicians consider the lower economic standard of living among people with IDs and prescribe paracetamol rather than recommend over-the-counter purchases. However, the increased prescription of COX(1+2) and COX2 inhibitors as well as weak opioids may also reflect differences in healthcare access between the two cohorts. While paracetamol is often prescribed in primary health care, the drugs prescribed in the gPop cohort were most commonly done so by pain specialists rather than primary health care physicians. Therefore, the results may be an indication of better access to specialist care for people in the general population than people with IDs. Lastly, the fact that people in the general population were prescribed a greater range of drugs for pain treatment may be a reflection of a better follow-up of treatment effects and potential side effects in this group.

Even though only 1% of the people in the ID cohort were prescribed fentanyl during the study period, this was markedly more than in the general population. There is no "specific" pharmacological treatment for chronic pain, and unfortunately, strong opioids such as fentanyl are sometimes used as a last resort when nothing else helps. The problem with this is that the pain-relieving effect of strong opioids is temporary, while the cognitive and visceral side effects are ever present [47] and may well create a situation of general worsening of an ID patient's symptoms of pain. Further studies should be performed to investigate if the prescription of fentanyl among older people with IDs truly is justified.

## 5. Conclusions

Compared with the general population, older people with IDs were more likely to be prescribed paracetamol and fentanyl and were less likely to be prescribed other drugs for pain. Whether this is due to physicians trying to avoid polypharmacy in a population that is known to have prescriptions to a multitude of drugs or if there are other reasons not to prescribe a greater range of pain treatments needs to be further investigated. However, it is important to closely evaluate all pharmacological treatments for pain among older patients with IDs as well as in all patient groups and to stop them if no significant effect can be recognized.

In Sweden, the use of fentanyl outside of operations and intensive care is mainly as plasters developed for cancer pain, but it is suspected that it has been overused in chronic, non-malignant cases during the last decade. This needs to be further investigated.

**Author Contributions:** A.A. contributed to the design of the study, conducted the analysis, and drafted the article. The project leader, G.A., was the recipient (PI) of the national research grant. G.A. applied for ethical permission, contributed to the design of the study, and performed a critical revision of the article. H.W. contributed to the design of the project and performed a critical revision of the manuscript. All of the authors contributed to the content of the manuscript and approved the final manuscript.

**Funding:** This research was funded by Forte, the Swedish Research Council for Health, Working Life and Welfare grant number 2014-4753.

**Acknowledgments:** We would like to acknowledge the cooperation of the FUB (The Swedish National Association for People with Intellectual Disability).

## References

1.    IASP Task Force on Taxonomy. Classification of chronic pain. In *Part III: Pain Terms, a Current List with Definitions and Notes on Usage*; Merskey, H., Bogduk, N., Eds.; IASP Press: Seattle, WA, USA, 1994.

2.    International Association for the Study of Pain. IASP Terminology. Available online: https://www.iasp-pain.org/terminology (accessed on 10 April 2018).

3.    Treede, R.-D.; Rief, W.; Barke, A.; Aziz, Q.; Bennett, M.I.; Benoliel, R.; Cohen, M.; Evers, S.; Finnerup, N.B.; First, M.B.; et al. A classification of chronic pain for ICD-11. *Pain* **2015**, *156*, 1003–1007. [CrossRef] [PubMed]

4.    Tsang, A.; von Korff, M.; Lee, S.; Alonso, J.; Karam, E.; Angermeyer, M.C.; Borges, G.L.; Bromet, E.J.; Demytteneare, K.; de Girolamo, G.; et al. Common chronic pain conditions in developed and developing countries: Gender and age differences and comorbidity with depression-anxiety disorders. *J. Pain* **2008**, *9*, 883–891. [CrossRef] [PubMed]

5.    Hooten, W.M. Chronic pain and mental health disorders: Shared neural mechanisms, epidemiology, and treatment. *Mayo Clin. Proc.* **2016**, *91*, 955–970. [CrossRef] [PubMed]

6.    Fillingim, R.B.; Bruehl, S.; Dworkin, R.H.; Dworkin, S.F.; Loeser, J.D.; Turk, D.C.; Widerstrom-Noga, E.; Arnold, L.; Bennett, R.; Edwards, R.R.; et al. The acttion-american pain society pain taxonomy (AAPT): An evidence-based and multidimensional approach to classifying chronic pain conditions. *J. Pain* **2014**, *15*, 241–249. [CrossRef] [PubMed]

7.    Gibson, S.J.; Lussier, D. Prevalence and relevance of pain in older persons. *Pain Med.* **2012**, *13* (Suppl. 2), S23–S26. [CrossRef] [PubMed]

8.    Stubbs, B.; Binnekade, T.; Eggermont, L.; Sepehry, A.A.; Patchay, S.; Schofield, P. Pain and the risk for falls in community-dwelling older adults: Systematic review and meta-analysis. *Arch. Phys. Med. Rehabil.* **2014**, *95*, 175–187. [CrossRef] [PubMed]

9.    Horgas, A.L. Pain assessment in older adults. *Nurs. Clin. N. Am.* **2017**, *52*, 375–385. [CrossRef] [PubMed]

10.    Murdoch, J.; Larsen, D. Assessing pain in cognitively impaired older adults. *Nurs. Stand.* **2004**, *18*, 33–39. [CrossRef] [PubMed]

11.    Curtiss, C.P. Challenges in pain assessment in cognitively intact and cognitively impaired older adults with cancer. *Oncol. Nurs. Forum* **2010**, *37*, 7–16. [CrossRef] [PubMed]

12. Breivik, H.; Collett, B.; Ventafridda, V.; Cohen, R.; Gallacher, D. Survey of chronic pain in europe: Prevalence, impact on daily life, and treatment. *Eur. J. Pain* **2006**, *10*, 287–333. [CrossRef] [PubMed]

13. Breivik, H.; Eisenberg, E.; O'Brien, T. The individual and societal burden of chronic pain in europe: The case for strategic prioritisation and action to improve knowledge and availability of appropriate care. *BMC Public Health* **2013**, *13*. [CrossRef] [PubMed]

14. Fain, K.; Alexander, G.C.; Dore, D.D.; Segal, J.B.; Zullo, A.R.; Castillo-Salgado, C. Frequency and predictors of analgesic prescribing in U.S. Nursing home residents with persistent pain. *J. Am. Geriatr. Soc.* **2017**, *65*, 286–293. [CrossRef] [PubMed]

15. Shipton, E.A.; Shipton, E.E.; Shipton, A.J. A review of the opioid epidemic: What do we do about it? *Pain Ther.* **2018**, *7*, 23–36. [CrossRef] [PubMed]

16. de Knegt, N.; Lobbezoo, F.; Schuengel, C.; Evenhuis, H.M.; Scherder, E.J. Self-reporting tool on pain in people with intellectual disabilities (stop-id!): A usability study. *Augment. Altern. Commun.* **2016**, *32*, 1–11. [CrossRef] [PubMed]

17. Walsh, M.; Morrison, T.G.; McGuire, B.E. Chronic pain in adults with an intellectual disability: Prevalence, impact, and health service use based on caregiver report. *Pain* **2011**, *152*, 1951–1957. [CrossRef] [PubMed]

18. Turk, V.; Khattran, S.; Kerry, S.; Corney, R.; Painter, K. Reporting of health problems and pain by adults with an intellectual disability and by their carers. *J. Appl. Res. Intell. Disabil.* **2012**, *25*, 155–165. [CrossRef] [PubMed]

19. de Knegt, N.; Scherder, E. Pain in adults with intellectual disabilities. *Pain* **2011**, *152*, 971–974. [CrossRef] [PubMed]

20. Boerlage, A.A.; Valkenburg, A.J.; Scherder, E.J.; Steenhof, G.; Effing, P.; Tibboel, D.; van Dijk, M. Prevalence of pain in institutionalized adults with intellectual disabilities: A cross-sectional approach. *Res. Dev. Disabil.* **2013**, *34*, 2399–2406. [CrossRef] [PubMed]

21. McGuire, B.E.; Daly, P.; Smyth, F. Chronic pain in people with an intellectual disability: Under-recognised and under-treated? *J. Intell. Disabil. Res.* **2010**, *54*, 240–245. [CrossRef]

22. Amor-Salamanca, A.; Menchon, J.M. Pain underreporting associated with profound intellectual disability in emergency departments. *J. Intell. Disabil. Res.* **2017**. [CrossRef] [PubMed]

23. Baldridge, K.H.; Andrasik, F. Pain assessment in people with intellectual or developmental disabilities. *Am. J. Nurs.* **2010**, *110*, 28–35. [CrossRef] [PubMed]

24. Findlay, L.; Williams, A.C.; Scior, K. Exploring experiences and understandings of pain in adults with intellectual disabilities. *J. Intell. Disabil. Res.* **2014**, *58*, 358–367. [CrossRef] [PubMed]

25. Kankkunen, P.; Janis, P.; Vehvilainen-Julkunen, K. Pain assessment among non-communicating intellectually disabled people described by nursing staff. *Open Nurs. J.* **2010**, *4*, 55–59. [CrossRef] [PubMed]

26. Turk, V.; Kerry, S.; Corney, R.; Rowlands, G.; Khattran, S. Why some adults with intellectual disability consult their general practitioner more than others. *J. Intell. Disabil. Res.* **2010**, *54*, 833–842. [CrossRef] [PubMed]

27. Moriarty, O.; McGuire, B.E.; Finn, D.P. The effect of pain on cognitive function: A review of clinical and preclinical research. *Prog. Neurobiol.* **2011**, *93*, 385–404. [CrossRef] [PubMed]

28. Passmore, P.; Cunningham, E. Pain assessment in cognitive impairment. *J. Pain Palliat. Care Pharmacother.* **2014**, *28*, 305–307. [CrossRef] [PubMed]

29. Zis, P.; Daskalaki, A.; Bountouni, I.; Sykioti, P.; Varrassi, G.; Paladini, A. Depression and chronic pain in the elderly: Links and management challenges. *Clin. Interv. Aging* **2017**, *12*, 709–720. [CrossRef] [PubMed]

30. Snowden, M.B.; Steinman, L.E.; Bryant, L.L.; Cherrier, M.M.; Greenlund, K.J.; Leith, K.H.; Levy, C.; Logsdon, R.G.; Copeland, C.; Vogel, M.; et al. Dementia and co-occurring chronic conditions: A systematic literature review to identify what is known and where are the gaps in the evidence? *Int. J. Geriatr. Psychiatry* **2017**, *32*, 357–371. [CrossRef] [PubMed]

31. Wranker, L.S.; Rennemark, M.; Berglund, J. Pain among older adults from a gender perspective: Findings from the swedish national study on aging and care (SNAC-blekinge). *Scand. J. Public Health* **2016**, *44*, 258–263. [CrossRef] [PubMed]

32. Kaye, A.D.; Baluch, A.; Scott, J.T. Pain management in the elderly population: A review. *Ochsner J.* **2010**, *10*, 179–187. [PubMed]

33. Jones, M.R.; Ehrhardt, K.P.; Ripoll, J.G.; Sharma, B.; Padnos, I.W.; Kaye, R.J.; Kaye, A.D. Pain in the elderly. *Curr. Pain Headache Rep.* **2016**, *20*, 23. [CrossRef] [PubMed]

34. Coppus, A. People with intellectual disability: What do we know about adulthood and life expectancy? *Dev. Disabil. Res. Rev.* **2013**, *18*, 6–16. [CrossRef] [PubMed]

35. Fisher, K.; Kettl, P. Aging with mental retardation: Increasing population of older adults with mr require health interventions and prevention strategies. *Geriatrics* **2005**, *60*, 26–29. [PubMed]

36. Axmon, A.; Sandberg, M.; Ahlström, G.; Midlöv, P. Prescription of potentially inappropriate medications among older people with intellectual disability: A register study. *BMC Pharmacol. Toxicol.* **2017**, *18*. [CrossRef] [PubMed]

37. Wettermark, B.; Hammar, N.; Fored, C.M.; Leimanis, A.; Otterblad Olausson, P.; Bergman, U.; Persson, I.; Sundström, A.; Westerholm, B.; Rosén, M. The new swedish prescribed drug register—Opportunities for pharmacoepidemiological research and experience from the first six months. *Pharmacoepidemiol. Drug Saf.* **2007**, *16*, 726–735. [CrossRef] [PubMed]

38. WHO Collaborating Centre for Drug Statistics Methodology. *Guidelines for Atc Classification and Ddd Assignment 2018*; WHO: Oslo, Norway, 2017.

39. Pergolizzi, J.; Boger, R.H.; Budd, K.; Dahan, A.; Erdine, S.; Hans, G.; Kress, H.G.; Langford, R.; Likar, R.; Raffa, R.B.; et al. Opioids and the management of chronic severe pain in the elderly: Consensus statement of an international expert panel with focus on the six clinically most often used world health organization step III opioids (buprenorphine, fentanyl, hydromorphone, methadone, morphine, oxycodone). *Pain Pract.* **2008**, *8*, 287–313. [PubMed]

40. Driscoll, M.; Kerns, R.D. Integrated, team-based chronic pain management: Bridges from theory and research to high quality patient care. *Adv. Exp. Med. Biol.* **2016**, *904*, 131–147. [PubMed]

41. Palomba, S.; Di Cello, A.; Riccio, E.; Manguso, F.; La Sala, G.B. Ovarian function and gastrointestinal motor activity. *Min. Endocrinol.* **2011**, *36*, 295–310.

42. Heitkemper, M.M.; Chang, L. Do fluctuations in ovarian hormones affect gastrointestinal symptoms in women with irritable bowel syndrome? *Gend. Med.* **2009**, *6* (Suppl. 2), 152–167. [CrossRef] [PubMed]

43. Wicksell, R.K.; Ahlqvist, J.; Bring, A.; Melin, L.; Olsson, G.L. Can exposure and acceptance strategies improve functioning and life satisfaction in people with chronic pain and whiplash-associated disorders (wad)? A randomized controlled trial. *Cogn. Behav. Ther.* **2008**, *37*, 169–182. [CrossRef] [PubMed]

44. Casey, M.; Smart, K.; Segurado, R.; Hearty, C.; Gopal, H.; Lowry, D.; Flanagan, D.; McCracken, L.; Doody, C. Exercise combined with acceptance and commitment therapy (exact) compared to a supervised exercise programme for adults with chronic pain: Study protocol for a randomised controlled trial. *Trials* **2018**, *19*. [CrossRef] [PubMed]

45. Polatin, P.; Bevers, K.; Gatchel, R.J. Pharmacological treatment of depression in geriatric chronic pain patients: A biopsychosocial approach integrating functional restoration. *Expert Rev. Clin. Pharmacol.* **2017**, *10*, 957–963. [CrossRef] [PubMed]

46. Peklar, J.; Kos, M.; O'Dwyer, M.; McCarron, M.; McCallion, P.; Kenny, R.A.; Henman, M.C. Medication and supplement use in older people with and without intellectual disability: An observational, cross-sectional study. *PLoS ONE* **2017**, *12*. [CrossRef] [PubMed]

47. Trescot, A.M.; Helm, S.; Hansen, H.; Benyamin, R.; Glaser, S.E.; Adlaka, R.; Patel, S.; Manchikanti, L. Opioids in the management of chronic non-cancer pain: An update of american society of the interventional pain physicians' (ASIPP) guidelines. *Pain Physician* **2008**, *11*, S5–S62. [PubMed]

# 14

# A Comparative Study of Oral Health Status between International and Japanese University Student Patients in Japan

Ai Ohsato [1,2], Masanobu Abe [1,3,*], Kazumi Ohkubo [3], Hidemi Yoshimasu [2], Liang Zong [4,5], Kazuto Hoshi [3], Tsuyoshi Takato [3], Shintaro Yanagimoto [1] (ID) and Kazuhiko Yamamoto [1]

[1] Division for Health Service Promotion, the University of Tokyo, 7-3-1 Hongo, Bunkyo-ku, Tokyo 113-0033, Japan; osato.ai@mail.u-tokyo.ac.jp (A.O.); yanagimoto@hc.u-tokyo.ac.jp (S.Y.); yamamoto-tky@umin.ac.jp (K.Y.)

[2] School of Oral Health Sciences, Faculty of Dentistry, Tokyo Medical and Dental University, Tokyo 113-8549, Japan; h-yoshimasu.ocsh@tmd.ac.jp or phyoshimasu@outlook.jp

[3] Oral and Maxillofacial Surgery, Dentistry and Orthodontics, the University of Tokyo Hospital, Tokyo 113-8655, Japan; okubok-ora@h.u-tokyo.ac.jp (K.O.); hoshi-ora@h.u-tokyo.ac.jp (K.H.); t-takato@jreast.co.jp (T.T.)

[4] Graduate School of Medicine, the University of Tokyo, Tokyo 113-8655, Japan; zl20014111@163.com

[5] Key Laboratory of Carcinogenesis and Translational Research (Ministry of Education), Department of Gastrointestinal Surgery, Peking University Cancer Hospital & Institute, Beijing 100142, China

[*] Correspondence: abem-ora@h.u-tokyo.ac.jp

**Abstract:** *Background:* The number of international students enrolled in universities in Japan is increasing. To provide better oral care services for international students, we have to understand their oral environment and dental health behaviors. However, few studies have investigated the oral health status of international university students. The object of the present study was to clarify the current oral status of international university students. *Methods:* The subjects were students who visited the dental department at the University of Tokyo's Health Services Center between April 2012 and March 2013. Our medical records were reviewed with regard to the following items: attributes (nationality, gender, and age); chief complaint (reason for visit); history of dental treatment; mean number of decayed (D), missing (M) or filled (F) teeth as a single (DMFT) index; degree of calculus deposition; gingival condition; and oral hygiene status. *Results:* The records of 554 university students (138 international and 416 non-international students) were analyzed; 88.4% of the 138 international students were from Asian countries ($n = 122$), of which 47.1% were from China and 10.9% from Korea, followed by North America (5.8%), Europe (4.3%), and Africa (1.5%). Although no significant differences were found regarding the history of dental treatment between international and non-international students (49.3% and 48.8%, respectively), international students had a significantly higher dental caries morbidity rate (60.1%) than non-international students (49.0%). The international students showed a significantly higher DMFT value compared with the non-international students: 5.0 and 4.0 per individual, respectively. Severe calculus deposition was observed in international students compared with non-international students (51.9% and 31.7%, respectively). *Conclusions:* The international university students had poorer oral health status than the non-international students, even though the result might include many uncertainties and possible biases.

**Keywords:** oral health; university student; check-up; DMFT

## 1. Introduction

The present study was conducted to clarify the oral environment and dental health behaviors of university students who visited the dental clinic at the University of Tokyo's Health Services Center. Oral diseases, particularly periodontal disease, are evidently the leading cause of tooth loss in adolescence and subsequent life stages [1]. Current evidence suggests that poor oral health status influences systemic disorders, such as cardiovascular disease, diabetes mellitus, etc. [2–7]. Therefore, strengthening regular oral check-ups for young people is considered necessary to prevent not only oral diseases but also systemic diseases [8–10].

According to the Japan Student Services Organization (JASSO), an independent administrative institution under the aegis of the Japanese Ministry of Education, Culture, Sports, Science and Technology (MEXT), the number of international university students in Japan has increased by 18% in the past 5 years, with students from Asian countries comprising the largest portion of the international student population. To provide better oral care services for international students, we have to understand the features of their oral health status, which might be affected by many social factors such as cultural differences, health insurance system differences, dental access differences, etc. However, few studies have compared the oral status between international and non-international university students [11].

The present study was conducted to clarify the oral environment and dental health behaviors of international university students who visited the dental clinic in Health Services Center in University.

## 2. Methods

### 2.1. Ethics Approval and Consent to Participate

This research was approved by Institutional Review Board of the University of Tokyo (the approval number 13-146). Because this was a retrospective observational study and included no therapeutic intervention, the need for informed consent has been waived by the Institutional Review Board.

### 2.2. Subjects

Our subjects consisted of 554 students (138 international students and 416 non-international students) who visited the dental department at the university's Health Service Center between April 2012 and March 2013. All accessible data were collected. Students who held Japanese nationality ($n = 414$) or who were permanent residents of Japan ($n = 2$) were classified into the group of non-international students. Among 138 international students, 60.1% and 39.9% were male and female, and among the 416 non-international students, 74.5% and 25.5% were male and female, respectively. We reviewed the students' medical records available at the Health Service Center with regard to the following items: attributes (nationality, gender, and age), chief complaint (reason for visit), history of dental treatment, and mean number of decayed, missing or filled teeth in a single (DMFT) index, degree of calculus deposition and oral hygiene status. Calculus grading scale was as follows, NO: No calculus; MILD: calculus deposits less than one second of the tooth surface; SEVERE: Calculus deposits greater than one second of the tooth surface and/or extends subgingival. Categories of oral hygiene status was as follows, GOOD: No or slight dental plaque deposits on the several teeth; POOR: heavy dental plaque deposits extending to all the teeth.

### 2.3. Analytical Procedures

The retrospectively obtained survey results were anonymized from the original dental charts and converted to numeric data, which were statistically analyzed using the chi-square test, question-specific simple tabulation, and cross tabulation. As a rule, the level of significance was set at $p < 0.05$.

## 3. Results

The mean age was $28 \pm 3$ years for the 138 international students and $25 \pm 4$ years for the 416 non-international students, with an overall mean age of $26 \pm 4$ years. The international students tended to be older than the non-international students, but the difference was not significant. The most common home origin of the international students was Asia, accounting for 88.4%, followed by North America (5.8%), Europe (4.3%), and Africa (1.5%). Of the students from Asia the percentages from China and Korea were particularly high (47.1% and 10.9%, respectively) (Figure 1).

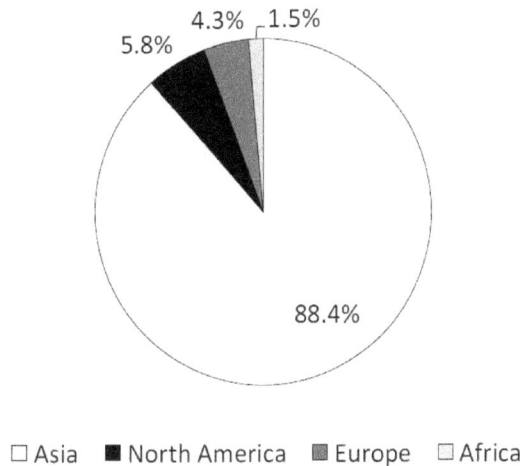

**Figure 1.** Home countries of the international students visiting our university dental clinic. The most common origin of the international students was Asia, followed by North America, Europe, and Africa.

Our subject classification by chief complaint (reason for visit) showed that 48.6% of the non-international students wanted a dental checkup, 20.8% wanted dental cleaning, 17.1% wanted dental caries treatment, and 8.6% wanted a dental consultation. Among the international students, 30.1% wanted a dental checkup, 28.2% wanted dental caries treatment, 19.9% wanted a dental consultation, and 17.9% wanted dental cleaning. A higher percentage of international students complained of specific oral symptoms compared to the non-international students (Supplementary Figure S1).

Dental caries occurred at significantly higher rates in the international students than in non-international students ($p < 0.05$). The dental caries morbidity rates were 60.1% and 49.0% in international and non-international students, respectively. However, the rate of past dental treatment was similar between international and non-international students: 49.3% and 48.8%, respectively (Figure 2).

Compared with the international students, the non-international students had significantly lower mean numbers of DMFT (4.0 vs. 5.0 per individual; $p < 0.05$) and decayed teeth (D) (1.8 vs. 2.2; $p < 0.05$). Missing teeth (M) and filled teeth (F) showed no significant differences between international and non-international students (Figure 3).

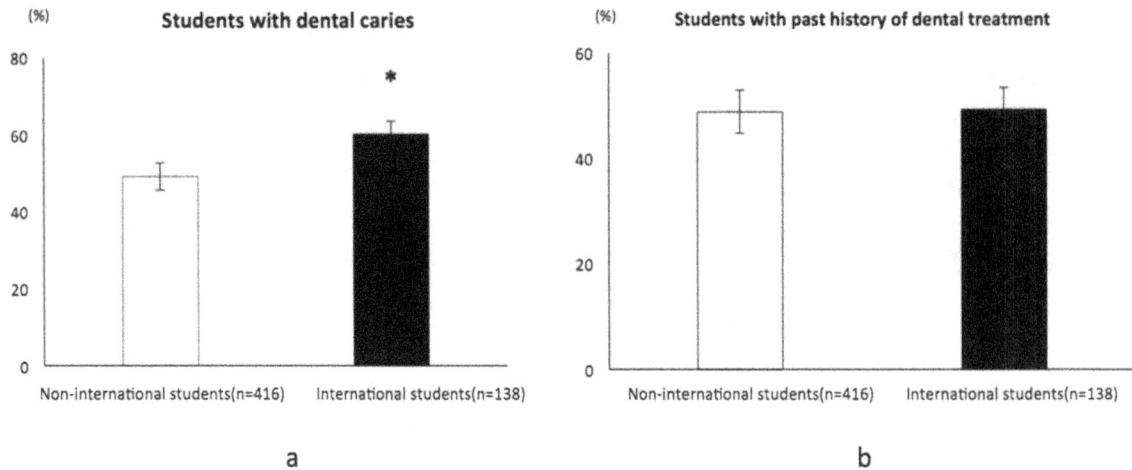

a

b

**Figure 2.** Comparison of morbidity of dental caries, past history of tooth extraction and dental treatment between international and non-international students in Japan. (**a**) Non-international students had a significantly lower dental caries morbidity rate than the international students ($p < 0.05$); * $p < 0.05$. (**b**) The rate of dental treatment was similar between international and non-international students in Japan.

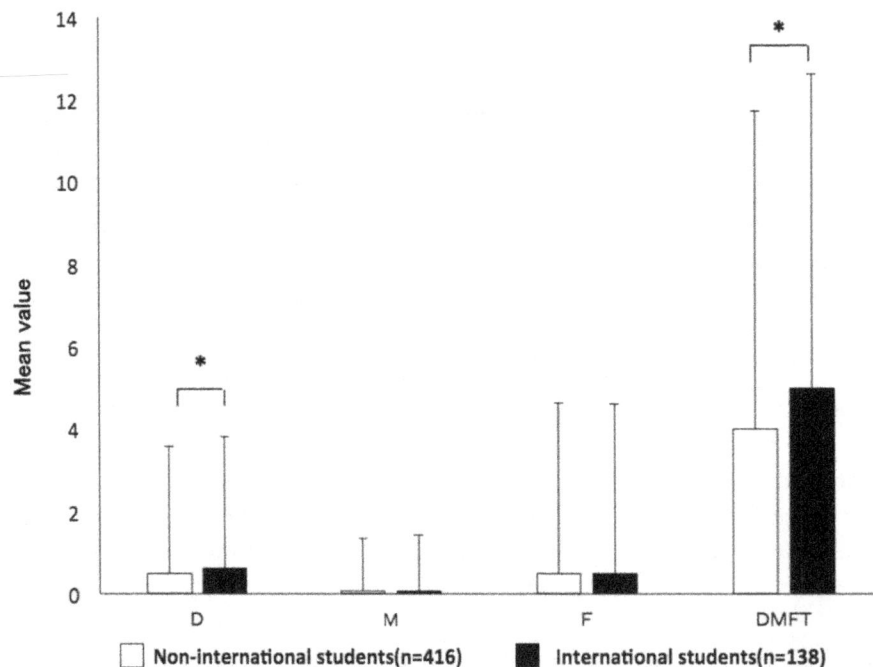

**Figure 3.** Comparison of the decayed, missing or filled teeth (DMFT) index between international and non-international students. Compared with the international students, the non-international students had a significantly lower value of DMFT, lower number of decayed teeth (D). Missing teeth (M) and filled teeth (F) showed no significant differences between international and non-international students in Japan. * $p < 0.05$.

The calculus deposition was severe in 51.9% of the international students and in 31.7% of the non-international students. The international students were significantly more likely than the non-international students to have severe dental conditions (Figure 4).

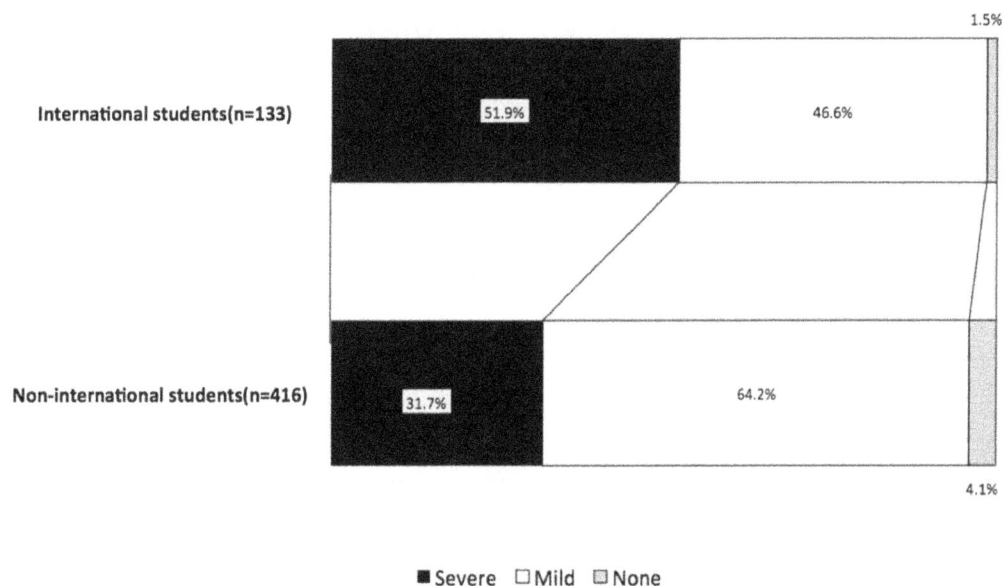

**Figure 4.** Comparison of the calculus deposition by severity. The calculus deposition was more severe in the international students than the non-international students in Japan.

The dental hygiene status at the first visit was rated good or average for 40.9% for the international students and 66.2% of the non-international students. The percentage of international students with poor dental hygiene status was 59.0%; that of the non-international students was 33.8% ($p < 0.05$, Supplementary Figure S2).

## 4. Discussion

The number of foreign university students in Japan increased by 18% in the past 5 years. Enhanced promotion of dental hygiene practices is necessary for foreign university students. The number of international university students is increasing year by year in Japan. The total number of university students at the University of Tokyo was 56,319, of which only 554 visited the dental department at the university's Health Services Center from April 2012 to March 2013. Of these 554 students, 138 (24.9%) were from foreign countries. The large fraction of international university students who visited the department of dentistry had poorer dental health status than non-international students, although the current result might include a selection bias because our target is "student patients", not "students". We analyzed "student patients" instead of "students" in this study. Therefore, the validation of the data in another population of "students" is necessary. The majority of the international students were from Asia (88.4%); in particular, students from China accounted for a large fraction of the international students (47.1%). The comparative investigation between international students from Asia and non-international students was performed. The outcomes of analyses were not largely changed even if the students from North America, Europe and Africa were excluded (data was not shown).

The ratio of people to dentists in China is much lower (10,000:1.1) than that in Japan (10,000:7.1) (Working Together for Health—The World Health Report 2006, WHO). This might mean that people have less chance to access adequate treatment from the dentists in China [12]. This could be one of the reasons for the differences in oral health status we found. The difference of the programs of health insurance coverage between China and Japan (affordability of dental care) might be also important. There are two major types of insurance programs available in Japan: Employee Health Insurance and National Health Insurance, and both programs cover basic dental treatments.

On the other hand, Chu et al. emphasized the importance of oral health education [8]. They pointed out that the level of awareness and knowledge about dental erosion is generally low in Chinese urban areas even though most such residents receive regular dental check-ups. Ohshima et al. compared periodontal health status and oral health behavior between Japanese and Chinese dental students, and found that periodontal disease rates were much higher in Chinese students than Japanese students, even though dental students may not represent the general university population [11]. They concluded that this might result from different lifestyles and oral hygiene habits. Peltzer et al. investigated the oral health behavior of university students in 26 countries and concluded that the behavior was affected by the social and health factors [13]. In our present study, although international students showed poorer oral health status than the non-international students, there was no significant difference between the two groups in the history of dental treatment. The previous studies indicate the importance of awareness and knowledge of oral health issues. Accordingly, the establishment and the strengthening of oral hygiene education are urgently needed to prevent periodontal and dental diseases [8–10].

Early detection of life-threatening diseases is considered a preferential issue, with dental care considered of lower priority. However, emerging evidence suggests that poor oral health influences not only oral diseases such as dental caries and periodontitis but also systemic disorders such as cardiovascular disease, diabetes mellitus, rheumatoid arthritis, Alzheimer's disease, metabolic syndrome, preterm delivery, and osteoporosis, to name a few [2–7]. We have also shown that the imbalance of oral bacterial flora deriving from poor oral health can lead to several systemic diseases [14–19]. Therefore, maintaining good oral health is crucial for not only prevention of local oral diseases but also prevention and management of systemic diseases [20].

To prevent oral and systemic diseases, the most important step is encouraging students to have regular check-ups and cleanings. In addition, improving self-efficacy has been reported to be beneficial for maintaining good oral health in university students [21]. The number of international university students in Japan increased by 18% in the past 5 years. Enhanced promotion of dental hygiene practices is necessary for international university students.

## 5. Conclusions

International students presented poorer oral health statuses than non-international students in Japan, even though the result might include many uncertainties and possible biases. Encouraging regular oral check-ups and cleanings and education for self-efficacy are necessary to improve oral health and prevent systemic diseases.

**Author Contributions:** A.O. and M.A. conceived and designed this study. A.O. and M.A. wrote the manuscript. K.O. and L.Z. reviewed the manuscript. H.Y., K.H., T.T., S.Y. and K.Y. supervised the study. All authors have read and approved the final manuscript.

**Funding:** This research received no external funding.

## References

1.    Nibali, L.; Sun, C.; Akcali, A.; Meng, X.; Tu, Y.K.; Donos, N. A retrospective study on periodontal disease progression in private practice. *J. Clin. Periodontol.* **2017**. [CrossRef] [PubMed]

2.    Han, Y.W.; Wang, X. Mobile microbiome: Oral bacteria in extra-oral infections and inflammation. *J. Dent. Res.* **2013**, *92*, 485–491. [CrossRef] [PubMed]

3.    Kaur, S.; White, S.; Bartold, P.M. Periodontal disease and rheumatoid arthritis: A systematic review. *J. Dent. Res.* **2013**, *92*, 399–408. [CrossRef] [PubMed]

4.   Barnes, C.M. Dental hygiene intervention to prevent nosocomial pneumonias. *J. Evid. Based Dent. Pract.* **2014**, *14*, 103–114. [CrossRef] [PubMed]

5.   Lamster, I.B.; Pagan, M. Periodontal disease and the metabolic syndrome. *Int. Dent. J.* **2017**. [CrossRef] [PubMed]

6.   Scannapieco, F.A.; Cantos, A. Oral inflammation and infection, and chronic medical diseases: Implications for the elderly. *Periodontology 2000* **2016**, *72*, 153–175. [CrossRef] [PubMed]

7.   Su, L.; Liu, W.; Xie, B.; Dou, L.; Sun, J.; Wan, W.; Fu, X.; Li, G.; Huang, J.; Xu, L. Toothbrushing, Blood Glucose and HbA1c: Findings from a Random Survey in Chinese Population. *Sci. Rep.* **2016**, *6*, 28824. [CrossRef] [PubMed]

8.   Chu, C.H.; Pang, K.K.; Lo, E.C. Dietary behavior and knowledge of dental erosion among Chinese adults. *BMC Oral Health* **2010**, *10*, 13. [CrossRef] [PubMed]

9.   Zhu, L.; Petersen, P.E.; Wang, H.Y.; Bian, J.Y.; Zhang, B.X. Oral health knowledge, attitudes and behaviour of adults in China. *Int. Dent. J.* **2005**, *55*, 231–241. [CrossRef] [PubMed]

10.  Gambhir, R.S.; Brar, P.; Singh, G.; Sofat, A.; Kakar, H. Utilization of dental care: An Indian outlook. *J. Nat. Sci. Biol. Med.* **2013**, *4*, 292–297. [CrossRef] [PubMed]

11.  Ohshima, M.; Zhu, L.; Yamaguchi, Y.; Kikuchi, M.; Nakajima, I.; Langham, C.S.; Lin, W.; Otsuka, K.; Komiyama, K. Comparison of periodontal health status and oral health behavior between Japanese and Chinese dental students. *J. Oral Sci.* **2009**, *51*, 275–281. [CrossRef] [PubMed]

12.  Hou, R.; Mi, Y.; Xu, Q.; Wu, F.; Ma, Y.; Xue, P.; Xiao, G.; Zhang, Y.; Wei, Y.; Yang, W. Oral health survey and oral health questionnaire for high school students in Tibet, China. *Head Face Med.* **2014**, *10*, 17. [CrossRef] [PubMed]

13.  Peltzer, K.; Pengpid, S. Oral health behaviour and social and health factors in university students from 26 low, middle and high income countries. *Int. J. Environ. Res. Public Health* **2014**, *11*, 12247–12260. [CrossRef] [PubMed]

14.  Abe, M.; Mori, Y.; Saijo, H.; Hoshi, K.; Ohkubo, K.; Ono, T.; Takato, T. The efficacy of dental therapy for an adult case of Henoch-Schönlein Purpura. *Oral Sci. Int.* **2012**, *9*, 59–62. [CrossRef]

15.  Abe, M.; Mori, Y.; Inaki, R.; Ohata, Y.; Abe, T.; Saijo, H.; Ohkubo, K.; Hoshi, K.; Takato, T. A Case of Odontogenic Infection by Streptococcus constellatus Leading to Systemic Infection in a Cogan's Syndrome Patient. *Case Rep. Dent.* **2014**, *2014*, 793174. [CrossRef] [PubMed]

16.  Inaki, R.; Igarashi, M.; Abe, M.; Saijo, H.; Hoshi, K.; Takato, T. A case of infective endocarditis by Streptococcus mutans bacteremia induced by asymptomatic chronic dental caries in a wisdom tooth. *Oral Sci. Jpn.* **2014**, *9*, 95–96.

17.  Itai, S.; Yonenaga, K.; Uchiyama, T.; Suenaga, H.; Abe, M.; Saijo, H.; Hoshi, K.; Takato, T. Management oral care of a case of bullous pemphigoid with oral hemorrhage and oral dyskinesia. *Oral Sci. Jpn.* **2015**, 97–98.

18.  Inagaki, Y.; Abe, M.; Inaki, R.; Zong, L.; Suenaga, H.; Abe, T.; Hoshi, K. A Case of Systemic Infection Caused by Streptococcus pyogenes Oral Infection in an Edentulous Patient. *Diseases* **2017**, *5*. [CrossRef] [PubMed]

19.  Abe, M.; Abe, T.; Mogi, R.; Kamimoto, H.; Hatano, N.; Taniguchi, A.; Saijo, H.; Hoshi, K.; Takato, T. Cervical necrotizing fasciitis of odontogenic origin in a healthy young patient without pre-systemic disorders. *J. Oral Maxillofac. Surg. Med. Pathol.* **2017**, *29*, 341–344. [CrossRef]

20.  Chapple, I.L.; Van der Weijden, F.; Doerfer, C.; Herrera, D.; Shapira, L.; Polak, D.; Madianos, P.; Louropoulou, A.; Machtei, E.; Donos, N.; et al. Primary prevention of periodontitis: Managing gingivitis. *J. Clin. Periodontol.* **2015**, *42* (Suppl. S16), S71–S76. [CrossRef] [PubMed]

21.  Mizutani, S.; Ekuni, D.; Furuta, M.; Tomofuji, T.; Irie, K.; Azuma, T.; Kojima, A.; Nagase, J.; Iwasaki, Y.; Morita, M. Effects of self-efficacy on oral health behaviours and gingival health in university students aged 18- or 19-year-old. *J. Clin. Periodontol.* **2012**, *39*, 844–849. [CrossRef] [PubMed]

# 15

# Anger and Aggression in UK Treatment-Seeking Veterans with PTSD

**David Turgoose** [1,*] **and Dominic Murphy** [1,2]

[1]   Combat Stress, Surrey KT22 0BX, UK

[2]   King's Centre for Military Health Research, King's College London, London WC2R 2LS, UK; dominic.murphy@combatstress.org.uk

*   Correspondence: david.turgoose@combatstress.org.uk

**Abstract:** Prevalence rates of anger and aggression are often higher in military personnel. Therefore, it is important to understand more about why this is, and the factors with which it is associated. Despite this, there is little evidence relating to anger and aggression in UK veterans who are seeking treatment for mental health difficulties such as post-traumatic stress disorder (PTSD). This study investigated the prevalence rates of anger and aggression in this population, as well as the associations between anger and aggression, and various sociodemographic, functioning and mental health variables. A cross-sectional design was used, with participants completing a battery of self-report questionnaires. Prevalence rates for significant anger and aggression were 74% and 28% respectively. Both women and those over 55 were less likely to report difficulties. Those with high levels of PTSD and other mental health difficulties were more likely to report anger and aggression. Other factors related to anger and aggression included unemployment due to ill health, and a perceived lack of family support. Findings showed that veterans who are seeking support for mental health are likely to be experiencing significant difficulties with anger and aggression, especially if they have comorbid mental health difficulties. The associations between anger, aggression, and other variables, has implications for the assessment and treatment of military veterans.

**Keywords:** military; veterans; anger; aggression; PTSD; mental health

---

## 1. Introduction

Research has suggested that military personnel are likely to experience difficulties with anger and aggressive behaviours [1,2]. Prevalence rates in military populations have been estimated at 29% for all types of physical assault, 12% for violent behaviour, and 10% for physical assault [1,3]. Anger in military populations is strongly associated with a range of other variables, including mental health issues such as post-traumatic stress disorder (PTSD) [4]. Specifically, anger and aggression in US veterans have been associated with PTSD hyperarousal [5], PTSD re-experiencing [6], and depression [7]. The relationship between anger and mental health is complex, and there is considerable overlap, with some research showing that anger in military personnel is substantially accounted for by mental ill health [2].

Anger and aggression have also been related to an individual's history, such as childhood adversity, childhood antisocial behaviour [2], and issues relating to their military service, such as having a combat role and experiencing multiple traumas whilst on deployment [1,2]. The extent of anger and aggression problems in military personnel is concerning given the challenges that this population faces in readjusting following deployment [8], with ex-service personnel often over-represented in prisons for violent offences and more likely to report committing violent crimes after combat exposure [9,10].

There have been several large-scale studies of anger and aggression using general military samples, often including those who have recently served in Iraq and Afghanistan. However, comparatively little research has investigated the specific mental health needs of military veterans who are seeking help for such difficulties. A recent study showed that 46% of UK veterans waited for more than five years to seek help for their mental health difficulties, and that this was related to greater mental health difficulties [11], strengthening the notion that there can be a long delay between deployment and veterans seeking support for their mental health [12]. In this sample, the second most commonly reported mental health issue was anger (76%), which has been strongly correlated with PTSD in US and UK veterans [5–7,11]. Given the apparently high prevalence rate of anger in treatment-seeking veterans, and the potential implications for veterans' well-being, it is important to further our understanding of these issues to help shape mental health services and improve treatments for veterans. By investigating factors associated with anger and aggression, clinicians could be assisted in identifying risk factors in veterans seeking support for mental health difficulties.

The aims of the present study were firstly to investigate prevalence rates of anger and aggression in a sample of treatment-seeking UK veterans. Secondly, we explored the relationships between anger and aggression, and a range of sociodemographic, functioning and mental health variables. Given the past evidence showing rates and associations of anger and aggression in the wider military population, it is pertinent to investigate such links in treatment-seeking veterans as our understanding of this group is limited.

## 2. Materials and Methods

### 2.1. Procedure

A cross-sectional design was used, with questionnaire responses collected from a random sample of treatment-seeking UK veterans recruited from Combat Stress (CS), a national charity providing specialist mental health services to military veterans. Questionnaire data was collected pertaining to anger and aggression, as well as a number of mental health and sociodemographic variables.

The questionnaire contained instructions informing participants that participation was voluntary, that the research was being conducted independently from clinical services at CS, and that participant input would not affect their treatment in any way. Questionnaires were sent to participants in the post using a three-wave mail out strategy between April and August 2016. Individuals from whom a response was not received were followed up by telephone. A research assistant made three attempts to contact these individuals by telephone.

### 2.2. Participants

Data for the present study was taken from a wider investigation of the needs of treatment-seeking veterans [11]. A sample of participants was randomly taken from a population of veterans who had sought support from CS over a 12-month period, between 31st January 2015 and 1st February 2016. The sample was drawn from the total number of veterans who had attended an initial assessment and at least one further appointment during this period ($N = 3335$). From this group, a random 20% sample was taken ($N = 667$), 67 of whom were removed prior to data collection either due to participant death or not having sufficient contact information. The final sample size was 600. Of these, 403 (67%) were recruited into the study by returning completed questionnaires. As demonstrated in a previous paper, there were no significant differences between those who took part in the study and those who did not [11].

### 2.3. Outcomes

#### 2.3.1. Anger and Aggression

Data on anger was collected using the *Dimensions of Anger Reactions* measure (DAR-5) [13]. This five-item measure gives an overall score to assess anger, with items including: 'I often find myself getting angry at people or situations', and 'When I get angry, I get really mad'. Items are scored on a

Likert scale ranging from 0–4 and a total score is calculated by adding these together, with scores of 12 and above indicating significant difficulties with anger.

In order to assess aggressive behaviours, we used a measure developed by the Walter Reed Army Institute of Research [14], based on the Interpersonal Conflict Scale [15] and the State/Trait Anger Scale [16]. This measure has been used previously in military samples [2,14]. For the purposes of this study, we termed this four-item measure the *Walter Reed Four* (WR-4). The WR-4 included the following items: 'How often did you get angry at someone and yell or shout', 'How often did you get angry with someone and kick or smash something, slam the door, punch the wall etc.', 'How often did you get into a fight with someone not in your family and hit the person' and 'How often did you threaten someone with physical violence'. Respondents were asked to rate each question with five options (never, once, twice, three or four times or five or more). These were scored between 0–4 and a total score calculated by adding these together. Caseness was defined if participant total scores were in the highest tertile.

### 2.3.2. Socio-Demographic Outcomes

Participants completed questionnaires relating to sociodemographic variables, including age, sex, relationship status and employment status. Participants were also asked to state how many years had passed between leaving the Armed Forces and seeking help. This was divided into <5 years and >5 years, and the date they left service, which was used to determine if they were an early service leaver, defined as leaving with under four years of continuous service.

Data was collected on childhood adversity, whereby participants rated 16 true or false statements relating to events from childhood, e.g., 'I regularly used to see or hear physical fighting or verbal abuse between my parents'. These items were taken from a previous epidemiological study of health and well-being in the UK military [17]. Participants responded on a binary yes/no scale to each item. Total scores were added and those in the top tertile deemed as having high levels of childhood adversity.

### 2.3.3. Functioning

A number of factors relating to general functioning were measured, including relationship and employment status. Data was also collected about social support, with participants asked to complete items on whether they felt supported by friends and family members.

The *Work and Social Adjustment Scale* (WSAS) [18] was used as a basic measure of functional impairment, i.e., the extent to which health difficulties interfere with the ability to carry out day-to-day tasks such as work and relationships. Totalled scores on this measure are categorised as mild (1–10), moderate (11–20) or severe (21+).

### 2.3.4. Health

A number of mental health outcomes were assessed. PTSD was measured using the *PTSD Checklist* [19] (PCL-5); a validated, 20-item measure assessing all domains of PTSD. Items are scored on a Likert scale from 0–4, with total scores of 34+ indicating caseness for PTSD. Common mental health difficulties (CMD) of anxiety and depression were assessed using the 12-item *General Health Questionnaire-12* [20] (GHQ-12). Scores on the GHQ-12 range from 0–12, with caseness defined as a score of 6+.

Data on alcohol use was collected using the *Alcohol Use Disorders Identification Test* [21] (AUDIT). This ten-item measure gives an overall score to assess alcohol-related risk. Harmful drinking levels were defined by scores of 16+.

Traumatic brain injury (TBI) was measured using the *Brain Injury Screening Index* [22]. Participants were deemed to meet criteria for TBI if they reported experiencing a serious blow to the head plus one of a series of symptoms as a result, such as alteration of mental state (e.g., dazed), gaps in memory of over one hour, or loss of consciousness.

*2.4. Analysis*

The first stage of the analysis was to calculate prevalence rates for the DAR-5 and WR-4. Following this, logistical regression models were fitted to explore associations between the DAR-5 and WR-4, and sociodemographic factors. These were adjusted for variables found to be significant (age, sex and childhood adversity) in order to control for any mediating or moderating effects. This analysis was repeated to explore associations between the DAR-5 and WR-4, and outcomes of functioning and health. All analyses were conducted using STATA 13.0 (College Station, TX, USA).

## 3. Results

*3.1. Demographics*

Of the sample of 600 veterans who were sent the questionnaire, 403 (67.2%) responded. The majority were male (95.8% vs. 4.2% female). Most participants were over 45 years old (68.2%), and just over two-thirds of participants were unemployed (68.1%). More were currently in a relationship (60.8%) than not (39.2%). Regarding their time spent in the Armed Forces, 12.6% were classified as early service leavers, and 45.7% had a period of five years or more since leaving the military and seeking help from CS. Based on established cut-off scores, 74% of participants reported significant difficulties with anger on the DAR-5. For aggressive behaviours, 28% of participants reported significant difficulties as indicated by scores on the WR-4.

*3.2. Relationships between Anger, Aggression and Other Variables*

3.2.1. Sociodemographic Variables

Table 1 contains sociodemographic variables and their associations with anger and aggression. Although only a small minority of participants were female, results suggest that women were less likely to report issues with anger (DAR-5: Odds Ratio 0.34, 95% Confidence Interval 0.12–0.92). Similarly, participants who were over the age of 55 were less likely to report aggressive behaviours (WR-4: OR 0.34, 95% CI 0.16–0.72). Participants who reported a high number of childhood adversity events were more likely to report difficulties with both anger and aggression (DAR-5: OR 3.43, 95% CI 1.68–7.00; WR-4: OR 2.22, 95% CI 1.34–3.69), although this association may be explained by other variables, such as PTSD (see Table 1).

3.2.2. Functioning

Table 2 presents functioning variables and their associations with anger and aggression. Social support was a significant factor, with those reporting that they did not feel supported by their family more likely to report problems with aggressive behaviours (WR-4: OR 3.10, 95% CI 1.59–6.01). This was not replicated in those not feeling supported by friends. Employment status was also a significant factor, with unemployment due to ill health associated with higher rates of both anger and aggression (DAR-5: OR 2.80, 95% CI 1.58–4.96; WR-4: OR 2.62, 95% CI 1.51–4.55). Unemployment not due to ill health was not a significant factor. Also, those participants who reported severe levels of functional impairment were more likely to be experiencing high levels of both anger and aggression (DAR-5: OR 2.89, 95% CI 1.77–4.74; WR-4: OR 1.01, 95% CI 1.00–2.79), although this association may be explained by other variables, such as PTSD (see Table 2).

3.2.3. Health

Table 3 presents associations between anger, aggression and different health variables. The most strongly associated variable was PTSD, with those meeting case criteria for PTSD being more likely to report difficulties with both anger and aggressive behaviours (DAR-5: OR 10.70, 95% CI 5.79–19.60; WR-4: OR 8.71, 95% CI 2.99–25.40). The same associations were true of common mental health difficulties such as depression and anxiety (DAR-5: OR 4.14, 95% CI 2.47–6.94; WR-4: OR 6.00,

CI 2.97–12.10), and difficulties with alcohol misuse (DAR-5: OR 2.08, 95% CI 1.08–4.01; WR-4: OR 2.05, 95% CI 1.21–3.47).

**Table 1.** Factors associated with anger and aggression.

| Demographic Variable | Anger (DAR-5) | | Aggression (WR-4) | |
|---|---|---|---|---|
| | n (%) | OR (95% CI) | n (%) | OR (95% CI) |
| *Sex* | | | | |
| Male | 286 (75.1) | 1.00 | 112 (29.0) | 1.00 |
| Female | 8 (47.1) | 0.34 (0.12–0.92) * | 2 (11.8) | 0.38 (0.08–1.73) |
| *Age group* | | | | |
| <35 | 37 (75.5) | 1.00 | 21 (42.9) | 1.00 |
| 35–44 | 72 (76.6) | 1.10 (0.48–2.54) | 27 (28.4) | 0.54 (0.26–1.14) |
| 45–54 | 83 (76.9) | 1.19 (0.52–2.75) | 36 (32.7) | 0.68 (0.33–1.42) |
| 55+ | 102 (69.4) | 0.80 (0.36–1.81) | 30 (20.1) | 0.34 (0.16–0.72) * |
| *Years to seek help* | | | | |
| <5 years | 153 (72.9) | 1.00 | 58 (27.6) | 1.00 |
| >5 years | 141 (75.0) | 1.25 (0.76–2.07) | 56 (29.0) | 1.35 (0.84–2.19) |
| *Childhood adversity* | | | | |
| Low group | 214 (69.5) | 1.00 | 75 (24.0) | 1.00 |
| High group | 80 (88.9) | 3.43 (1.68–7.00) * | 39 (43.3) | 2.22 (1.34–3.69) * |
| *Early service leaver* | | | | |
| No | 262 (74.0) | 1.00 | 100 (28.0) | 1.00 |
| Yes | 32 (72.7) | 0.89 (0.42–1.88) | 14 (30.4) | 1.00 (0.49–2.04) |

Note. * $p \leq 0.05$. OR = Odds Ratio. 95% CI = 95% Confidence Intervals. Odds Ratios adjusted for all other variables in table.

**Table 2.** Associations between factors related to functioning and anger and aggression.

| Functioning Variable | Anger (DAR-5) | | Aggression (WR-4) | |
|---|---|---|---|---|
| | n (%) | OR (95% CI) | n (%) | OR (95% CI) |
| *Feeling supported by friends* | | | | |
| Yes | 195 (73.3) | 1.00 | 77 (28.6) | 1.00 |
| No | 76 (81.7) | 1.69 (0.90–3.16) | 30 (31.9 | 1.16 (0.69–1.97) |
| *Feeling supported by family* | | | | |
| Yes | 238 (72.3) | 1.00 | 83 (25.0) | 1.00 |
| No | 38 (82.6) | 1.97 (0.86–4.51) | 23 (50.0) | 3.10 (1.59–6.01) * |
| *Relationship Status* | | | | |
| In relationship | 196 (72.9) | 1.00 | 69 (25.3) | 1.00 |
| Single | 98 (76.0) | 1.37 (0.81–2.31) | 45 (34.6) | 1.62 (1.01–2.62) * |
| *Employment status* | | | | |
| Working | 83 (67.5) | 1.00 | 27 (21.4) | 1.00 |
| Not working | 65 (65.7) | 0.97 (0.50–1.89) | 20 (20.0) | 1.31 (0.64–2.68) |
| Ill not working | 146 (83.0) | 2.80 (1.58–4.96) * | 67 (37.9) | 2.62 (1.51–4.55) * |
| *Functional impairment (WSAS)* | | | | |
| Mild/moderate | 80 (59.7) | 1.00 | 28 (20.7) | 1.00 |
| Severe (21+) | 214 (81.1) | 2.89 (1.77–4.74) * | 86 (32.1) | 1.01 (1.00–2.79) * |

Note. * $p \leq 0.05$. OR = Odds Ratio. 95% CI = 95% Confidence Intervals. Odds Ratios adjusted for age, sex and childhood adversity.

Further analysis was conducted to explore these associations, whilst adjusting for all other significant variables, to see which variables were still significant after controlling for all others. Findings are presented in Table 4. Childhood adversity, severe functional impairment and being single were no longer associated with anger or aggression following these adjustments.

**Table 3.** Health factors associated with anger and aggression.

| Health Variable | Anger (DAR-5) | | Aggression (WR-4) | |
|---|---|---|---|---|
| | *n* (%) | OR (95% CI) | *n* (%) | OR (95% CI) |
| *PTSD (PCL-5)* | | | | |
| Not a case | 23 (31.9) | 1.00 | 4 (5.6) | 1.00 |
| Case (38+) | 271 (83.1) | 10.7 (5.79–19.6) * | 110 (33.2) | 8.71 (2.99–25.4) * |
| *CMD (GHQ-12)* | | | | |
| Not a case | 60 (55.1) | 1.00 | 11 (10.0) | 1.00 |
| Case (4+) | 234 (81.0) | 4.14 (2.47–6.94) * | 103 (35.5) | 6.00 (2.97–12.1) * |
| *Alcohol (AUDIT)* | | | | |
| Not a case | 225 (71.2) | 1.00 | 79 (24.8) | 1.00 |
| Case (16+) | 69 (84.2) | 2.08 (1.08–4.01) * | 35 (41.7) | 2.05 (1.21–3.47) * |
| *Brain Injury* | | | | |
| Negative | 148 (71.5) | 1.00 | 58 (27.5) | 1.00 |
| Positive | 146 (76.4) | (1.24 (0.78–1.98) | 56 (29.2) | 1.04 (0.66–1.65) |

* $p \leq 0.05$.

**Table 4.** Exploring associations with anger and aggression adjusting for all other significant variables previously identified.

| Variable | Anger (DAR-5) | Aggression (WR-4) |
|---|---|---|
| | OR (95% CI) | OR (95% CI) |
| *Sex* | | |
| Male | 1.00 | 1.00 |
| Female | 0.20 (0.06–0.65) * | 0.32 (0.07–1.57) |
| *Age group* | | |
| <35 | 1.00 | 1.00 |
| 35–44 | 1.38 (0.54–3.54) | 0.59 (0.26–1.32) |
| 45–54 | 1.14 (0.46–2.86) | 0.59 (0.27–1.28) |
| 55+ | 0.98 (0.39–2.46) | 0.31 (0.14–0.70) * |
| *Childhood adversity* | | |
| Low group | 1.00 | 1.00 |
| High group | 1.35 (0.72–2.53) | 1.37 (0.81–2.33) |
| *Feeling supported by family* | | |
| Yes | 1.00 | 1.00 |
| No | 1.36 (0.52–3.53) | 2.54 (1.20–5.36) * |
| *Relationship status* | | |
| In relationship | 1.00 | |
| Single | 0.88 (0.47–1.66) | 0.85 (0.47–1.53) |
| *Employment status* | | |
| Working | 1.00 | 1.00 |
| Not working | 0.88 (0.40–1.94) | 1.34 (0.60–3.03) |
| Ill not working | 1.31 (0.66–2.60) | 1.94 (1.05–3.59) * |
| *Functional impairment (WSAS)* | | |
| Mild/moderate | 1.00 | 1.00 |
| Severe | 1.64 (0.91–2.95) | 1.11 (0.61–2.03) |
| *PTSD (PCL-5)* | | |
| Not a case | 1.00 | 1.00 |
| Case (38+) | 6.06 (3.12–11.77) * | 3.45 (1.14–10.43) * |
| *CMD (GHQ-12)* | | |
| Not a case | 1.00 | 1.00 |
| Case (4+) | 1.87 (1.03–3.38) * | 3.35 (1.63–6.90) * |
| *Alcohol (AUDIT)* | | |
| Not a case | 1.00 | 1.00 |
| Case (16+) | 1.51 (0.73–3.13) | 1.83 (1.02–3.28) * |

Note. * $p \leq 0.05$. CMD = Common Mental Health Disorders. OR = Odds Ratio. 95% CI = 95% Confidence Intervals. Odds Ratios adjusted for age, sex, childhood adversity, family support, relationship status, employment status, functional impairment (WSAS), post-traumatic stress disorder (PTSD; PCL-5), CMD (GHQ-12), Alcohol (AUDIT).

## 4. Discussion

This study observed that nearly three quarters of treatment-seeking veterans in this sample reported significant difficulties with anger, and more than a quarter reported problems with aggressive behaviour. Furthermore, anger and aggression were strongly associated with PTSD, and also associated with common mental health difficulties, and alcohol misuse. Links between anger and PTSD and other mental health disorders have been found previously [4], but this is the first study to show this relationship in veterans who are seeking help for their mental health.

One possible explanation may be that some PTSD, depression or anxiety symptoms overlap with anger and aggression. For example, irritability is a common feature of PTSD, which, given the association between anger and PTSD, raises the question of whether anger in treatment-seeking veterans is a separate construct, or can be explained by its relation to other mental health difficulties. Indeed, past research has suggested that the strong association between anger and mental health difficulties is due to the overlap of these conditions within the individual [2].

Previous research has found that after deployment, military personnel who experienced more traumatic events had higher levels of anger [1], which might partly explain the high prevalence rates of anger and aggression in the current sample, if we are to assume that they had experienced traumas that were related to the fact that they were seeking support. The prevalence of anger and aggression might also be explained in part by the military culture in which veterans might have been required to use acts of aggression in their work. Furthermore, most of the participants in this sample were men, and past research has illustrated the existence of a 'macho' culture within the armed forces [23], in which the expression of anger and aggression might be a more readily accepted method of displaying emotion.

An association was observed between problems with anger and aggression and higher rates of childhood adversity. Previous large-scale research has shown strong relationships between adverse childhood experiences (ACEs) and an array of difficulties in later life, including for mental health and violent behaviours [24,25]. It has also been suggested that recruits into the military are often from disadvantaged backgrounds [10]. In this study, the links between childhood adversity, anger and aggression were explained by other factors such as severity of PTSD. This perhaps indicates that those with high levels of childhood adversity were more likely to develop PTSD, which in turn was the risk factor for anger and aggression. Indeed, there are some commonalities between anger and PTSD symptoms, such as irritability and hypervigilance which could make some more prone to acting aggressively.

The finding that those who were unemployed due to ill health were more likely to report anger and aggression was notable, particularly because those who were unemployed not due to ill health did not report such difficulties. This could in part be explained if the illnesses in question were related to mental health, given the association here between anger, aggression and mental health. Similarly, those who had the most severe interference with day-to-day functioning might be those who have the biggest mental health difficulties which might explain the association between WSAS scores and anger and aggression.

Participants were more likely to report problems with aggressive behaviour if they did not feel supported by their family. Past research has suggested that social support can help to reduce anger in people with PTSD [26], although the results in the present study relate to aggression, not anger. The fact that perceived support of family but not friends was significant here, could suggest that there is something important about families in the role of aggression in the context of treatment-seeking veterans. Similar findings have been reported elsewhere in a sample of POWs [27], and in an adolescent sample, where anger expression was more likely in those who did not perceive support from family, which was not replicated for support from friends [28]. There is evidence for the notion that social support and family support are important in overcoming PTSD and other mental health difficulties [29–32], plus there is evidence that social support improves treatment efficacy for PTSD [33]. This finding suggests that those who are not in a relationship or do not feel supported by family are more likely to act on their anger. It may be that close family support is a protective factor stopping some from acting out on their anger, or that those who do not perceive support have been alienated from partners or family members due to their aggressive behaviours.

Results here suggested that women were less likely to report difficulties with anger, although only a small minority of this sample were female. Common narratives exist around the increased likelihood of men to feel anger and act out aggressively, which is supported by some research [34,35], although evidence in some instances is mixed [36].

### 4.1. Limitations

Due to the cross-sectional design of this study, it is not possible to determine causality relating to the associations found. For example, is it the case that veterans display aggression because they do not have support from family, or is it the case that their aggression has caused strain in family relationships? With other variables, such as childhood adversity, we know little from the present study about the mechanisms by which this might relate to anger and aggression. Although, theories from elsewhere in the wider literature might offer suitable explanations, such as the role of childhood adversity on the development of emotional regulation [37]. This study found that some variables were associated with anger but not aggression, or vice versa. It was beyond the scope of the present study to investigate why this occurred, and future research might adopt different designs such as qualitative methods in order to explore this. Furthermore, some evidence suggests an important neurobiological role in PTSD which could help explain the role of some of these variables [38].

The current sample was taken from a population of veterans who were actively seeking treatment from a national veterans mental health charity. CS receives approximately 2500 new referrals per year [12], so the current sample represents a significant number of treatment-seekers but may not be generalisable to all. While the response rate was high, the present study did not conduct a power calculation to determine a sample size required to find significant differences in the given analyses. The relatively large confidence intervals in some of the statistics may point to a lack of power in some instances.

### 4.2. Implications

Findings from the present study suggest that anger and aggression are a significant part of the difficulties faced by the treatment-seeking veteran population. Also, both anger and aggression are strongly related to other comorbid mental health difficulties, such as PTSD. This could be important in identifying mental health difficulties in veterans, if for example a veteran presents with anger, this could be used as a starting point to discuss other difficulties they may be experiencing. Research has shown that there can be a long gap between a veteran completing military service and seeking help for mental health [39], so increasing our knowledge of the main signs and symptoms could help increase the number who are identified and then able to access appropriate support. These findings suggest that anger and aggression should be routinely screened for in mental health assessments of veterans and appropriate treatments offered. Also, it may be pertinent in mental health settings to assess for risk of aggressive behaviours.

## 5. Conclusions

This study showed that veterans who are seeking support with their mental health are likely to be having significant difficulties with anger and aggression, especially if they have other comorbid mental health difficulties. Being unemployed due to ill health, and a lack of perceived family support were also related to higher levels of anger and/or aggression. Being female and over 55 years old were associated with reduced anger and aggression respectively.

Given the high prevalence rates of anger and aggression in treatment-seeking veterans, there is a need to ensure that appropriate forms of assessment and support are available, and the presence of anger or aggression could provide a useful bridge for discussing wider mental health difficulties, given their strong association. While the present study is limited by its cross-sectional design, it provides useful insights into the needs of this population.

**Author Contributions:** Conceptualization, D.M.; Methodology, D.M.; Validation, D.M., D.T.; Formal Analysis, D.M.; Data Curation, D.M.; Writing-Original Draft Preparation, D.T.; Writing-Review & Editing, D.M., D.T.; Visualization, D.T.; Project Administration, D.M., D.T.

**Funding:** This research received no external funding.

**Acknowledgments:** The authors acknowledge the contributions of all participants in this study and the work of Combat Stress clinical and research staff in supporting the study.

## References

1.  MacManus, D.; Dean, K.; Al Bakir, M.; Iversen, A.C.; Hull, L.; Fahy, T.; Wessely, S.; Fear, N.T. Violent behaviour in UK military personnel returning home after deployment. *Psychol. Med.* **2012**, *42*, 1663–1673. [CrossRef] [PubMed]
2.  Rona, R.J.; Jones, M.; Hull, L.; MacManus, D.; Fear, N.T.; Wessely, S. Anger in the UK Armed Forces: Strong association with mental health, childhood antisocial behavior, and combat role. *J. Nerv. Ment. Dis.* **2015**, *203*, 15–22. [CrossRef] [PubMed]
3.  MacManus, D.; Rona, R.; Dickson, H.; Somaini, G.; Fear, N.; Wessely, S. Aggressive and violent behavior among military personnel deployed to Iraq and Afghanistan: Prevalence and link with deployment and combat exposure. *Epidemiol. Rev.* **2015**, *37*, 196–212. [CrossRef] [PubMed]
4.  Gonzalez, O.I.; Novaco, R.W.; Reger, M.A.; Gahm, G.A. Anger intensification with combat-related PTSD and depression comorbidity. *Psychol. Trauma* **2016**, *8*, 9–16. [CrossRef] [PubMed]
5.  Elbogen, E.B.; Wagner, H.R.; Calhoun, P.S.; Fuller, S.R.; Kinneer, P.M. Mid-Atlantic Mental Illness Research Education and Clinical Center Workgroup; Beckham, J.C. Correlates of Anger and Hostility among Iraq and Afghanistan War Veterans. *Am. J. Psychiatry* **2010**, *167*, 1051–1058. [CrossRef] [PubMed]
6.  Hellmuth, J.C.; Stappenbeck, C.A.; Hoerster, K.D.; Jakupcak, M. Modeling PTSD symptom clusters, alcohol misuse, anger, and depression as they relate to aggression and suicidality in returning veterans. *J. Trauma Stress* **2012**, *25*, 527–534. [CrossRef] [PubMed]
7.  Taft, C.T.; Weatherill, R.P.; Woodward, H.E.; Pinto, L.A.; Watkins, L.E.; Miller, M.W.; Dekel, R. Intimate partner and general aggression perpetration among combat veterans presenting to a posttraumatic stress disorder clinic. *Am. J. Orthopsychiatr.* **2009**, *79*, 461–468. [CrossRef] [PubMed]
8.  Sayers, S.L.; Farrow, V.A.; Ross, J.; Oslin, D.W. Family problems among recently returned military veterans referred for a mental health evaluation. *J. Clin. Psychiatry* **2009**, *70*, 163–170. [CrossRef] [PubMed]
9.  Booth-Kewley, S.; Larson, G.E.; Alderton, D.L.; Farmer, W.L.; Highfill-McRoy, R. Risk factors for misconduct in a navy sample. *Mil. Psychol.* **2009**, *21*, 252–269. [CrossRef]
10. MacManus, D.; Wessely, S. Why do some ex-armed forces personnel end up in prison? New report emphasises the role of alcohol, social exclusion, and financial problems. *BMJ* **2011**, *342*. [CrossRef] [PubMed]
11. Murphy, D.; Ashwick, R.; Palmer, E.; Busuttil, W. Describing the profile of a population of UK veterans seeking support for mental health difficulties. *J. Ment. Health* **2017**. Epub ahead of print. [CrossRef] [PubMed]
12. Murphy, D.; Weijers, B.; Palmer, E.; Busuttil, W. Exploring patterns in referrals to Combat Stress for UK veterans with mental health difficulties between 1994 and 2014. *Int. J. Emerg. Ment. Health* **2015**, *17*, 652–658.
13. Forbes, D.; Alkemade, N.; Mitchell, D.; Elhai, J.D.; McHugh, T.; Bates, G.; Novaco, R.W.; Bryant, R.; Lewis, V. Utility of the Dimensions of Anger reactions-5 (DAR-5) scale as a brief anger measure. *Depress. Anxiety* **2014**, *31*, 166–173. [CrossRef] [PubMed]
14. Wilk, J.E.; Bliese, P.D.; Thomas, J.L.; Wood, M.D.; McGurk, D.; Castro, C.A.; Hoge, C.W. Unethical battlefield conduct reported by soldiers serving in the Iraq war. *J. Nerv. Ment. Dis.* **2013**, *201*, 259–265. [CrossRef] [PubMed]
15. Spector, P.E.; Jex, S.M. Development of four self-report measures of job stressors and strain: Interpersonal Conflict at Work Scale, Organizational Constraints Scale, Quantitative Workload Inventory, and Physical Symptoms Inventory. *J. Occup. Health Psychol.* **1998**, *3*, 356–367. [CrossRef] [PubMed]

16. Spielberger, C. *Manual for the State Trait. Anger Expression Inventory (STAXI-2)*, 2nd ed.; Psychological Assessment Resources: Odessa, FL, USA, 1999.

17. Iversen, A.; Fear, N.T.; Simonoff, E.; Hull, L.; Horn, O.; Greenberg, N.; Hotopf, M.; Rona, R.; Wessely, S. Influence of childhood adversity on health among male UK military personnel. *Brit. J. Psychiatry* **2007**, *191*, 506–511. [CrossRef] [PubMed]

18. Mundt, J.C.; Marks, I.M.; Shear, M.K.; Greist, J.H. The Work and Social Adjustment Scale: A simple measure of impairment in functioning. *Brit. J. Psychiatry* **2002**, *180*, 461–464. [CrossRef]

19. Weathers, F.W.; Litz, B.T.; Keane, T.M.; Palmieri, P.A.; Marx, B.P.; Schnurr, P.P. *The PTSD Checklist for DSM-5 (PCL-5)*; Scale available from the National Center for PTSD; 2013. Available online: www.ptsd.va.gov (accessed on 30 January 2015).

20. Goldberg, D.; William, P. *A Users' Guide to the General Health Questionnaire*; NFER-Nelson Windsor: Berkshire, UK, 1998.

21. Babor, T.F.; Higgins-Biddle, J.C.; Saunders, J.B.; Monteiro, M.G. *AUDIT: The Alcohol Use Disorders Identification Test*; Department of Mental Health and Substance Dependence, World Health Organization: Geneva, Switzerland, 2001.

22. Pitman, I.; Haddelsey, C.; Ramos, S.; Oddy, M.; Fortescue, D. The association between neuropsychological performance and self-reported traumatic brain injury in a sample of adult male prisoners in the UK. *Neuropsychol. Rehabil.* **2015**, *25*, 763–779. [CrossRef] [PubMed]

23. Keats, P.A. Soldiers working internationally: Impacts of masculinity, military culture, and operational stress on cross-cultural adaptation. *Int. J. Adv. Couns.* **2010**, *32*, 290–303. [CrossRef]

24. Duke, N.N.; Pettingell, S.L.; McMorris, B.J.; Borowsky, I.W. Adolescent violence perpetration: Associations with multiple types of adverse childhood experiences. *Pediatrics* **2010**, *125*, 778–786. [CrossRef] [PubMed]

25. Hughes, K.; Bellis, M.A.; Hardcastle, K.A.; Sethi, D.; Butchart, A.; Mikton, C.; Jones, L.; Dunne, M.P. The effect of multiple adverse childhood experiences on health: A systematic review and meta-analysis. *Lancet Pub. Health* **2017**, *2*. [CrossRef]

26. Kotler, M.; Iancu, I.; Efroni, R.; Amir, M. Anger, impulsivity, social support, and suicide risk in patients with Posttraumatic Stress Disorder. *J. Nerv. Ment. Dis.* **2001**, *189*, 162–167. [CrossRef] [PubMed]

27. Schützwohl, M.; Maercker, A. Anger in former East German political prisoners: Relationship to posttraumatic stress reactions and social support. *J. Nerv. Ment. Dis.* **2000**, *188*, 483–489. [CrossRef] [PubMed]

28. Arslan, C. Anger, self-esteem, and perceived social support in adolescence. *Soc. Behav. Personal.* **2009**, *37*, 555–564. [CrossRef]

29. Peirce, R.S.; Frone, M.R.; Russell, M.; Cooper, M.L.; Mudar, P. A longitudinal model of social contact, social support, depression, and alcohol use. *Health Psychol.* **2000**, *19*, 28–38. [CrossRef] [PubMed]

30. Ozer, E.J.; Best, S.R.; Lipsey, T.L.; Weiss, D.S. Predictors of posttraumatic stress disorder and symptoms in adults: A meta-analysis. *Psychol. Bull.* **2003**, *129*, 52–73. [CrossRef] [PubMed]

31. Amaresha, A.C.; Venkatasubramanian, G. Expressed emotion in schizophrenia: An overview. *Indian J. Psychol. Med.* **2012**, *34*, 12–20. [PubMed]

32. Koutra, K.; Simos, P.; Triliva, S.; Lionis, C.; Vgontzas, A.N. Linking family cohesion and flexibility with expressed emotion, family burden and psychological distress in caregivers of patients with psychosis: A path analytic model. *Psychiatr. Res.* **2016**, *240*, 66–75. [CrossRef] [PubMed]

33. Tarrier, N.; Humphreys, A.L. PTSD and the social support of the interpersonal environment: The development of Social Cognitive Behavior Therapy. *J. Cognitive Psychother.* **2003**, *17*, 187–198. [CrossRef]

34. Jakupcak, M.; Lisak, D.; Roemer, L. The role of masculine ideology and masculine gender role stress in men's perpetration of relationship violence. *Psychol. Men Masc.* **2002**, *3*, 97–106. [CrossRef]

35. Archer, J. Sex differences in aggression between heterosexual partners: A meta-analytic review. *Psychol. Bull.* **2000**, *126*, 651–680. [CrossRef] [PubMed]

36. Melton, H.; Belknap, J. He hits, she hits: Assessing gender differences and similarities in officially reported intimate partner violence. *Crim. Justice Behav.* **2003**, *30*, 328–348. [CrossRef]

37. Kim, J.; Cicchetti, D. Longitudinal pathways linking child maltreatment, emotion regulation, peer relations, and psychopathology. *J. Child Psychol. Psychiatry* **2010**, *51*, 706–716. [CrossRef] [PubMed]

38. Pitman, R.K.; Rasmusson, A.M.; Koenen, K.C.; Shin, L.M.; Orr, S.P.; Gilbertson, M.W.; Milad, M.R.; Liberzon, I. Biological studies of post-traumatic stress disorder. *Nat. Rev. Neurosci.* **2012**, *13*, 769–787. [CrossRef] [PubMed]

39. Murphy, D.; Busuttil, W. PTSD, stigma and barriers to help-seeking within the UK Armed Forces. *J. R. Army Med. Corps* **2014**, *18*. [CrossRef] [PubMed]

# 16

# Chief Nursing Officers' Views on Meeting the Needs of the Professional Nurse: How This Can Affect Patient Outcomes

Charlene Ingwell-Spolan

School of Nursing, University of Maine, Orono, ME 04469, USA; Charlene.ingwellspolan@maine.edu

**Abstract:** Chief Nursing Officers (CNOs) have a demanding, complex role that commands accountability in leading the nursing profession and achieving quality patient outcomes. The purpose of this study was to understand the CNO's view of meeting the needs of the Registered Nurse (RN) at point of care and how this could affect quality patient outcomes. In two qualitative studies twenty-five CNOs were individually interviewed in eight states including: Florida, Tennessee, Kentucky, Maine, New Hampshire, Vermont, Massachusetts, and New Jersey. The majority of these CNOs interviewed believed they were doing the best for their nurses and their healthcare facility. After analyzing their responses, it was apparent that some CNOs actually encouraged peer pressure among nurses to achieve compliance and felt patient acuity is being addressed adequately, since most patients were discharged within three to four days and those that were more critical were admitted to the critical care units. The average length of stay, which is the number of paid days a patient remained in the hospital, was an important metric. A large amount of nurses felt they were unable to deliver the care needed for their patients due to patient load, lack of collaboration among the health care team, higher patient acuity and absence of decision-making and autonomy. Many of the CNOs trusted that patient care outcomes, meaning relatively short hospital stays, demonstrated that the nursing practice was successful; rather than first having the nurse being set up for success to provide the best care possible to their patients.

**Keywords:** leadership; nursing leadership; patient outcomes; healthy work environment; nurse education

## 1. Introduction

The demanding, complex role of Chief Nursing Officers (CNOs) today commands accountability in leading the professional nurse to help achieve consistent quality patient outcomes. Twenty-five CNOs were interviewed individually in two qualitative research studies from eight states including: Florida, Tennessee, Kentucky, Maine, New Hampshire, Vermont, Massachusetts, and New Jersey. These phenomenological inquiries examined the CNOs' perspectives of meeting the needs of the Registered Nurse (RN) at point of care and how they felt this affected quality patient outcomes.

Today's RNs' experiences often include: job dissatisfaction; high patient acuity; lack of autonomy and decision making; plus bullying in the workplace [1–4]. These barriers in the acute care setting result in a less supportive work environment and may prevent the RN from delivering quality patient care [5–9]. The CNO is the leader of the professional nurse and is ultimately responsible for the actions and interventions of the RN at point of care [10]. Metrics are in place to measure patient care outcomes; e.g., The Hospital Consumer Assessment of Healthcare Providers and Systems (HCAHPS), physician/health care colleagues' reactions/complaints, and patient incident reports. There is intense pressure for the CNO to maintain high scores on these measures; all required for the ultimate success of the CNO [9,11–13].

## 2. Background

In prior studies, RNs describe their jobs as stressful [2,7]. Negative perceptions of the work environment can be predictors of the desire to leave nursing [2,7] and can also be a cause for an even lower commitment to the institution and profession by newly licensed RNs, affecting nurse retention, overall attrition rates, and patient outcomes [1,6]. Likewise, these additional factors negatively affect the success and length of CNO employment [14].

Nurse-assessed quality of care and better RN job satisfaction at point of care [9,12] are influenced by strong leadership, organizational culture, and group cohesiveness [9,12]. A cross sectional survey [6] showed that there is a relationship between a transformational leadership style and quality of care; facilitated through organizational and peer support, autonomy, and workload of the RN.

A mixed method study [11] showed a linkage between organizational climate and nurses' performance of caring practices in hospitals showing consistency with the Quality Caring Model [15,16]. This model promotes caring with relationship building concepts that nurses demonstrate within their daily clinical practice. These relationship centered encounters are with patients, families, and the health care team and are related to improved patient care outcomes [16]. The workload of the RN is the most obvious factor influencing caring practices and patient outcomes [11,15,16]. Leadership and teamwork linked to role clarity for nurses and characteristics of patients/families such as relationships, support systems, and past history have distinct influences on RNs caring and quality patient outcomes [11,15,16].

The CNO is the leader of the RN at point of care. Remarkable leaders keep themselves informed on what is going on in the workplace, welcoming ideas and opinions that are intended for the improvement of performance. They also see the significance in knowing the truth within the current experiences of the daily work environment. Finding the truth and making people feel comfortable and safe in communicating relevant information are attributes of successful and renowned leaders [17].

The CNO needs to move beyond dependence on current clinical models in which the RN at point of care implements physicians' orders, is a subordinate member of the health care team and is not comfortable in voicing their observations in regards to their patients' care. Rather, professional nurses, under the direction of the CNO need to become more skilled and interdisciplinary team members. This requires high-level communication and advocacy for nurses to become equal partners in health care. Speaking up about organizational issues and suggesting changes to operating procedures may cause risk to the person speaking; however, when spoken effectively this could be viewed as constructive [18,19]. Research has found that CNOs do not have consistent, standardized leadership education that facilitates success in these areas regarding the RN at point of care in the healthcare industry [9,10,17].

Professional barriers in the workplace, fragmentation of clinical systems, and administrative disconnect can prevent the professional nurse from articulating new models for patient care. Many times nurses are systematically excluded from contributing information crucial to patient decision-making and quality of care [6,8,18]. Nurses must find a way, institutionally, to overcome the barriers that prevent them from enacting their professional model of care. This will involve nursing staff communicating and negotiating interpersonally, socially, and organizationally, as well as clinically; which are imperative to further the trust of patients, families, and the wider population [18,19].

For example; a platform for change at patient point of care focusing on the CNO and Chief Financial Officer's (CFO) relationship in addressing challenges of quality patient care, safety, and financial performance found that CNOs communicating with CFOs and Chief Executive Officers (CEO) involves understanding financial constraints and balancing them with expected quality patient outcomes [13]. This financial knowledge from the nursing perspective should be communicated by the CNO to the CFO as well as to the professional nurses. With ever-increasing pressure to cut costs the partnership between nursing and finance needs to tackle these new challenges. This collaboration has historically been strained and does not always come easily due to differences in focus, priorities, and disparate communication. In this case, effective communication between the CNO and CFO resulted in the development of benchmarks, a functional nurse staff council, an evaluation process of patient acuity, and classification systems to prevent inequitable assignments [13]. These sorts of proven effective models of communication and collaboration are imperative not only for the success of the CNO but for the RN at point of care and most importantly for quality patient outcomes.

Therefore, from the literature it is known that a healthy work environment including effective communication, advocacy, and interdisciplinary cooperation facilitates consistent quality patient outcomes [20,21]. Since the CNO is the highest nursing decision maker, communicator, and collaborator she/he is best able to set the required standards to achieve a healthy work environment for nursing that provides the catalyst for consistent quality patient outcomes.

During the literature review there were no qualitative studies of CNOs' perceived work experiences in the acute care setting. As a result two qualitative studies, an initial study and a replication study, were completed and combined by this author in which CNOs voiced their views on meeting the needs of the professional nurse and its effect on patient care outcomes.

## 3. Materials and Methods

The purpose of this author's initial and replicated study was to explore the lived experience of the CNO as the lead voice for the professional nurse. The substance of the interviews consisted of "what" they experienced and "how" they experienced it. Following the expansive, overarching research questions were the follow-up interview questions and prompts in which this portion of both studies explored the CNOs' view on meeting the needs of the RN at point of care and how they felt this affected quality patient outcomes. The researcher's own prejudgments were set aside through epoch. Trustworthiness is equated to validity in quantitative research [22]. This was implemented through one-on-one interviews and member checks which provided the participants an opportunity to give feedback on the identified themes. Trustworthiness is not established as it is created and cultivated. This is accomplished through methodical collection of data and in-depth analysis of the data; yielding, thick, rich descriptions of the phenomenon of studies that has been clearly saturated. The continuous bracketing of the researcher served as evidence of the researcher's honesty. Dependability was achieved as each participant reviewed his or her verbatim transcript along with confirmability as the results were confirmed or collaborated by others showing details of the methodology used.

CNO participants were accessed through professional nursing leadership organizations and through purchased targeted contact lists. Email invitations were sent to future participants advising them of the general scope of the studies.

Institutional Review Board (IRB) approval was received for both the initial study and the replicated study. Inclusion criteria for the two studies included: CNOs within an acute setting, a hospital which has facilities and all personnel including medical staff appropriate to diagnose, treat and care for acute conditions, including injuries, located within the Southeastern and Northeastern United States. CNOs were identified as the highest ranking administrative registered nurse in the acute care organization, responsible for the practice of nursing throughout their healthcare system. Exclusion criteria included anyone not meeting the inclusion criteria. Department directors, division directors, unit or service managers, supervisors, charge nurses and other senior nurses who have non-nursing, executive positions in hospitals were also excluded.

Both studies were explained to the participants prior to the interviews, in which all questions were answered in regards to the informed consent. All the participants who met the inclusion criteria and who agreed to participate in the study then signed the informed consent. Twenty-five CNOs were interviewed using Moustakas' transcendental phenomenological inquiry approach, determining the overall essence of the CNOs' lived experience as the lead voice for the RN in the acute care setting.

The two research questions viewed appropriate for this portion of the two studies in accordance with Moustakas' design were: (1) How do you meet the needs of the RN at point of care? and (2) Does meeting the needs of the RN affect patient care outcomes?

A naturalistic inquiry research approach was integrated through the direct experience of the CNOs. This model-included context, perspectives, experiences, underlying motivations and factors that influence decision making and opinions of CNOs.

The studies included six male and nineteen female CNOs actively practicing in Florida, Tennessee, Kentucky, Maine, New Hampshire, Massachusetts, Vermont, and New Jersey. The participants' ages ranged from early forties to late sixties. They were educated to at least a master's level up to a PhD degree and were primarily Caucasian. The CNOs in these studies generally held several CNO positions in the last decade. The types of hospitals represented included; corporate system, community, government, academic health center and rural facilities. The number of beds per hospital ranged from less than 50 to over 1000.

In accordance with Moustakas' Transcendental Phenomenology, there were multiple reviews of transcriptions following each interview with member checks. These reviews led to identification through horizontalization and delimited meanings of the invariant qualities in which patterns and themes emerged. From these patterns and themes, an integrated textural and structural description was completed per participant.

## 4. Results

After careful and studied consideration and analysis of the phenomenon being studied, two essential themes emerged in regards to meeting the needs of the RN at point of care and how this affects quality patient care outcomes. These two themes were advocating and conflicting. The CNOs were continuously advocating for the patient and many times this advocacy for the patient could be conflicting with the needs of the nurse. Following are examples of the transcriptions obtained in these two studies.

The Chief Nursing Officer, by virtue of the title, might be assumed to chiefly represent nursing. However, all CNOs interviewed in this study noted their primary goal and responsibility was to the patient. According to these CNOs, this may or may not coincide with the best interest and objectives of the nurses. This is the conflict that is one of the primary themes that emerged from these two studies.

As one CNO described this conflict:

"People know that I have the patient's best interests at heart. Because I have to think what's best for the patient, not best for the nurses. What's best for the patients right now might be what's best for the nurse's today. But it might not be … "

Another CNO explained their role as an advocate for the patient even though they are the Chief Nursing Officer:

"That is why I round on patients, because that reminds me why I do what I do every day. … because I am a nurse first … I'm doing it for the patient in the bed … because my priority is the patient's safety."

Even though patient care and patient care outcomes are the primary goal of the CNOs interviewed, many were apprehensive and some even cautioned by their executive teams to not foster dissension among nurses which might result in outcomes detrimental to the organization including; nurse turnover, loss of reputation, and union activity. This at times caused the CNO to feel frustrated in bringing new ideas and processes to the workplace for concern this would cause discord among the RNs.

As one CNO stated this conflicting dilemma:

"No one wants the nurses trying to bring in a union … picketing in front of the hospital. So, you got to keep the nurses happy … but there is also this extreme pressure to get the largest workforce in the hospital to perform well for everyone else."

In order to be an effective leader, the individuals you lead must have a work environment conducive to success, feel valued, have opportunities to advance professionally and have a voice.

Only one of the CNOs interviewed seemed less conflictive and was an advocate for the nurse as they identified this connection; that if the nurses are allowed to self-actualize, the patient will be the ultimate beneficiary. The CNO stated: "If my nurses are well taken care of, my patients will be taken care of."

Many of the CNOs talked about having better work processes, documentation systems, and call systems for the RN at point of care. In practice, evidence of meeting goals and objectives of the non-nursing leadership team took priority. For example, peer pressure among nurses was utilized to meet staffing needs. Another example of a CNO's conflict between believing they are an advocate for the professional nurse is that they were actually influencing nurses to work overtime by encouraging nurses to coerce other nurses to do so:

> "We never pressure for overtime, it's just not a good work environment . . . you do a neutral approach and people contribute if they're part of a team . . . there are always some that do more than others . . . if you have somebody who never does it that brings the team down . . . you address it more from a team performance . . . after a while the peers will look and resent it . . . If they see the team doing it everybody pitches in . . . "

Many of the CNOs were concerned about length of patient stay, since this affects revenue. However, they were generally not concerned if, e.g., nursing assessments were not being done since they are not evaluated on this standard. Yet, assessments are being documented as always being completed, even though they are not always fully or even substantially completed. As one CNO noted, patient assessments were not important, however, RN's at point of care feel they do not have the ability to give best patient care such as assessments. They also feel they do not have adequate time to spend with each patient. This CNO expressed continuous conflict; such as revenue versus patient care and advocating for nurses without providing appropriate time for assessment and other interventions at point of care:

> "I don't think (assessments) are very thorough . . . I mean the length of stay is 4 days. The median is probably 3.1. I don't know how important it is, you know? I will tell you that there are a lot of things I would like to improve in terms of having nurses spend more time at the bedside . . . if they had more time, they would probably do more things . . . for patients . . . but within a few days . . . they go home."

When asked about patient acuity and if this is factored into the success of the RN, one CNO stated using the term "nursing acuity" that this may not be an issue as nurses do have enough time for even the most complex patient interventions. However, most RNs at point of care feel they do not have the time to give the best care to their patients which contributes to an unhealthy work environment. This CNO did not perceive the conflict, instead felt that nurses are adequately advocated for, stating:

> "When you think about nursing acuity systems, even if patient load . . . is about 20 percent more than what you would expect . . . on the patient load of four patients . . . what are you going to need, eight and a half hours on your shift? . . . So I am not believer that we're that nuanced . . . Teaching and talking to them, talking to the family, I mean, that's about it. Even the most complex dressing change doesn't take very long . . . the nursing things are 1000 one minute things."

Another CNO discussed that patient care outcomes revolve around having enough resources for the nurses. This CNO explained how advocating for nurses helped achieve good results for the patient:

> "I got great outcomes because we didn't have a lot of resources, . . . because I was in a position as a COO, I ratcheted down all the non-nursing departments and ran them lean as anything, but ran nursing at a higher level of nursing hours per patient per day. And that did give great outcomes for the hospital . . . when nursing has a voice at the table at the board level and at the senior executive level, you can do good things. The key is getting well-trained people . . . however, if you have folks like here, that . . . are getting what they're getting because they're

compromising and, you know, Ms. Nicey-nice and stuff ... that can be to the detriment of nursing ... they don't want to take the risks and fight the fight. And you've—got to—you've got to be a fighter to be a—a successful nurse executive. You can't sit back ... "

## 5. Discussion

These two studies found are groundbreaking in the area of qualitative research on the lived experiences of CNOs. There were no comparable studies prior to these.

The majority of CNOs interviewed for these two studies were considered highly clinically competent early in their careers. The skills required later at the executive level were not the focus of their undergraduate and graduate level of education. A two-year initiative by the Robert Wood Johnson Foundation (RWJF) and the Institute of Medicine (IOM) found that the undergraduate and graduate education of nurses in the academic setting does not address the realities of health care [23]. The need for highly educated nurses to manage complex healthcare systems, build relationships with healthcare teams in order to collaborate and coordinate across all specialties and professions within the healthcare industry is paramount to achieve better patient outcomes. This will be accomplished by reinventing the nursing curriculum to include all aspects of competency in leadership, health policy, systems, research, and evidence based practice [23]. In order to deliver high quality patient care and the nurses' expanding role, nursing curricula needs to be reexamined and updated to prepare future nurses to be highly competent in the present complex health care industry [23]. Many schools of nursing keep adding more knowledge and information due to the expanding growth of research. The timeline of nursing education remains the same and yet the content for students to learn is increased resulting in more student memorization, less retention of knowledge and ability to critically analyze within the clinical environment [23]. One school of nursing had implemented an active learning approach to leadership in which reflection and observation of leadership is promoted to provide a baseline for future leadership development after graduation [24]. The philosophy behind this approach is to promote leadership awareness as nurses are expected to have leadership skills within their practice. A quantitative comparative study examining transformational leadership among graduating baccalaureate nursing students (BSN) and practicing nurses showed that the BSN nursing students had significantly lower scores in transformational leadership components than the practicing nurses and the practicing nurses in leadership positions did not consider themselves better transformational leaders than the staff nurses [25]. Overall, the educational methods in preparing undergraduate and graduate nurses in academia for the present and future healthcare industry is not adequate to provide continuous success for the nurse and nurse leader [23–25].

In nursing, the primary focus is always the patient. At the undergraduate level of nursing studies all the skills, learning the disease entities, and being able to apply this knowledge safely at the bedside is the nucleus of nursing. Nursing work environments, turnover, retention, and interdisciplinary collaboration are not generally discussed with nursing students at a high level of understanding. Therefore, new nurses are not fully aware of the discontent within the profession of nursing. In fact, most of the time novice nurses are quite surprised that these types of issues are commonplace in the hospital work environment [2,5,9]. Many times they are confused and resort to a comfort zone of focusing on their clinical abilities and patients. Some actually leave the profession [2]. For those that stay, often they are not sure if these conditions are isolated events, temporary, or being perceived incorrectly [2,26]. Various behaviors of "settling" become the standard way of coping with these numerous circumstances of discord [26]. Eventually these methods of adjustment are not long lasting, especially if it affects patient care outcomes. Nurses, including CNOs, are all about the patient; this is their nature and to some their calling. If most of the time nurses feel they are unable to deliver the care needed for their patients, then the nurse may feel inadequate, unhappy, and unsure if they represent the caring nurse they have been taught to be [11]. The instinctual need to defend the care delivered to their patients is customary within the nursing culture.

Most of these CNOs are very good to excellent leaders despite these obstacles within their environments. This takes persistence, intelligence, communication, and courage to be successful within these circumstances. In spite of their challenges, they continued to set themselves apart from their colleagues. They were promoted without much mentoring or additional education. This additional education would have allowed them to be even more effective leaders by changing the healthcare system in a global aspect, rather than in fragments [10,12]. Nurses generally do not have a personal agenda. If allowed to be taught the true infrastructure in both the clinical and financial realms they would be the best likely change agent for healthcare. In doing so, they would broaden the inevitable process of developing beyond one's scope.

Most of these CNOs are self-learners and highly flexible. They have had role models that were either non-nursing business executives, non-clinical nurse executives or, as most of these CNOs were, a highly clinical nurse executive. More often than not, these CNOs were being mentored by someone who may not have fully understood the nursing profession, its thinking, or processes. Knowing the whole healthcare industry is how a nurse would optimally function; it is the holistic approach and most of them are being educated in parts mixed with nursing philosophy. However, many of them believed that patient care outcomes will promote the success of the nurse, rather than first having the nurse being set up for success in order to have consistent successful patient care outcomes. How can they do this easily if the core of their profession is all about the patient and not about the nurse and the patient since they are interrelated.

## 6. Conclusions

Many of these CNOs interviewed believed they were doing the best for their nurses and healthcare facility. These interviews though, showed conflict of CNOs choosing between being an advocate for the patient or being an advocate for the nurse. Looking at their responses it was apparent that inadvertently some actually encouraged peer pressure among nurses to achieve compliance in the name of being a team player, which could make the RN feel pressured and in some cases bullied to work extra shifts. Other CNOs concluded that most nursing bedside interventions take very little time and thus the work load of an acute care RN is fairly reasonable, even though research has found many nurses believe they do not have enough time or staff to give the best care to their patients [1–3]. In some cases, CNOs believed that patient acuity is being addressed adequately, as critically ill patients are in the critical care areas in spite of the research stating that the workload of the RN even in Medical/Surgical units has increased due to patients being more acutely ill and their conditions more complex [1,2]. One CNO did believe that being an advocate for the nurse by making sure the nurse was set up for success would contribute greatly to the quality outcomes of patients. This CNO understood how the nurse and the patient are connected and the needs of both are required to be met in order for success in obtaining quality patient outcomes. One CNO advocated for resources for nurses in the work environment and found that not only did the nurses feel successful but quality patient outcomes were realized. As a nurse leader being an advocate for the patient involves first being an advocate for the nurse to succeed in obtaining consistent patient outcomes. A conflict between nurse productivity standards and nursing satisfaction was a concern raised by another CNO, as senior executives do not want to see unionization or poor public relations in the media concerning their facilities.

## 7. Implications

The majority of the CNOs in these two studies experienced conflict between advocacy for the patient versus advocacy for the nurse. However, they are interrelated. Being an advocate for the nurse results in better advocacy and outcomes for the patients. Therefore, the CNO of the twenty-first century needs to have the undergraduate to graduate nursing educational foundation incorporating fundamental dynamics and relevance of the true nature of nursing, the nurse and the patient. This would include the relationship between the successful nursing environment and consistent patient care outcomes. Primary to advanced leadership development, infrastructure of the healthcare environment, financial management of healthcare systems, along with assessment, critical thinking, clinical skills, analysis and interventions of patient centered care are subjects that should be taught throughout the curriculum. The prerequisites for a BSN degree could be more inclusive of these important areas of development. The graduate level of the nursing curriculum would continue these concepts in more depth and help further hone critical thought processes for even more successful nurse executives. The results would be extremely effective for the future of nursing in all levels of leadership by performing the skills of listening, understanding, analytical reasoning, relational development, persistence, and courage within the decision making and delegating processes of nursing. The results based on the strengths and areas of potential development evidenced in these two studies across various hospital settings reveal the need to update leadership development in all levels of academia (Figure 1). This will provide the sustainability, vision, and consistency of quality patient outcomes. Knowledge is a form of power and this will promote the ability, confidence, and innovation to a profession that has had turmoil and discord for more than a century [27–29].

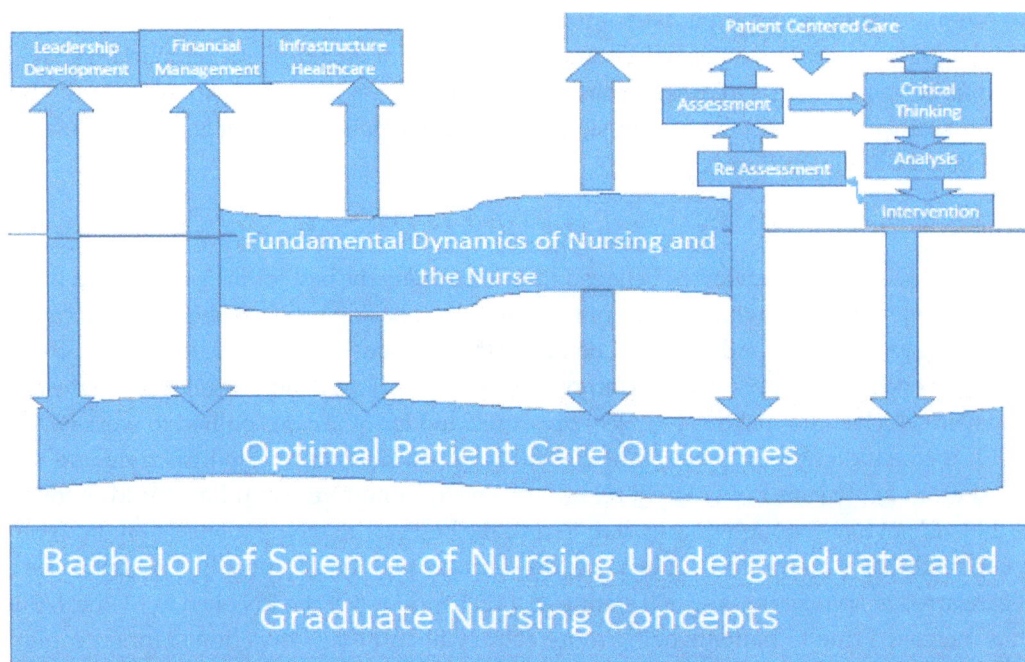

**Figure 1.** An adaption of universal Leadership and Nursing components combined by Ingwell-Spolan (2017) into the Nursing undergraduate and graduate nursing concepts.

Change is difficult, but inevitable and necessary. Adapting to ever changing initiatives in healthcare systems, reacting to situations rather than being proactive, all lead to less than optimally effective patient care outcomes. For nursing to attain its true position in the healthcare industry, we must pursue these endeavors; moving forward with cohesive purpose, starting in academia, both undergraduate and graduate levels, threading through professional practice while respecting all nursing specialties and health care disciplines. The Nursing collaboration with academia and private sector are key for the future success of our profession's achieving optimal patient care outcomes.

**Author Contributions:** C.I.-S., conceived and designed the experiments; performed the experiments; analyzed the data; and wrote the paper.

## References

1. Copanitsanou, P.; Fotos, N.; Brokalaki, H. Effects of work environment on patient and nurse outcomes. *Br. J. Nurs.* **2017**, *26*, 172–176. [CrossRef] [PubMed]

2. Chiang, H.Y.; Hsiao, Y.C.; Lee, H.F. Predictors of hospital nurse's safety practices: Work environment, workload, job satisfaction, and error reporting. *J. Nurs. Care Qual.* **2017**, *32*, 359–368. [CrossRef] [PubMed]

3. Johansen, M.; Cadmus, E. Conflict management style, supportive work environments and the experience of work stress in emergency nurses. *J. Nurs. Manag.* **2016**, *24*, 211–218. [CrossRef] [PubMed]

4. McHugh, M.; Rochman, M.; Sloane, D.; Berg, R.; Mancine, M.; Nadkarmi, V.; Merchant, R.; Aiken, L. Better nurse staffing and nurse work environments associated with increased survival of in-hospital cardiac arrest patients. *Med. Care* **2016**, *54*, 74–80. [CrossRef] [PubMed]

5. Flynn, L.; Liang, Y.; Dickson, G.; Xie, M.; Dong-Churl, S. Nurse's practice environments, error interception on practices, and impatient medication errors. *J. Nurs. Sch.* **2012**, *44*, 180–186. [CrossRef] [PubMed]

6. Lacher, S.; Degeest, S.; Denhaerynck, K.; Trede, I.; Ausserhofer, D. The quality of nurses' work environment and workforce outcomes from the perspective of swiss allied healthcare assistants and registered nurses: A cross-sectional survey. *J. Nurs. Sch.* **2015**, *47*, 458–467. [CrossRef] [PubMed]

7. Unruh, L.; Zhang, N.J. The role of work environment in keeping newly licensed RNS in nursing: A questionnaire survey. *Int. J. Nurs Stud.* **2013**, *50*, 1678–1688. [CrossRef] [PubMed]

8. Wheeler, R.; Foster, J.; Hepburn, K. The experience of discrimination by US and internationally educated nurses in hospital practice in the USA: A qualitative study. *J. Adv. Nurs.* **2013**, *70*, 350–359. [CrossRef] [PubMed]

9. Westerberg, K.; Tafrelin, S. The importance of leadership style and psychosocial work environment to staff-assessed quality of care: Implications for home help services. *Health Soc. Care Community* **2014**, *22*, 461–468. [CrossRef] [PubMed]

10. American Organization of Nurse Executives (AONE). Nurse Executive Competencies. 2018. Available online: http://www.aone.org/resource/system-core-competencies (accessed on 20 March 2018).

11. Roch, G.; Dubois, C.; Clarke, S. Organizational climate and hospital nurses' caring practices: A mixed methods study. *Res. Nurs. Health* **2014**, *37*, 229–240. [CrossRef] [PubMed]

12. Shirey, M. Leadership practices for healthy work environments. *Nurs. Manag.* **2017**, *48*, 42–50. [CrossRef] [PubMed]

13. Valentine, N.; Kirby, K.; Wolf, K. The CNO/CFO partnership: Navigating the changing landscape. *Nurs. Econ.* **2011**, *29*, 201–210. [PubMed]

14. American Organization of Nurse Executive Foundation (AONE). Interview: Donna Havens. 2018. Available online: http://www.Aone.org/aone-foundation/research/havens.shtml (accessed on 20 March 2018).

15. Duffy, J.; Hoskins, L. The quality caring model: Blending dual paradigms. *Adv. Nurs. Sci.* **2003**, *2*, 77–88. [CrossRef]

16. O'Nan, C.; Jenkins, K.; Morgan, L.; Adams, T. Evaluation of duffy's quality caring model on patients' perceptions of nurse caring in a community hospital. *Int. J. Hum. Caring* **2014**, *18*, 27–34. [CrossRef]

17. Aguayo, R. *Dr. Demming, the American Who Taught the Japanese Quality*; Simon & Schuster: New York, NY, USA, 1991.

18. Gausvik, C.; Lautar, H.; Miller, L.; Palleria, H.; Schlaudecker, J. Structured nursing communication on interdisciplinary acute care teams improves perceptions of safety, efficiency, understanding of care plan and teamwork as well as job satisfaction. *J. Multidiscip. Healthc.* **2015**, *8*, 33–37. [CrossRef] [PubMed]

19. Whiting, S.; Maynes, T.; Podsakoff, N.; Podsakoff, P. Effects of message, source and context on evaluations of employee voice behavior. *J. Appl. Psychol.* **2012**, *97*, 159–182. [CrossRef] [PubMed]

20. Suhonen, R.; Stolt, M.; Gustafsson, M.; Katajisto, J.; Charalambous, S. The associations among the ethical climate, the professional practice environment and individualized care in care settings for older people. *J. Adv. Nurs.* **2013**, *70*, 1356–1368. [CrossRef] [PubMed]

21. Selanders, L.; Crane, P. The voice of Florence nightingale on advocacy. *Online J. Issues Nurs.* **2012**, *17*, 1–10. [PubMed]

22. Lincoln, Y.S.; Guba, E.G. *Naturalistic Inquiry*; Sage: Newbury Park, CA, USA, 1985.

23. Robert Wood Johnson Foundation & Institute of Medicine. *The Future of Nursing: Leading Change, Advancing Healthcare*; The National Academies Press: Washington, DC, USA, 2011.

24. Middleton, R. Active learning and leadership in an undergraduate curriculum: How effective is it for student learning and transition to practice? *Nurse Educ. Pract.* **2013**, *13*, 83–88. [CrossRef] [PubMed]

25. Lizy, M. An examination of transformational leadership among graduating baccalaureate nursing students and practicing nurses. *Open J. Nurs.* **2014**, *4*, 737–742.

26. Dubrosky, R. Iris young's five faces of oppression applied to nursing. *Nurs. Forum* **2013**, *48*, 205–209. [CrossRef] [PubMed]

27. Helmstadter, C.; Godden, J. *Nursing before Nightingale, 1815–1899*; Ashgate: Burlington, VT, USA, 2011.

28. Keddy, B.; Jones, G.; Bulton, H.; Rogers, M. The doctor-nurse relationship: An historical perspective. *J. Adv. Nurs.* **1986**, *11*, 745–753. [CrossRef] [PubMed]

29. University of Virginia School of Nursing Center for Historical Inquiry. Binghamton is over-crowded. *Am. J. Nurs.* **1930**, *30*, 344.

# 17

# Rational Use of Medicines in Neonates: Current Observations, Areas for Research and Perspectives

Karel Allegaert [1,2]

[1]   Department of Pediatrics, Division of Neonatology, Erasmus MC-Sophia Children's Hospital, Doctor Molenwaterplein 40, 3015 GD Rotterdam, The Netherlands; k.allegaert@erasmusmc.nl or karel.allegaert@uzleuven.be

[2]   Department of Development and Regeneration, KU Leuven, Herestraat 49, 3000 Leuven, Belgium

**Abstract:** A focused reflection on rational medicines use in neonates is valuable and relevant, because indicators to assess rational medicines use are difficult to apply to neonates. Polypharmacy and exposure to antibiotics are common, while dosing regimens or clinical guidelines are only rarely supported by robust evidence in neonates. This is at least in part due to the extensive variability in pharmacokinetics and subsequent effects of medicines in neonates. Medicines utilization research informs us on trends, on between unit variability and on the impact of guideline implementation. We illustrate these aspects using data on drugs for gastroesophageal reflux, analgesics or anti-epileptic drugs. Areas for additional research are drug-related exposure during breastfeeding (exposure prediction) and how to assess safety (tools to assess seriousness, causality, and severity tailored to neonates) since both efficacy and safety determine rational drug use. To further improve rational medicines use, we need more data and tools to assess efficacy and safety in neonates. Moreover, we should facilitate access to such data, and explore strategies for effective implementation. This is because prescription practices are not only rational decisions, but also have psychosocial aspects that may guide clinicians to irrational practices, in part influenced by the psychosocial characteristics of this population.

**Keywords:** newborn; rational drug utilization; perinatal pharmacology; clinical pharmacology; effective implementation

---

## 1. Introduction

*"Why a focused reflection on rational use of medicines in neonates is valuable and relevant."*

The World Health Organization (WHO) defines the rational use of medicines as the use of medicines so that individual patients receive medicines that are appropriate to their clinical needs, in doses in accordance with their own individual requirements, for the appropriate period of time, and at the lowest or reasonable cost to both the individual and the community [1]. Rational use of medicines relates to: (i) an *accurate strategy and monitoring on medicines use* (advocating rational medicines use, identifying and promoting successful strategies, and securing responsible medicines promotion); (ii) *rational use of medicines by health professionals* (develop and update national guidelines, essential medicines list, and training on rational medicines use); and (iii) *rational use of medicines by consumers/patients* (develop and support effective systems of medicines information and empower consumers/patients to take responsible and well-educated decisions regarding medicines use) [1].

The WHO estimate that more than 50% of the medicines are prescribed, dispensed or sold inappropriately and that about 50% of patients fail to take their medicines correctly. These inaccuracies result in wastage of resources, additional health risks, suboptimal management or failure to use proven more effective interventions (failed opportunity cost). Commonly used indicators of potential irrational practices are the incidence of polypharmacy, inappropriate use of antibiotics (dose, indication, duration, and route of administration), inappropriate self-medication, or failure to adhere to clinical guidelines or dosing regimens [1]. Consequently, irrational use of medicines is a major and global problem, but has specific issues when we focus on rational medicines use in neonates [1–3]. These issues relate to current practices and areas in need of additional research.

As documented in the latest Pediatrix analysis (2005–2010, $n$ = 450,386 neonates), only 35% of the medicines were FDA-approved. Polypharmacy in neonates turned out to be common, with a mean number of medicines courses of 4 (1–14) per infant, raising up to 17 (2–45) courses in extreme low birth weight (ELBW < 1 kg) infants. Moreover, 16 antibiotics were observed in the Top 50, and 3 (ampicillin, gentamicin, and vancomycin) in the Top 5 most commonly administered drugs [4]. The majority of drugs in neonates are prescribed and administered in a hospital setting. Consequently, inaccurate exposure to medicines almost exclusively relates to organizational issues and drug errors within health care facilities. Dosing errors were identified as the most common error, with computerized physician order entry and interventions by clinical pharmacists as most common interventions suggested to reduce drug errors in neonates [2,5]. The risk for errors in neonates is further increased because of the absence of sufficient evidence on pharmacotherapy and the lack of formulations tailored to neonates [2].

Compared to the available data on benefits and risks to make rational decisions on medicine use in adults, the existing information to make such informed decisions in neonates is much more limited. Off-label or unlicensed use of drugs remains most prevalent in neonates [6]. Medicines utilization research serves as a tool to assess if medicines use is rational. In neonates, this goal is largely hampered because of the extensive off-label and unlicensed medicines use. *Quality* (compare practices to guidelines and local drug formularies), *patterns* (extent or profiles of drug use and trends), *outcomes* (health outcomes and both benefits and adverse effects) or *determinants* (prescriber characteristics and impact of interventions) can still be explored as potential indicators of irrational practices [7,8].

In this narrative review on rational medicines use in neonates, we highlight trends on anti-reflux drugs (Section 2.1), analgesics (Section 2.2) and anti-epileptics (Section 2.3) as Anatomical Therapeutic Chemical (ATC) Classification System classes to illustrate issues related to implementation of rational medicine use in this population. This is preceded by a short topical introduction on the specific characteristics of neonatal clinical pharmacology, and followed by highlighting some areas for future research (breastfeeding (Section 3.1) and drug safety assessment in neonates (Section 3.2)). We deliberately do not cover aspects related to antibiotics, since patterns of empiric antibiotic administration, the extensive variability in practices, the limited evidence to support practices, and strategies to implement antimicrobial stewardship have recently been described [9–14].

## 2. Neonatal Clinical Pharmacology

*"Extensive variability in dosing and effects are the key characteristics of neonatal clinical pharmacology. The impact of medicines to improve outcome and rational medicines use in neonates remains underexplored."*

When clinicians prescribe medicines to neonates, it is with the intention to provide the newborn an effective intervention, avoiding disproportional side-effects. Clinical pharmacology aims to estimate the effects of such interventions, using pharmacokinetics (PK) and pharmacodynamics (PD) to generate predictions, including a grade of certainty and confidence intervals. PK (absorption, distribution and elimination, through either metabolism or renal elimination) estimates the concentration–time relationship. PD aims to estimate (side-)effects of a specific medicine (concentration–effect relationship). Very specific to newborns are the fast maturational changes in neonatal life with weight and age as main drivers of this maturation, resulting in extensive between- and within-individual variability in PK and subsequent PD [15]. Non-maturational changes further add to the variability. Observed non-maturational changes relate to co-medication such as ibuprofen, pharmacogenetics or co-morbidity (sepsis snf asphyxia) [16]. At best, this means that dosing regimens of medicines in newborns should be based on integrated knowledge concerning the specific diseases to be treated, the maturational and non-maturational characteristics of the newborn, and the PK and PD estimates of the medicine.

Consequently, the potential health impact of neonatal pharmacotherapy remains underexplored. It is still very common practice to administer medicines outside their authorization. Although off-label is not necessarily equal to off-knowledge, this does result in the fact that clinicians commonly lack the crucial information to make the best possible, informed decision. Unfortunately, history repeatedly provided evidence that newborns are more prone to specific adverse reactions to drugs, although some of these adverse reactions may have been anticipated based on the available knowledge on developmental pharmacology illustrated in Table 1 [2,3].

**Table 1.** Illustrations of clinical relevant adverse drug reactions in neonates, with the mechanisms involved.

| Compound | Clinical Syndrome | Mechanisms Involved | Potential Similarities |
|---|---|---|---|
| Sulfisoxazole | "kernicterus" | Highly albumin bound antibiotic, competitive with endogenous compounds, including bilirubin. This results in higher free bilirubin concentrations and subsequent kernicterus. | Similar effects can be anticipated for other high protein bound medicines such as ceftriaxone or diphantoine. |
| Chloramphenicol | "grey baby syndrome" | Impaired glucuronidation capacity, results in chloramphenicol accumulation and subsequent mitochondrial dysfunction, circulatory collapse and death. | Similar effects can be anticipated for other glucuronidation dependent drug metabolism compounds, such as paracetamol or propofol. |
| Kaletra (lopinavir/ritonavir) | "alcohols" | Kaletra syrup contains both ethanol and propylene glycol. Impaired metabolic clearance results in accumulation, and subsequent hyperosmolality, lactic acidosis, renal toxicity, central nervous system impairment, cardiac arrhythmia, hemolysis and collapse. | Explained by ethanol/propylene glycol, competition for hepatic metabolic elimination. |
| Codeine by breastfeeding | "SIDS" | Exposure to morphine after conversion from codeine, related to an ultrafast metabolizer maternal genotype. The newborn has a poor glucuronidation and renal elimination capacity, resulting in accumulation, sedation, and sudden infant death syndrome. | Similar effects can be anticipated by other analgesics, such as oxycodone. |
| Ceftriaxone + Calcium | "collaps" | Simultaneous administration of calcium containing infusions and ceftriaxone results in intravascular precipitate, as observed during autopsy. | May be similar for other "mixtures" with calcium containing formulations. |
| Topical iodide | "hypothyroidism" | More pronounced skin permeability and higher body surface area results in more effective absorption of iodine with subsequent suppression of thyroid function. | Similar for other topical compounds, e.g., steroids and hexachlorophene. |

In the current narrative review, we focus on drug utilization of specific ATC groups, such as drugs for peptic ulcer and gastroesophageal reflux (Section 2.1), analgesics (Section 2.2) or anti-epileptics (Section 2.3), in neonates; drug utilization studies to illustrate how such studies can inform us on trends over time; between unit variability; and the impact of implementation of guidelines on drug utilization patterns.

### 2.1. Drugs for Peptic Ulcer and Gastroesophageal Reflux Disease (ATC Class A02B)

*"We should be aware that a shift in practices because of a documented safety issue may result in a subsequent irrational practice with another drug."*

Gastroesophageal reflux is commonly defined as the passage of acid or non-acid gastric fluids back into the esophagus. This diagnosis is frequently made during neonatal stay, and is claimed to be link to apnea-bradycardia events [17]. While cisapride decreases the incidence of GOR events, the impact on reflux-related apnea was much weaker [18]. Once this compound was withdrawn from the market because of cardiac arrhythmia events, there was a shift to acid reducing drugs and other pro-kinetics. This occurred despite the lack of evidence that gastric acid reducing drugs are effective to reduce gastric acid production, reflux and apnea. More recently and following this shift, there was also emerging evidence on relevant harm (higher incidence of necrotizing enterocolitis or late onset sepsis) [17,19].

Using the analyses on trends as published in two consecutive Pediatrix (1997–2004 and 2005–2010) cohorts, the impact of these findings into clinical practices are reflected [4,20]. In the first (1997–2004) cohort, there was a significant decrease for cisapride (7.5% to 0%, neonates exposed during neonatal stay). However, this decrease was mirrored by a significant increase in metoclopramide (2.2% to 10%) and ranitidine (5.5% to 8%) between 1997 and 2004, while proton pump inhibitors (PPIs, omeprazole and pantoprazole) were not yet present in the Top 30 list of most commonly administered drugs in neonates. In the second (2005–2010) time interval, Hsieh et al. observed a subsequent decrease in metoclopramide (−84%, from 88 to 14/1000 neonates) and ranitidine (−61%, from 80 to 31/1000 neonates), mirrored by an increase in lanzoprazole (+58%, from 9.8 to 16/1000 neonates) exposure. The stable prescription of erythromycin (27th and 24th most commonly prescribed drug in the consecutive cohorts) also illustrates the limitations of such analysis without simultaneous collection of data on indications (infection related or as prokinetic) [4,20]. A strategy how to implement a guideline (set at target, plan–do–study–act, feedback and education) to decrease the use of acid-suppressing medicines in a neonatal intensive care unit has recently been described [21].

## 2.2. Analgesics (ATC Class N02)

*"Increased exposure to analgesics and the extensive variability observed in drug prescription practices is concerning given the limited evidence of benefit and potential harm. Implementation strategies to structure rational use of analgesics are effective."*

Effective analgesia in neonates is relevant not only because of ethics or empathy, but also since a crucial and valid part of contemporary nursing and medical practice. However, and resulting in the need for a balanced approach, there is also emerging evidence on the extent of exposure to analgesics and poorer neurodevelopmental outcome in neonates. Consequently, the increased exposure to analgesics over time and the extensive variability observed in drug prescription practice is concerning given the limited evidence of benefit and the potential harm [4,20,22–24].

The Pediatrix consortium reported on medication use in two consecutive time intervals (1997–2004 and 2005–2010). When we compare these cohorts, fentanyl and morphine were in the Top 30 list (19th and 25th) with an estimated exposure of 56 and 35/1000 admitted neonates in the 1997–2004 cohort, respectively, and were observed seventh and 14th (estimated exposure of 70 and 51/1000 neonates, respectively) in the 2005–2010 cohort [4,20,24]. Using the same Pediatrix dataset (1997–2012) with focus on the use of analgesics, sedatives and paralytics in ventilated preterms (<1500 g, <32 weeks, $n = 8591$), Zimmerman et al. documented that—despite the meta-analytical evidence [25]—opioid exposure increased from 5% to 32% of ventilation days [24]. In the Canadian network, extensive between unit variability in prescriptions was observed (3–41% analgesics), not explained by clinical characteristics [23]. A similar pattern (common (26%) opioid exposure and extensive variability) has been reported in the EUROPAIN cohort [22].

Implementation exercises of guidelines on opioid use are effective to reduce the utilization of these drugs and its variability [26]. This reduction in exposure was reflected in the number of patients (from 63% to 33%) and the cumulative morphine dose (from 1.64 to 0.51 mg/kg, −68%). Interestingly, this implementation effort also resulted in a significant reduction in the number of cases (from 10/205 to 3/250 cases, $p < 0.05$) requiring methadone treatment for iatrogenic NAS syndrome [26].

## 2.3. Anti-Epileptic Drugs (ATC Class N03A)

*"Rational use of AED medicines necessitates the development of more advanced tools to improve the accuracy of the diagnosis, while better knowledge on pathways involved in the 'seizures' phenotype in neonates is needed to further individualize treatment."*

The Pediatrix consortium reported on the prescription of anti-epileptic drugs (AED) in two consecutive time periods (1997–2004 compared to 2005–2010), analyzing the same administrative database. Phenobarbital was prescribed in 4.5% and 3.8% of cases in these time intervals, and midazolam in 3.8% and 6.1%. [4,20]. More recently, but using the same Pediatrix database (2005–2014, $n = 9134/778,395$, 1.1% with seizures), Ahmad et al. confirmed that neonates with seizures are still overwhelmingly exposed to phenobarbital with a very minor decease over the studied time interval (from 99% to 96%), a decrease in phenytoin use (from 15% to 11%), and a very relevant increase in levetiracetam (from 1.4% to 14%) with carbamazepine, lidocaine or topiramate as rarely administered AEDs in neonates (all < 1%) [27]. Similar to the earlier mentioned issue on erythromycin use, it is also difficult to assess trends in the prescription of benzodiazepines when either seizures or sedation is aimed for. Despite this comment, we can still reflect about the available data.

First, the still overwhelming use of phenobarbital as first line AED is suboptimal and unique to neonates, since cumulative phenobarbital exposure is associated with a decrease in cognitive and motor Bayley scores (8 and 9 IQ points, respectively, for every 100 mg phenobarbital/kg body weight), and a higher risk for cerebral palsy (2.3-fold) [28]. Second, different approaches have been considered to proceed to better evidence and rational drug utilization. These strategies included more advanced technology with bedside neuro-physiological monitoring (*reduce the number of inaccurate diagnoses*) instead of clinical observations based on motor or autonomic events, and strategies to reduce the mean phenobarbital burden and reduction in the incidence of AED exposure at discharge (*reduce the duration of exposure in treated newborns*) [29]. Even more promising, better insights into the variety of mechanisms (asphyxia, infarction, channelopathies, and metabolic syndromes) involved in the "seizure phenotype" should enable us to shift from a "one drug fits all" approach to individualized pharmacotherapy (*better mechanism driven medicine selection*) [30].

## 3. Areas in Need of Research on Perinatal Drug Exposure

### 3.1. Breastfeeding

*"It is a misconception that a 'when in doubt, do not provide breastfeeding' approach has no negative effects. We need new tools to quantify breastfeeding related exposure and tools to provide access to this information."*

Lactating women regularly take medicines, and are commonly advised to interrupt or even stop nursing while taking medicines, even though only a limited number of medicines have been identified as (likely) harmful. Since breastfeeding itself also provides clinically relevant benefits to both mother and infant, it is a misconception that *"when in doubt, do not provide breastfeeding"* has no negative effects [31,32]. Consequently, the overarching intention of maternal intake of medicines during nursing should fulfill two criteria: (i) provide effective and safe medicines for the mother; and (ii) assure safety of nursing newborns from adverse events related to these medicines following breastfeeding related exposure as well as the adverse events related to the interruption of breastfeeding [31,32]. The relevance of these balanced decisions is illustrated with the impact of breastfeeding on neonatal abstinence syndrome (NAS) and the neurodevelopment outcome following breastfeeding related exposure to anti-epileptic drugs (AED) following fetal exposure.

The effects of breastfeeding on the incidence and severity of opioid-related NAS have been quantified. In essence, there is a significant reduction in the incidence (number needed to treat 5–6) and the severity of NAS during breastfeeding [33]. Similarly, the impact of breastfeeding on neurocognitive outcome following AED exposure during pregnancy and lactation has been documented by the

Neurodevelopmental Effects of antiepileptic drugs (NEAD) group. At six years, children of mothers on AEDs had a higher (11.5% instead of 4.8%) risk of impaired fine motor skills compared with controls and a lower and dose dependent IQ (from −6 to −9 IQ point) following fetal valproate exposure when compared to other AEDs. Building on these background characteristics, subsequent breastfeeding in infants of women using AEDs was associated with *improved* neurodevelopment outcome compared with those with either no breastfeeding or breastfeeding for less than six months [34,35]. Overall, the adjusted IQ was higher by four points for children who were breastfed compared to those who were not. The difference in IQ was most pronounced in the valproate group (+12, range, 1–24 IQ) [35]. To facilitate more rational decisions on this topic, we need more advanced tools to generate knowledge, and we should subsequently ensure access to this evolving knowledge.

Physiologically-based pharmacokinetic (PB and PK) modeling tools are evolving and have been used to assess fetal or infant exposure to toxic compounds such as perfluoro-alkyl substances or mercury [36]. These models can also be applied to convert observations on drug levels in human milk into a population distribution to assess drug exposure and subsequent safety in newborns. Using a rather small dataset of 18 breastfeeding women on escitalopram, PB and PK methods served as tool to generate an average estimate (1.7%, range 0.5–5.9%) of the maternal plasma area under the curve [37]. However, such approaches mainly estimate population average exposure, not necessary covering all individual outlier patterns due to, e.g., polymorphisms [38].

There are different initiatives to subsequently ensure access to these data. LactMed is a free, easily accessible online database with information on drugs and lactation as one of the newest additions to the National Library of Medicine's TOXNET system [39]. Such an online tool facilitates updates when additional information becomes available. Along the same line, and related to the Pregnancy and Lactation Labeling Final Rule, the FDA requests a more narrative description of the available evidence on medicines use during pregnancy in three subsections, including "lactation". The "lactation" section hereby aims to provide information about the use of medicines while breastfeeding, such as the amount of medicines observed in human milk and effects on the nursing infant [40].

### 3.2. How to Assess Drug Safety in Neonates

*"How to retrieve, qualify and quantify the drug safety signal in the noise."*

An adverse event is any untoward medical occurrence in a patient or trial participant exposed to a medicine. Adverse event assessment relates to seriousness, causality and severity, but all have their issues when applied to neonates. *Seriousness* is a regulatory concept, but prolongation of existing hospitalization in a (preterm) newborn is sometimes difficult to assess. *Causality* necessitates the disentangling of adverse drug events from confounding events such as organ dysfunction, maturational changes or co-morbidity. The more commonly used tools such as the Naranjo algorithm do not sufficiently reliably document causality in neonates, and none of these tools has been validated in this setting. A specific tool to assess causality in neonates has been suggested, but has not yet undergone prospective validation in the clinical setting [41]. The same holds true for *severity* (mild, moderate, severe, life threating or death) grading. Severity scales exist, but none of these grading scores is fully tailored to neonates. The generic criteria (instrumental activities of daily life (ADL), or self-care) are not applicable to neonates, and typical neonatal adverse events are still lacking. This necessitates development in a consensus approach, with subsequent prospective validation. At least, harmonization of the adverse event assessment enables clinicians, parents and regulatory bodies to compare treatment modalities on their effects and side-effects.

### 4. Discussion: Perspectives to Further Improve Rational Use of Medicines in Neonates

*"We like to believe that decisions on medicines use in neonates are driven by rational processes, but we should also explore the psychosocial aspects that guide our decisions."*

Using a narrative approach, we illustrate that a focused reflection on rational medicines use in neonates is valuable and relevant. We hereby documente that polypharmacy and exposure to antibiotics are very common, while dosing regimens or clinical guidelines are only rarely supported by robust evidence in neonates. Consequently, extensive variability in practices is observed. Medicines utilization research informs us on trends, on between unit variability and on the impact of guideline implementation. This utilization research is not limited to exposure to antibiotics [4,9–14,20], but has been illustrated using data on drugs for gastroesophageal reflux, analgesics or anti-epileptic drugs [4,17–21]. We hereby illustrate how a shift in practices can result in another irrational practice with another compound (shift from prokinetics to anti-acid drugs to treat reflux associated-apnea). Extensive variability in the use of analgesics is observed. For both ATC groups, research on implementation strategies proved to be effective [21,26]. For AEDs, we use the data on the minor shifts in drug utilization patterns to illustrate the relevance to develop tools for more accurate diagnosis, and guidelines to reduce the duration of exposure [27]. Finally, we need more data on the mechanisms involved in the "neonatal seizures phenotype" to shift away from the currently "one drug fits all" approach to a more individualized AED use [30].

The need to develop more tailored tools to assess exposure, efficacy and safety of medicines in neonates is not limited to these ATCs or clinical syndromes. This was subsequently illustrated by the need to generate additional tools to predict medicine related exposure through breastfeeding and to facilitate access to data (online tools and regulatory initiatives). Similarly, tailored tools are needed to assess all aspects of safety (seriousness, causality, and severity tailored to neonates) since both efficacy and safety determine rational medicine use: *How can the signal in the noise be recognized?*

However, we should be aware that clinical decision making and drug utilization practices are not only just rational decisions, but also have psychosocial aspects that may guide clinicians, parents and stakeholders: *people in general do not make choices by acting only as rational balancers of risk (safety) and reward (efficacy)* [42]. These drivers, patterns and irrational practices may also be different due to the specific characteristics of this vulnerable population. This is at present still a poorly explored area in medicine, even more when we focus on perinatal or neonatal medicine.

This means that progress on rational use of medicines in neonates will not only depend on the generation of high-quality data on efficacy and safety (*"knowledge"*) and the related new tools (*"methods"*) to assess these outcome variables, but also on the subsequent approaches to facilitate access to such data and the development of implementation strategies. Data access and implementation strategies should not only facilitate technical access to data or guidelines, but should also consider the most effective strategies (*"skills"*) to approach caregivers not only as rational decision makers, but also cover the psychosocial aspects involved in the decision process of medicines prescription.

In conclusion, to further improve rational medicines use, we need more data, and tools to assess efficacy and safety in neonates. Moreover, we should facilitate access to such data, and explore strategies for effective implementation. This is because prescription practices are not only rational decisions, but also have psychosocial aspects that may guide clinicians to irrational practices, in part influenced by the psychosocial characteristics of this population.

**Funding:** This research was funded by the agency for innovation by Science and Technology in Flanders (IWT) Safepedrug grant number (IWT/SBO 130033).

## References

1.    World Health Organization. Essential Medicines and Health Products. The Pursuit of Responsible Use of Medicines. Available online: https://www.who.int/medicines/areas/rational_use/en (accessed on 20 August 2018).

2.    Allegaert, K.; Van den Anker, J.N. Adverse drug reactions in neonates and infants: A population-tailored approach is needed. *Br. J. Clin. Pharmacol.* **2015**, *80*, 788–795. [CrossRef] [PubMed]

3.    Choonara, I. Educational paper: Aspects of clinical pharmacology in children—Pharmacovigilance and safety. *Eur. J. Pediatr.* **2013**, *172*, 577–580. [CrossRef] [PubMed]

4.    Hsieh, E.M.; Hornik, C.P.; Clark, R.H.; Laughon, M.M.; Benjamin, D.K., Jr.; Smith, P.B. On behalf of the Best Pharmaceuticals for Children Act—Pediatric Trials Network. Medication use in the neonatal intensive care unit. *Am. J. Perinatol.* **2014**, *31*, 811–821. [CrossRef] [PubMed]

5.    Chedoe, I.; Molendijk, H.A.; Dittrich, S.T.; Jansman, F.G.; Harting, J.W.; Brouwers, J.R.; Taxis, K. Incidence and nature of medication errors in neonatal intensive care with strategies to improve safety: A review of the current literature. *Drug. Saf.* **2007**, *30*, 503–513. [CrossRef] [PubMed]

6.    Ward, R.M.; Benjamin, D.; Barrett, J.S.; Allegaert, K.; Portman, R.; Davis, J.M.; Turner, M.A. Safety, dosing, and pharmaceutical quality for studies that evaluate medicinal products (including biological products) in neonates. *Pediatr. Res.* **2017**, *81*, 692–711. [CrossRef] [PubMed]

7.    Rosli, R.; Dali, A.F.; Abd Aziz, N.; Abdullah, A.H.; Ming, L.C.; Manan, M.M. Drug utilization on neonatal wards: A systematic review of observational studies. *Front. Pharmacol.* **2017**, *8*, 27. [CrossRef] [PubMed]

8.    Osokogu, O.U.; Verhamme, K.; Sturkenboom, M.; Kaguelidou, F. Pharmacoepidemiology in pediatrics: Needs, challenges and future directions for research. *Thérapie* **2018**, *73*, 151–156. [CrossRef] [PubMed]

9.    Oliver, E.A.; Reagan, P.B.; Slaughter, J.L.; Buhimschi, C.S.; Buhimschi, I.A. Patterns of empiric antibiotic administration for presumed early-onset neonatal sepsis in neonatal intensive care units in the United States. *Am. J. Perinatol.* **2017**, *34*, 640–647. [CrossRef] [PubMed]

10.   Nzegwu, N.I.; Rychalsky, M.R.; Nallu, L.A.; Song, X.; Deng, Y.; Natusch, A.M.; Baltimore, R.S.; Paci, G.R.; Bizzarro, M.J. Implementation of an antimicrobial stewardship program in a neonatal intensive care unit. *Infect. Control. Hosp. Epidemiol.* **2017**, *38*, 1137–1143. [CrossRef] [PubMed]

11.   Esaiassen, E.; Fjalstad, J.W.; Juvet, L.K.; van den Anker, J.N.; Klingenberg, C. Antibiotic exposure in neonates and early adverse outcomes: A systematic review and meta-analysis. *J. Antimicrob. Chemother.* **2017**, *72*, 1858–1870. [CrossRef] [PubMed]

12.   Wilbaux, M.; Fuchs, A.; Samardzic, J.; Rodieux, F.; Csajka, C.; Allegaert, K.; Van den Anker, J.N.; Pfister, M. Pharmacometric approaches to personalize use of primarily renally eliminated antibiotics in preterm and term neonates. *J. Clin. Pharmacol.* **2016**, *56*, 909–935. [CrossRef] [PubMed]

13.   Allegaert, K.; Van den Anker, J. Neonates are not just little children and need more finesse in dosing of antibiotics. *Acta Clin. Belg.* **2018**. [CrossRef] [PubMed]

14.   Smits, A.; Kulo, A.; van den Anker, J.; Allegaert, K. The amikacin research program: A stepwise approach to validate dosing regimens in neonates. *Expert Opin. Drug. Metab. Toxicol.* **2017**, *13*, 157–166. [CrossRef] [PubMed]

15.   Allegaert, K.; Van den Anker, J. Neonatal drug therapy: The first frontier of therapeutics for children. *Clin. Pharmacol. Ther.* **2015**, *98*, 288–297. [CrossRef] [PubMed]

16.   Krekels, E.H.J.; van Hasselt, J.G.C.; Van den Anker, J.N.; Allegaert, K.; Tibboel, D.; Knibbe, C.A.J. Evidence-based drug treatment for special patient populations through model-based approaches. *Eur. J. Pharm. Sci.* **2017**, *109*, S22–S26. [CrossRef] [PubMed]

17.   Eichenwald, E.C. Committee on Fetus and Newborn. Diagnosis and management of gastroesophageal reflux in preterm infants. *Pediatrics* **2018**, *142*, e20181061. [CrossRef] [PubMed]

18.   Ariagno, R.L.; Kikkert, M.A.; Mirmiran, M.; Conrad, C.; Baldwin, R.B. Cisapride decreases gastroesophageal reflux in preterm infants. *Pediatrics* **2001**, *107*, e58. [CrossRef] [PubMed]

19.   Dermyshi, E.; Mackie, C.; Kigozi, P.; Schoonakker, B.; Dorling, J. Antacid therapy for gastroesophageal reflux in preterm infants: A systematic review. *BMJ Pediatr. Open* **2018**, *2*, e000287. [CrossRef] [PubMed]

20.   Clark, R.H.; Bloom, B.T.; Spitzer, A.R.; Gerstmann, D.R. Reported medication use in the neonatal intensive care unit: Data from a large national data set. *Pediatrics* **2006**, *117*, 1979–1987. [CrossRef] [PubMed]

21.   Angelidou, A.; Bell, K.; Gupta, M.; Tropea Leeman, K.; Hansen, A. Implementation of a guideline to decrease use of acid-suppressing medications in the NICU. *Pediatrics* **2017**, *140*, e20171715. [CrossRef] [PubMed]

22.   Carbajal, R.; Eriksson, M.; Courtois, E.; Boyle, E.; Avila-Alvarez, A.; Andersen, R.D.; Sarafidis, K.; Polkki, T.; Matos, C.; Lago, P.; et al. Sedation and analgesia practices in neonatal intensive care units (EUROPAIN): Results from a prospective cohort study. *Lancet Respir. Med.* **2015**, *3*, 796–812. [CrossRef]

23.   Borenstein-Levin, L.; Synnes, A.; Grunau, R.E.; Miller, S.P.; Yoon, E.W.; Shah, P.S. Canadian Neonatal Network Investigators. Narcotics and sedative use in preterm neonates. *J. Pediatr.* **2017**, *180*, 92–98. [CrossRef] [PubMed]

24. Zimmerman, K.O.; Smith, P.B.; Benjamin, D.K.; Laughon, M.; Clark, R.; Traube, C.; Stürmer, T.; Hornik, C.P. Sedation, analgesia, and paralysis during mechanical ventilation of premature infants. *J. Pediatr.* **2017**, *180*, 99–104. [CrossRef] [PubMed]

25. Bellù, R.; De Waal, K.; Zanini, R. Opioids for neonates receiving mechanical ventilation: A systematic review and meta-analysis. *Arch. Dis. Child. Fetal. Neonatal. Ed.* **2010**, *95*, F241–F251. [CrossRef] [PubMed]

26. Rana, D.; Bellflower, B.; Sahni, J.; Kaplan, A.J.; Owens, N.T.; Arrindell, E.L., Jr.; Talati, A.J.; Dhanireddy, R. Reduced narcotic and sedative utilization in a NICU after implementation of pain management guidelines. *J. Perinatol.* **2017**, *37*, 1038–1042. [CrossRef] [PubMed]

27. Ahmad, K.A.; Desai, S.J.; Bennett, M.M.; Ahmad, S.F.; Ng, Y.T.; Clark, R.H.; Tolia, V.N. Changing antiepileptic drug use for seizures in US neonatal intensive care units from 2005 to 2014. *J. Perinatol.* **2017**, *37*, 296–300. [CrossRef] [PubMed]

28. Maitre, N.L.; Smolinsky, C.; Slaughter, J.C.; Stark, A.R. Adverse neurodevelopmental outcomes after exposure to phenobarbital and levetiracetam for the treatment of neonatal seizures. *J. Perinatol.* **2013**, *33*, 841–846. [CrossRef] [PubMed]

29. Bashir, R.A.; Espinoza, L.; Vayalthrikkovil, S.; Buchhalter, J.; Irvine, L.; Bello-Espinosa, L.; Mohammad, K. Implementation of a neurocritical care program: Improved seizure detection and decreased antiseizure medication at discharge in neonates with hypoxic-ischemic encephalopathy. *Pediatr. Neurol.* **2016**, *64*, 38–43. [CrossRef] [PubMed]

30. Cornet, M.C.; Sands, T.T.; Cilio, M.R. Neonatal epilepsies: Clinical management. *Semin. Fetal. Neonatal. Med.* **2018**, *23*, 204–212. [CrossRef] [PubMed]

31. Sacker, A.; Kelly, Y.; Iacovou, M.; Cable, N.; Bartley, M. Breastfeeding and intergenerational social mobility: What are the mechanisms? *Arch. Dis. Child.* **2013**, *98*, 666–671. [CrossRef] [PubMed]

32. Bar, S.; Milanaik, R.; Adesman, A. Long-term neurodevelopmental benefits of breastfeeding. *Curr. Opin. Pediatr.* **2016**, *28*, 559–566. [CrossRef] [PubMed]

33. Lefevere, J.; Allegaert, K. Question: Is breastfeeding useful in the management of neonatal abstinence syndrome? *Arch. Dis. Child.* **2015**, *100*, 414–415. [CrossRef] [PubMed]

34. Veiby, G.; Bjørk, M.; Engelsen, B.A.; Gilhus, N.E. Epilepsy and recommendations for breastfeeding. *Seizure* **2015**, *28*, 57–65. [CrossRef] [PubMed]

35. Meador, K.J.; Baker, G.A.; Browning, N.; Cohen, M.J.; Bromley, R.L.; Clayton-Smith, J.; Kalayjian, L.A.; Kanner, A.; Liporace, J.D.; Pennell, P.B.; et al. Breastfeeding in children of women taking antiepileptic drugs: Cognitive outcomes at age 6 years. *JAMA Pediatr.* **2014**, *168*, 729–736. [CrossRef] [PubMed]

36. El-Masri, H.A.; Hong, T.; Henning, C.; Mendez, W., Jr.; Hudgens, E.E.; Thomas, D.J.; Lee, J.S. Evaluation of a physiologically based pharmacokinetic (PBPK) model for inorganic arsenic exposure using data from two diverse human populations. *Environ. Health Perspect.* **2018**, *126*, 077004. [CrossRef] [PubMed]

37. Delaney, S.R.; Malik, P.R.V.; Stefan, C.; Edginton, A.N.; Colantonio, D.A.; Ito, S. Predicting escitalopram exposure to breastfeeding infants: Integrating analytical and in silico techniques. *Clin. Pharmacokinet.* **2018**. [CrossRef] [PubMed]

38. Madadi, P.; Avard, D.; Koren, G. Pharmacogenetics of opioids for the treatment of acute maternal pain during pregnancy and lactation. *Curr. Drug Metab.* **2012**, *13*, 721–727. [CrossRef] [PubMed]

39. U.S. National Library of Medicine, National Institute of Health. Drugs and Lactation Database (LactMed). Available online: https://toxnet.nlm.nih.gov/newtoxnet/lactmed.htm (accessed on 20 August 2018).

40. U.S. Food and Drug Administration, U.S. Department of Health and Human Services. Pregnacy and Lactation Labeling (Drugs) Final Rule. Available online: https://www.fda.gov/drugs/developmentapprovalprocess/developmentresources/labeling/ucm093307.htm (accessed on 20 August 2018).

41. Du, W.; Lehr, V.T.; Lieh-Lai, M.; Koo, W.; Ward, R.M.; Rieder, M.J.; Van Den Anker, J.N.; Reeves, J.H.; Mathew, M.; Lulic-Botica, M.; et al. An algorithm to detect adverse drug reactions in the neonatal intensive care unit. *J. Clin. Pharmacol.* **2013**, *53*, 87–95. [CrossRef] [PubMed]

42. Avorn, J. The psychology of clinical decision making—Implications for medication use. *N. Engl. J. Med.* **2018**, *378*, 689–691. [CrossRef] [PubMed]

# 18

# Correlations of Self-Reported Androgen Deficiency in Ageing Males (ADAM) with Stress and Sleep among Young Adult Males

Camille M. Charlier [1], Makenzie L. Barr [2]⑩, Sarah E. Colby [3], Geoffrey W. Greene [4] and
Melissa D. Olfert [2],*⑩

1   Clinical & Translational Science, Health Sciences Center, West Virginia University,
    Morgantown, WV 26506, USA; ccharlie@hsc.wvu.edu
2   Davis College of Agriculture, Natural Resources and Design, Department of Animal & Nutritional Sciences,
    Agricultural Science Building, G025, West Virginia University, Morgantown, WV 26506, USA;
    mbarr6@mix.wvu.edu
3   Department of Nutrition, University of Tennessee, 1215 W Cumberland Ave, 229 Jesse Harris Building,
    Knoxville, TN 37996, USA; scolby@utk.edu
4   Department of Nutrition and Food Sciences, University of Rhode Island, Kingston, RI 02881, USA;
    ggreene@uri.edu
*   Correspondence: Melissa.olfert@mail.wvu.edu

**Abstract:** Androgen deficiency in males has traditionally been predominantly limited to older men aged 50+ years. However, little is known of the correlation between hormonal disruption, stress, and sleep in college-aged males. This cross-sectional study investigates lifestyle behavior patterns in young men and a screening for potential androgen deficiency. A survey of 409 male students, as part of a larger USDA-funded GetFruved study, was analyzed for this subproject. Survey instruments used include the Androgen Deficiency in the Aging Male Questionnaire (ADAM) to assess for inadequate ADAM scores, the Perceived Stress Scale to measure stress levels and the Pittsburgh Sleep Quality Index to evaluate sleep quality. In total, 144 male participants (35%) met criteria for potential androgen deficiency defined by the ADAM questionnaire. Correlation was found between having a positive ADAM score and both increased stress levels ($p < 0.001$) and poor sleep quality ($p < 0.001$), with stress displaying the strongest effect ($p < 0.001$ vs $p = 0.124$). An increased prevalence of having a positive ADAM score versus established norms for this age group was also noted. These findings highlight the need for investigation of endocrine disruptions in young men.

**Keywords:** androgen deficiency; ADAM score; low testosterone; young adult males; stress; sleep

## 1. Introduction

It is known that male androgen deficiency is more predominant among older-men, with prevalence rates of 34% for men in their 60s, 91% for men in their 80s, and less than 5% in males aged 20–29 [1]. Note that, due to testosterone being the primary male androgen hormone, the term male androgen deficiency, hypogonadism, male low testosterone, and male testosterone deficiency are used interchangeably in the literature. Additionally, hormone-based treatment is typically referred to as testosterone treatment for all of these conditions. However, the widespread rise of obesity, and its accompanying host of co-morbidities, including type 2 diabetes (T2DM), cardiovascular disease (CVD), and metabolic syndrome (MetS), is changing long-held assumptions about hormonal disruptions. Male hypogonadism has been found to positively correlate with all three of these co-morbid conditions [2–6]. Although prevalence rates are difficult to assess for individuals with CVD and MetS, in males with T2DM, hypogonadism prevalence is estimated to be 33–50% [7]. These trends are particularly concerning in younger demographics which have experienced significant increases in obesity rates in the past fifteen years. The Centers for Disease Control (CDC) reported that prevalence of obesity among American teenagers almost doubled from 2001 to 2015, going from 10.5% to 20% [8]. Additionally, nearly a third of young adults in the U.S. were considered obese in 2015 [8]. Interestingly, although treatment of hypogonadism remains challenging [9], medical management of androgen deficiency in males has displayed encouraging results. In obese men with low testosterone, testosterone replacement resulted in improved body composition and reduced waist circumference, leading to sustained weight loss and reduced body mass index (BMI) [10]. In male patients with androgen deficiency and T2DM, a disorder itself with a high prevalence of male hypogonadism [11,12], similar treatment not only yielded decreased subcutaneous fat and increased lean mass, it also improved insulin sensitivity [13].

In addition to specific medical diagnoses, certain lifestyle factors with well-established hormonal components can significantly affect health. Sleep and stress have been found to both be mediated by hormones and to have the capacity to alter normal endocrine function [14,15]. Indeed, male testosterone production appears to be linked to sleep cycles, including REM sleep [16]. Furthermore, young adults frequently experience poor sleep, with only approximately a third of college students reporting good sleep quality using the Pittsburgh Sleep Quality Index (PSQI) scale and 29.4% reporting getting the $\geq 8$ h of sleep recommended for this population [17]. Emerging evidence suggests that reduced sleep is a potential risk factor for obesity [18]. Stress (personal and academic) has been shown to significantly affect sleep quality in young adults [17]. Additionally, male teenagers with decreased stress resilience, or reduced ability to successfully cope with an issue, have been shown to be at increased risk of developing T2DM in adulthood, even when accounting for traditional risk factors such as BMI and family history [19]. Endocrine disruptions can result in a variety of physiological, cognitive and emotional conditions, which can each bring their own negative contribution to overall health, resulting in a snowballing effect damaging long-term quality of life and leading to increased healthcare costs.

The relationships among having a potential androgen deficiency, sleep, and stress in young adult males are unknown. This study investigated 409 male college students enrolled in the USDA-funded GetFruved study to examine if potential androgen deficiency, sleep, and stress are related via self-reported questionnaires.

## 2. Materials and Methods

Over 1200 college students across eight U.S. universities were surveyed as a part of a USDA-funded GetFruved study, a project aimed at identifying and improving lifestyle behaviors and environments associated with obesity prevention on university campuses. Male students (n = 409) were analyzed as a part of this subproject. Approval to use the dataset was granted by the University of Tennessee Institutional Review Board prior to study implementation. This material is based upon work that is supported by the National Institute of Food and Agriculture, U.S. Department of Agriculture, under award number 2014-67001-21851.

The validated survey instrument used included the Androgen Deficiency in the Aging Male Questionnaire (ADAM) to assess potential androgen deficiency [20,21]. This tool has been utilized to assess low bioavailable testosterone in older males aged 40–62 years and evaluated the change of these scores after administration of testosterone to those found to be low [21]. The ADAM tool was analyzed to have an 88% sensitivity and 60% specificity in capturing those males with lower testosterone. Specifically, 18 of the 21 men given testosterone treatment found improvement in their ADAM scores. Authors state the ADAM questionnaire poses an acceptable tool for screening tool for capturing males with low bioavailable testosterone.

The ADAM questionnaire was scored using the defined instructions listed in Figure 1, with a positive ADAM score being suggestive of a potential androgen deficiency [21]. A positive score was indicated as a "yes" answer to Question 1 or 7, or any other three variables. Per the scoring, the ADAM tool is then placed into a binary variable of "positive" or "negative". Note that participants with a positive ADAM score are henceforth labeled as "ADAM positive", with their negative counterparts being referred to as "ADAM negative".

Additional validated tools to assess these male's lifestyle traits included Cohen's 14-item Perceived Stress Scale (PSS) to measure stress levels [22] and the Pittsburgh Sleep Quality Index (PSQI) to evaluate sleep quality [23]. Sleep quality was further categorized per PSQI guidelines, with scores of 0–4 indicating good sleep quality and scores $\geq 5$ indicating poor or inadequate sleep quality [23].

Wilcoxon tests were used on nonparametric data to compare means for the following variables: height, weight, BMI, PSS scores, and PSQI scores. Pearson Chi-Squared test was used to assess the relationship between ADAM scores and PSQI categories. Logistic Regression Analysis and Agreement Analysis of the data were conducted to assess the effect of sleep and stress on ADAM scores. All analyses were completed using JMP [24] and SAS [25] software.

### Saint Louis University ADAM Questionnaire

1. Do you have a decrease in libido (sex drive)?
2. Do you have a lack of energy?
3. Do you have a decrease in strength and/or endurance?
4. Have you lost height?
5. Have you noticed a decreased "enjoyment of life"?
6. Are you sad and/or grumpy?
7. Are your erections less strong?
8. Have you noted a recent deterioration in your ability to play sports?
9. Are you falling asleep after dinner?
10. Has there been a recent deterioration in your work performance?

Scoring: A positive questionnaire result is defined as a "yes" answer to questions 1 or 7, or any 3 other questions.

*Note*: Reprinted from *Validation of a screening questionnaire for androgen deficiency in aging males*, by Morley et al. (2000).

**Figure 1.** Androgen Deficiency in the Aging Male Questionnaire (ADAM). This non-invasive screening tool was administered to all participants to assess androgen deficiency.

## 3. Results

There were 409 males from eight different states included in analysis (Table 1). Their average height, weight BMI and waist circumference were 176.06 $\pm$ 7.40 cm, 77.43 $\pm$ 15.98 kg, 24.90 $\pm$ 4.62 kg/m$^2$, and 82.94 $\pm$ 10.49 cm respectively (all Wilcoxon analyses non-significant between ADAM positive and ADAM negative groups; Table 1). The sample was predominantly composed of individuals identifying their race as 70.2% White, 17.1% Hispanic/Latino, 14.4% Asian, 12.0% Black only, 8.8% other (including Alaska Native/American Indian, Native Hawaiian/Pacific Islander and Other) (Table 1).

Overall, males had a PSS of 23.23 $\pm$ 7.40 and a PSQI score of 5.72 $\pm$ 2.64. Following PSQI categorization, good sleep quality was reported by 145 (36.16%) participants and poor sleep quality by 256 (63.84%) participants.

There were 144 (35.21%) male subjects that met the criteria for having a potential androgen deficiency as defined by positive ADAM questionnaire. Height, weight and BMI were not found to be significantly different between the ADAM positive and ADAM negative participants (Table 2).

**Table 1.** Demographics. Race, and state of the overall sample and the ADAM-positive sub-sample.

| Demographic | | Frequency (%) | |
|---|---|---|---|
| | | Male Sample | ADAM Positive Sub-Sample |
| | | N = 409 | N = 144 |
| Race * | Alaska Native/American Indian | 16 (3.91) | 5 (3.47) |
| | Asian | 59 (14.43) | 21 (14.58) |
| | Black/African-American | 49 (11.98) | 18 (12.50) |
| | Hispanic/Latino | 70 (17.11) | 21 (14.58) |
| | Native Hawaiian/Pacific Islander | 3 (0.73) | 1 (0.69) |
| | White | 287 (70.17) | 100 (69.44) |
| | Other or Choose not to answer | 17 (4.16) | 8 (5.56) |
| State | Alabama | 23 (5.62) | 9 (6.25) |
| | Florida | 79 (19.32) | 28 (19.44) |
| | Kansas | 35 (8.26) | 11 (7.64) |
| | Maine | 63 (15.40) | 14 (9.72) |
| | New York | 65 (15.89) | 20 (13.89) |
| | South Dakota | 15 (3.67) | 6 (4.17) |
| | Tennessee | 85 (20.78) | 33 (22.92) |
| | West Virginia | 40 (9.78) | 21 (14.58) |
| | Choose not to answer | 4 (0.98) | 2 (1.39) |

\* Individuals were able to classify themselves as more than one race (i.e. White and Hispanic/Latino) making the total percentage of race > 100%.

**Table 2.** Anthropometrics by ADAM scores. Height, weight, and BMI of the overall sample, including comparison between positive and negative ADAM scores with no statistically significant difference noted.

| Anthropometric | Total Male Sample | ADAM SCORES | | Significance |
|---|---|---|---|---|
| | | Positive | Negative | |
| Height (cm) | $176.06 \pm 7.40$ | $175.50 \pm 7.23$ | $176.36 \pm 7.48$ | $Z = -0.975$, $p = 0.3293$, Wilcoxon |
| Weight (kg) | $77.43 \pm 15.98$ | $77.95 \pm 16.67$ | $77.15 \pm 15.62$ | $Z = 0.323$, $p = 0.7460$, Wilcoxon |
| BMI (kg/m$^2$) | $24.90 \pm 4.62$ | $25.20 \pm 4.88$ | $24.74 \pm 4.48$ | $Z = 0.905$, $p = 0.3652$, Wilcoxon |
| Waist Circumference (cm) | $82.94 \pm 10.49$ | $82.46 \pm 9.66$ | $83.19 \pm 10.92$ | $Z = 0.7542$, $p = 0.7538$, Wilcoxon |

Wilcoxon test used on nonparametric height, weight, and BMI in relationship to ADAM positive and negative scores.

Figure 2 showing box plot of PSS among ADAM positive and negative males. Participants with positive ADAM scores self-reported higher levels of stress (PSS Mean = $26.82 \pm 6.91$) than participants with negative ADAM scores (PSS Mean = $21.26 \pm 6.91$) ($Z = 7.194$, $p < 0.001$, Wilcoxon).

Mean PSQI score of the ADAM positive males was $6.68 \pm 2.92$ versus $5.19 \pm 2.31$ for the ADAM negative participants ($Z = 5.177$, $p = 2.3 \times 10^{-7}$, Wilcoxon). Sleep findings were consistent following categorization, with poorer sleep quality observed in ADAM positive participants ($\chi^2 (1) = 12.621$, $p < 0.001$, Pearson Chi-Squared). In ADAM positives, categorized PSQI scores indicated that good sleep quality was reported by 35 (24.65%) participants and poor sleep quality by 107 (75.35%) participants. In ADAM negatives, categorized PSQI scores indicated that good sleep quality was reported by 110 (42.47%) participants and poor sleep quality by 149 (57.53%) participants. Conversely, ADAM positive subjects represented 42% of the "poor sleepers" but only 24% of the "good sleepers", as shown in Figure 3.

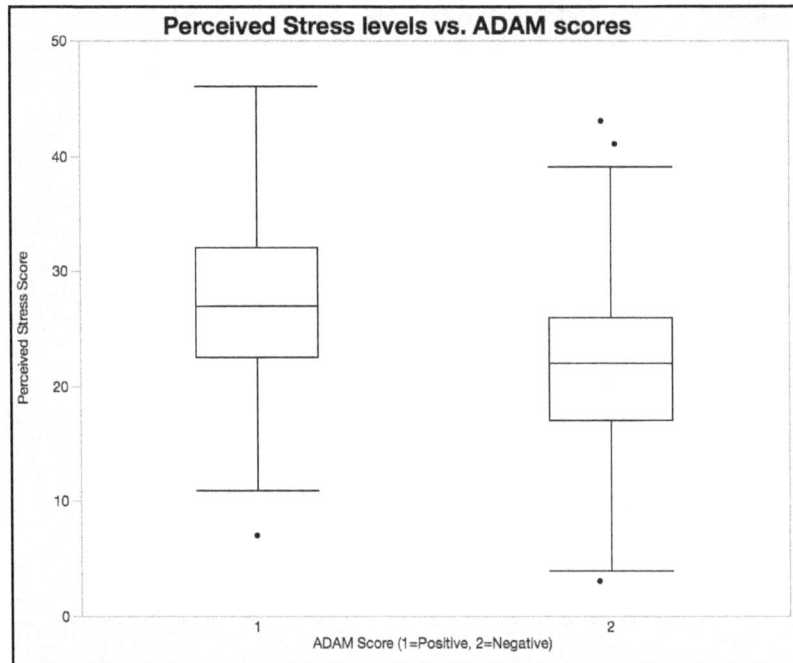

**Figure 2.** Perceived Stress levels vs. ADAM scores. Participants with positive ADAM scores self-reported higher levels of stress (PSS Mean = 26.82 ± 6.91) than participants with negative ADAM scores (PSS Mean = 21.26 ± 6.91).

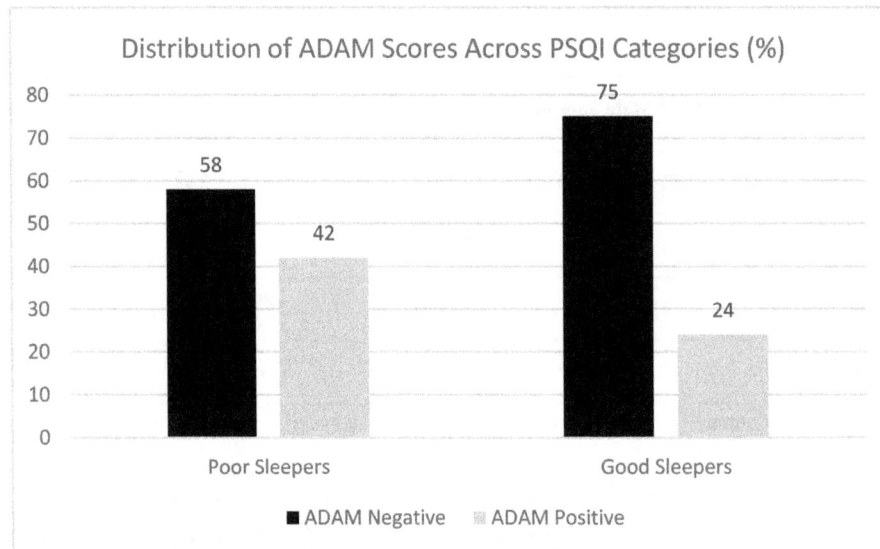

**Figure 3.** Distribution of ADAM Scores across PSQI Sleep Quality Categories. Participants with positive ADAM scores represented a larger percentage of the sample's "poor sleeper" group (42%) than it did the "good sleeper" group (24%).

Univariate logistic regression showed statistically significant effects of increased stress ($p < 0.001$) and poor sleep ($p = 0.0003$) on ADAM scores. When modeled together, stress showed a stronger effect than sleep on ADAM scores ($\chi^2$ (1) = 36.68, $p < 0.001$ versus $\chi^2$ (1) = 2.37, $p = 0.1235$ respectively).

## 4. Discussion

In young adult men, there was a correlation between a positive ADAM score indicating a potential androgen deficiency and both increased stress levels and poor sleep quality, with stress displaying the strongest effect on ADAM scores. These findings highlight the potential relationships within the testosterone–stress–sleep triad in young adult males. The observed connection between hypogonadism and sleep appears logical given the established role of testosterone in REM sleep cycles [16]. However, the stronger effect of stress than sleep on ADAM results was interesting and potentially suggestive of the co-depending nature of stress and sleep. As stress increases, sleep quality is likely to decrease thereby resulting in sleep as a compounding stressor. Similarly, decreased sleep quality itself may lead to increased stress levels. As such, true distinction between the two variables remains challenging.

Additionally, the high proportion of male subjects scoring positive on the ADAM questionnaire in this study appears to indicate a potentially higher prevalence of hypogonadism in young males than previously reported. Although this sample was a small convenience sample so nationwide prevalence conclusions cannot be made, an ADAM positivity rate of 35.21% was far greater than the estimated 5% androgen deficiency rate in young males [1]. One reason for such a large discrepancy could simply be an underestimation of androgen deficiency prevalence in young men in the current literature. Indeed, up to date estimates are not readily available and research in the field is primarily relying on the 2001 Baltimore Longitudinal Study on Aging. Several factors such as public health changes (i.e., increased obesity) could have reasonably affected the prevalence of androgen deficiency in young adult males over the past sixteen years. Most universities sampled in this study are located in states with high obesity rates. Obesity being linked to hormonal disruptions, this may have played a role in these findings. Indeed, four of the universities represented in this sample come from states ranked in the top ten for highest obesity rates. Furthermore, all but one institutions are located in a state ranked in the top 25 for highest obesity rates [26].

Another limitation of this study was the use of a screening questionnaire to assess for a potential androgen deficiency. By the very nature of its questions, the ADAM questionnaire may lead to a positive result independently of any androgen changes. For example, a patient's answer to question #2 ("Do you have a lack of energy") could have multiple potential causes, as could responses to Questions 3, 6, and 10. Furthermore, hormonal dysfunctions can be challenging to pinpoint and even the best screening tools have margins for errors. The ADAM questionnaire was designed for older men as androgen deficiency in males has conventionally predominantly been a concern in males ≥50 years old. This particular screening tool was selected as it is the most widely used one clinically and no young men focused instrument is currently available. However, it has not been specifically validated in younger males, representing a potential shortcoming of this study. Indeed, the ADAM questionnaire may not be valid in younger men. Further validation of the test in this population is strongly warranted. Specifically, when looking into the questions used for the ADAM questionnaire, potential shortening of the tool could be useful. For example, a question regarding loss of height in young adult college students may not be useful as muscle mass and structure tend to not deteriorate in males until after their fifth decade of life that encompasses hormonal deviations and reductions in exercise [27].

In light of our results and current obesity trends, further investigation, including laboratory bloodwork to test testosterone, is recommended: (1) to identify any significant changes to the historical prevalence of androgen deficiency in younger male demographics; and (2) to confirm relationships among clinically diagnosed androgen deficiency, stress, and sleep using physiological markers. Note that literature recommends testing of free or bioavailable testosterone as total testosterone levels can fail to reveal actual testosterone decline, particularly in individuals with milder forms of hypogonadism [28,29]. Unfortunately, with this multi-state sample of young males, we were unable to obtain these biochemical data. Indeed, bioavailable testosterone is the most widely used test in the literature pertaining to the screening for androgen deficiency [21] and should likely be used to ensure both accuracy and consistency [30]. Future studies should utilize this measure of testosterone, especially when validating this tool in a younger population. Overall, this study confirms the need for research to further examine hormonal disruptions and potential health ramifications in young adult males.

**Author Contributions:** C.M.C., M.L.B., S.E.C., G.W.G. and M.D.O. participated in the intellectual content of this manuscript. Manuscript draft was written by C.M.C. and M.L.B. Data Analysis was performed by C.M.C. and M.L.B. Conceptual framework of the project was completed by S.E.C., G.W.G. and M.D.O. All authors edited and approved final manuscript.

**Acknowledgments:** The authors thank Ida Holásková for help with data analysis. Approval to use the dataset was granted by the University of Tennessee Institutional Review Board prior to study implementation. This material is based upon work that is supported by the National Institute of Food and Agriculture, U.S. Department of Agriculture, under award number 2014-67001-21851.

# References

1.  Harman, S.M.; Metter, E.J.; Tobin, J.D.; Pearson, J.; Blackman, M.R. Longitudinal effects of aging on serum total and free testosterone levels in healthy men. *J. Clin. Endocrinol. Metab.* **2001**, *86*, 724–731. [CrossRef] [PubMed]

2.  Chiles, K.A. Hypogonadism and erectile dysfunction as harbingers of systemic disease. *Transl. Androl. Urol.* **2016**, *5*, 195–200. [CrossRef] [PubMed]

3.  Corona, G.; Rastrelli, G.; Monami, M.; Guay, A.; Buvat, J.; Sforza, A.; Forti, G.; Mannucci, E.; Maggi, M. Hypogonadism as a risk factor for cardiovascular mortality in men: A meta-analytic study. *Eur. J. Endocrinol.* **2011**, *165*, 687–701. [CrossRef] [PubMed]

4.  Grossmann, M.; Thomas, M.C.; Panagiotopoulos, S.; Sharpe, K.; MacIsaac, R.J.; Clarke, S.; Zajac, J.D.; Jerums, G. Low testosterone levels are common and associated with insulin resistance in men with diabetes. *J. Clin. Endocrinol. Metab.* **2008**, *93*, 1834–1840. [CrossRef] [PubMed]

5.  Guay, A.T.; Traish, A. Testosterone deficiency and risk factors in the metabolic syndrome: Implications for erectile dysfunction. *Urol. Clin.* **2011**, *38*, 175–183. [CrossRef] [PubMed]

6.  Traish, A.M.; Saad, F.; Feeley, R.J.; Guay, A. The dark side of testosterone deficiency: III. Cardiovascular disease. *J. Androl.* **2009**, *30*, 477–494. [CrossRef] [PubMed]

7.  Dandona, P.; Rosenberg, M. A practical guide to male hypogonadism in the primary care setting. *Int. J. Clin. Pract.* **2010**, *64*, 682–696. [CrossRef] [PubMed]

8.  Ogden, C.L.; Carroll, M.D.; Fryar, C.D.; Flegal, K.M. *Prevalence of Obesity among Adults and Youth: United States, 2011–2014*; US Department of Health and Human Services, Centers for Disease Control and Prevention, National Center for Health Statistics: Washington, DC, USA, 2015.

9.  Sterling, J.; Bernie, A.M.; Ramasamy, R. Hypogonadism: Easy to define, hard to diagnose, and controversial to treat. *Can. Urol. Assoc. J.* **2015**, *9*, 65–68. [CrossRef] [PubMed]

10. Traish, A.; Haider, A.; Doros, G.; Saad, F. Long-term testosterone therapy in hypogonadal men ameliorates elements of the metabolic syndrome: An observational, long-term registry study. *Int. J. Clin. Pract.* **2014**, *68*, 314–329. [CrossRef] [PubMed]

11. El Saghier, E.O.; Shebl, S.E.; Fawzy, O.A.; Eltayeb, L.M.; Bekhet, L.M.; Gharib, A. Androgen deficiency and erectile dysfunction in patients with type 2 diabetes. *Clin. Med. Insights Endocrinol. Diabetes* **2015**, *8*, 55–62. [CrossRef] [PubMed]

12. Ugwu, T.E.; Ikem, R.T.; Kolawole, B.A.; Ezeani, I.U. Clinicopathologic assessment of hypogonadism in men with type 2 diabetes mellitus. *Indian J. Endocrinol. Metab.* **2016**, *20*, 667–673. [CrossRef] [PubMed]

13. Dhindsa, S.; Ghanim, H.; Batra, M.; Kuhadiya, N.D.; Abuaysheh, S.; Sandhu, S.; Green, K.; Makdissi, A.; Hejna, J.; Chaudhuri, A. Insulin resistance and inflammation in hypogonadotropic hypogonadism and their reduction after testosterone replacement in men with type 2 diabetes. *Diabetes Care* **2016**, *39*, 82–91. [CrossRef] [PubMed]

14. Helmreich, D.L.; Parfitt, D.; Lu, X.-Y.; Akil, H.; Watson, S. Relation between the hypothalamic-pituitary-thyroid (HPT) axis and the hypothalamic-pituitary-adrenal (HPA) axis during repeated stress. *Neuroendocrinology* **2005**, *81*, 183–192. [CrossRef] [PubMed]

15. Leproult, R.; Van Cauter, E. Role of sleep and sleep loss in hormonal release and metabolism. In *Pediatric Neuroendocrinology*; Karger Publishers: Basel, Switzerland, 2010; Volume 17, pp. 11–21.

16. Mong, J.A.; Cusmano, D.M. Sex differences in sleep: Impact of biological sex and sex steroids. *Philos. Trans. R. Soc. B* **2016**, *371*, 20150110. [CrossRef] [PubMed]

17. Lund, H.G.; Reider, B.D.; Whiting, A.B.; Prichard, J.R. Sleep patterns and predictors of disturbed sleep in a large population of college students. *J. Adolesc. Health* **2010**, *46*, 124–132. [CrossRef] [PubMed]

18. Patel, S. Reduced sleep as an obesity risk factor. *Obes. Rev.* **2009**, *10*, 61–68. [CrossRef] [PubMed]

19. Crump, C.; Sundquist, J.; Winkleby, M.A.; Sundquist, K. Stress resilience and subsequent risk of type 2 diabetes in 1.5 million young men. *Diabetologia* **2016**, *59*, 728–733. [CrossRef] [PubMed]

20. Bernie, A.M.; Scovell, J.M.; Ramasamy, R. Comparison of questionnaires used for screening and symptom identification in hypogonadal men. *Aging Male* **2014**, *17*, 195–198. [CrossRef] [PubMed]

21. Morley, J.E.; Charlton, E.; Patrick, P.; Kaiser, F.; Cadeau, P.; McCready, D.; Perry, H. Validation of a screening questionnaire for androgen deficiency in aging males. *Metab. Clin. Exp.* **2000**, *49*, 1239–1242. [CrossRef] [PubMed]

22. Cohen, S.; Kamarck, T.; Mermelstein, R. A global measure of perceived stress. *J. Health Soc. Behav.* **1983**, 385–396. [CrossRef]

23. Buysse, D.J.; Reynolds, C.F., III; Monk, T.H.; Berman, S.R.; Kupfer, D.J. The Pittsburgh Sleep Quality Index: A new instrument for psychiatric practice and research. *Psychiatry Res.* **1989**, *28*, 193–213. [CrossRef]

24. JMP®. *V.S.I.I. [Statistical Software]*; A Business Unit of SAS; SAS Campus Drive: Cary, NC, USA, 1989–2007.

25. SAS Institute Inc. *Base SAS®9.3 Procedures Guide*; N.S.I.I.; SAS Institute Inc.: Cary, NC, USA, 2011.

26. Centers for Disease Control and Prevention. *Behavioral Risk Factor Surveillance System (BRFSS) Prevalence Data (2011 to present) | Chronic Disease and Health Promotion Data & Indicators*; Centers for Disease Control and Prevention: Atlanta, GA, USA, 2018.

27. Wells, J.C. Sexual dimorphism of body composition. *Best Pract. Res. Clin. Endocrinol. Metab.* **2007**, *21*, 415–430. [CrossRef] [PubMed]

28. Bhasin, S.; Cunningham, G.R.; Hayes, F.J.; Matsumoto, A.M.; Snyder, P.J.; Swerdloff, R.S.; Montori, V.M. Testosterone therapy in adult men with androgen deficiency syndromes: An endocrine society clinical practice guideline. *J. Clin. Endocrinol. Metab.* **2006**, *91*, 1995–2010. [CrossRef] [PubMed]

29. Mayo Clinic. *Test ID: TTFB—Testosterone, T., Bioavailable, and Free, Serum*; Mayo Medical Laboratories: Rochester, MN, USA, 2018.

30. Cabral, R.D.; Busin, L.; Rosito, T.E.; Koff, W.J. Performance of Massachusetts Male Aging Study (MMAS) and androgen deficiency in the aging male (ADAM) questionnaires in the prediction of free testosterone in patients aged 40 years or older treated in outpatient regimen. *Aging Male* **2014**, *17*, 147–154. [CrossRef] [PubMed]

# Permissions

# List of Contributors

**Daniel Leightley**
King's Centre for Military Health Research, Institute of Psychiatry, Psychology and Neuroscience, King's College London, London WC2R 2LS, UK

**Moi Hoon Yap**
School of Computing, Mathematics and Digital Technology, Manchester Metropolitan University, Manchester M15 6BH, UK

**Stephen M. Modell and Toby Citrin**
Department of Health Management and Policy, University of Michigan School of Public Health, 1415Washington Heights, Ann Arbor, MI 48109-2029, USA

**Sharon L. R. Kardia**
Department of Epidemiology, University of Michigan School of Public Health, M5174, SPH II, 1415Washington Heights, Ann Arbor, MI 48109-2029, USA

**Mohana Maddula, Laura Adams and Jonathan Donnelly**
Tauranga Hospital, Bay of Plenty District Health Board, Tauranga 3112, New Zealand

**Zahra Ezzat-Zadeh**
Department of Nutrition, Food and Exercise Sciences, Florida State University, Tallahassee, FL 32306-4310, USA

**Neda S. Akhavan, Lauren Ormsbee, Kelli S. George, Elizabeth M. Foley, Lynn B. Panton and Bahram H. Arjmandi**
Department of Nutrition, Food and Exercise Sciences, Florida State University, Tallahassee, FL 32306-4310, USA
Center for Advancing Exercise and Nutrition Research on Aging (CAENRA), College of Human Sciences, Florida State University, Tallahassee, FL 32306-4310, USA

**Sarah A. Johnson**
Department of Food Science and Human Nutrition, Colorado State University, Fort Collins, CO 80523-1571, USA

**Marcus L. Elam**
Department of Human Nutrition and Food Science, California State Polytechnic University, Pomona, CA 91768-2557, USA

**Radhika V. Seimon, Alice A. Gibson, Claudia Harper, Hamish A. Fernando and Michael R. Skilton**
Faculty of Medicine and Health, Charles Perkins Centre, The University of Sydney, the Boden Institute of Obesity, Nutrition, Exercise and Eating Disorders, Camperdown, NSW 2006, Australia

**Shelley E. Keating**
School of Human Movement and Nutrition Sciences, Centre for Research on Exercise, Physical Activity and Health, The University of Queensland, Brisbane, QLD 4072, Australia

**Nathan A. Johnson**
Faculty of Medicine and Health, Charles Perkins Centre, The University of Sydney, the Boden Institute of Obesity, Nutrition, Exercise and Eating Disorders, Camperdown, NSW 2006, Australia
Faculty of Health Sciences, The University of Sydney, Lidcombe, NSW 2141, Australia

**Felipe Q. da Luz and Amanda Sainsbury**
Faculty of Medicine and Health, Charles Perkins Centre, The University of Sydney, the Boden Institute of Obesity, Nutrition, Exercise and Eating Disorders, Camperdown, NSW 2006, Australia
Faculty of Science, School of Psychology, The University of Sydney, Camperdown, NSW 2006, Australia

**Tania P. Markovic and Ian D. Caterson**
Faculty of Medicine and Health, Charles Perkins Centre, The University of Sydney, the Boden Institute of Obesity, Nutrition, Exercise and Eating Disorders, Camperdown, NSW 2006, Australia
Metabolism and Obesity Services, Royal Prince Alfred Hospital, Camperdown, NSW 2050, Australia

**Phillipa Hay**
School of Medicine, Western Sydney University, Translational Health Research Institute (THRI), Locked Bag 1797, Penrith, NSW 2751, Australia

**Nuala M. Byrne**
School of Health Sciences, College of Health and Medicine, University of Tasmania, Launceston, TAS 7250, Australia

**Hiroto Ogi**
Department of Physical Therapy, Faculty of Health Sciences, Kobe University School of Medicine, 7-10-2 Tomogaoka, Suma-ku, Kobe 654-0142, Japan

Cardiovascular stroke Renal Project (CRP), 7-10-2 Tomogaoka, Suma-ku, Kobe 654-0142, Japan

**Daisuke Nakamura and Kazuhiro P. Izawa**
Cardiovascular stroke Renal Project (CRP), 7-10-2 Tomogaoka, Suma-ku, Kobe 654-0142, Japan
Department of International Health, Graduate School of Health Sciences, Kobe University, 7-10-2 Tomogaoka, Suma-ku, Kobe 654-0142, Japan

**Masato Ogawa**
Cardiovascular stroke Renal Project (CRP), 7-10-2 Tomogaoka, Suma-ku, Kobe 654-0142, Japan
Department of International Health, Graduate School of Health Sciences, Kobe University, 7-10-2 Tomogaoka, Suma-ku, Kobe 654-0142, Japan
Division of Rehabilitation Medicine, Kobe University Hospital, 7-5-2 Kusunoki-cho, Chuo-ku, Kobe 650-0017, Japan

**Teruhiko Nakamura**
Educational Corporation Tsukushi Gakuen, 2-3-11 Takadai, Chitose 066-0035, Japan

**Ganga S. Bey, Bill M. Jesdale, Christine M. Ulbricht, Eric O. Mick and Sharina D. Person**
Department of Quantitative Health Sciences, University of Massachusetts Medical School, Worcester, MA 01655, USA

**Shervin Assari**
Department of Psychology, University of California, Los Angeles (UCLA), Los Angeles, CA 90095, USA
Department of Psychiatry, University of Michigan, Ann Arbor, MI 48104, USA
Center for Research on Ethnicity, Culture and Health, School of Public Health, University of Michigan, Ann Arbor, MI 90095, USA

**Maryam Moghani Lankarani**
Department of Psychiatry, University of Michigan, Ann Arbor, MI 48104, USA

**Tom C. Zwart and Ingeborg M. van Geijlswijk**
Faculty of Veterinary Medicine, Pharmacy Department, Utrecht University, Utrecht 3584 CM, The Netherlands
Utrecht Institute for Pharmaceutical Sciences (UIPS), Department of Pharmacoepidemiology and Clinical Pharmacology, Faculty of Science, Utrecht University, Utrecht 3584 CG, The Netherlands

**Marcel G. Smits**
Department of Sleep-wake disorders and Chronobiology, Gelderse Vallei Hospital, Ede 6716 RP, The Netherlands
Governor Kremers Centre, Maastricht University, Maastricht 6229 GR, The Netherlands

**Toine C.G. Egberts**
Utrecht Institute for Pharmaceutical Sciences (UIPS), Department of Pharmacoepidemiology and Clinical Pharmacology, Faculty of Science, Utrecht University, Utrecht 3584 CG, The Netherlands
Department of Clinical Pharmacy, Division of Laboratory and Pharmacy, University Medical Centre Utrecht, Utrecht 3584 CX, The Netherlands

**Carin M.A. Rademaker**
Department of Clinical Pharmacy, Division of Laboratory and Pharmacy, University Medical Centre Utrecht, Utrecht 3584 CX, The Netherlands

**Prachi Syngal**
Pediatric Intensive Care Medicine, Yale-New Haven Children's Hospital, New Haven, CT 06520, USA

**John S. Giuliano Jr.**
Department of Pediatrics, Section Critical Care Medicine, Yale University School of Medicine, New Haven, CT 06520, USA

**Anna Axmon**
Division of Occupational and Environmental Medicine, Department of Laboratory Medicine, Lund University, SE-221 00 Lund, Sweden

**Gerd Ahlström**
Department of Health Sciences, Lund University, SE-221 00 Lund, Sweden

**Hans Westergren**
Department of Pain rehabilitation, Skane University hospital, 222 85 Lund, Sweden

**Ai Ohsato**
Division for Health Service Promotion, the University of Tokyo, 7-3-1 Hongo, Bunkyo-ku, Tokyo 113-0033, Japan
School of Oral Health Sciences, Faculty of Dentistry, Tokyo Medical and Dental University, Tokyo 113-8549, Japan

**Masanobu Abe**
Division for Health Service Promotion, the University of Tokyo, 7-3-1 Hongo, Bunkyo-ku, Tokyo 113-0033, Japan
Oral and Maxillofacial Surgery, Dentistry and Orthodontics, the University of Tokyo Hospital, Tokyo 113-8655, Japan

**Kazumi Ohkubo, Kazuto Hoshi and Tsuyoshi Takato**
Oral and Maxillofacial Surgery, Dentistry and Orthodontics, the University of Tokyo Hospital, Tokyo 113-8655, Japan

**Hidemi Yoshimasu**
School of Oral Health Sciences, Faculty of Dentistry, Tokyo Medical and Dental University, Tokyo 113-8549, Japan

**Liang Zong**
Graduate School of Medicine, the University of Tokyo, Tokyo 113-8655, Japan
Key Laboratory of Carcinogenesis and Translational Research (Ministry of Education), Department of Gastrointestinal Surgery, Peking University Cancer Hospital and Institute, Beijing 100142, China

**Shintaro Yanagimoto and Kazuhiko Yamamoto**
Division for Health Service Promotion, the University of Tokyo, 7-3-1 Hongo, Bunkyo-ku, Tokyo 113-0033, Japan

**David Turgoose**
Combat Stress, Surrey KT22 0BX, UK

**Dominic Murphy**
Combat Stress, Surrey KT22 0BX, UK
King's Centre for Military Health Research, King's College London, London WC2R 2LS, UK

**Charlene Ingwell-Spolan**
School of Nursing, University of Maine, Orono, ME 04469, USA

**Karel Allegaert**
Department of Pediatrics, Division of Neonatology, Erasmus MC-Sophia Children's Hospital, Doctor Molenwaterplein 40, 3015 GD Rotterdam, The Netherlands
Department of Development and Regeneration, KU Leuven, Herestraat 49, 3000 Leuven, Belgium

**Camille M. Charlier**
Clinical and Translational Science, Health Sciences Center, West Virginia University, Morgantown, WV 26506, USA

**Makenzie L. Barr and Melissa D. Olfert**
Davis College of Agriculture, Natural Resources and Design, Department of Animal and Nutritional Sciences, Agricultural Science Building, G025, West Virginia University, Morgantown, WV 26506, USA

**Sarah E. Colby**
Department of Nutrition, University of Tennessee, 1215 W Cumberland Ave, 229 Jesse Harris Building, Knoxville, TN 37996, USA

**Geoffrey W. Greene**
Department of Nutrition and Food Sciences, University of Rhode Island, Kingston, RI 02881, USA

# Index